Reforming India's Social Sector

Also from Social Science Press

Reforming India's Social Sector:

Poverty, Nutrition, Health and Gender

Edited by
K. Seeta Prabhu
and
R. Sudarshan

Social Science Press
New Delhi

Published by

Esha Béteille
Social Science Press
69 Jor Bagh, New Delhi 110003
E-mail: beteille@del3.vsnl.net.in

Distributed by

ORIENT LONGMAN PRIVATE LIMITED
Bangalore, Bhopal, Bhubaneshwar, Chennai, Ernakulam, Guwahati, Hyderabad, Jaipur, Kolkata, Lucknow, Mumbai, New Delhi, Patna

ISBN 81 87358 10 6

Set in Giovanni Book
Typeset by Eleven Art, Delhi-110 035
Printed by Yogesh Pracashan
at Ravindra Printing Press, Delhi-110 006.

Contents

Foreword

I am thankful to Dr K. Seeta Prabhu and Dr R. Sudarshan for asking me to write a foreword to their important collection of papers, *Reforming India's Social Sectors: Poverty, Nutrition, Health and Education*. Seeta Prabhu's pioneering work on the social sector in relation to human development is highly commendable. Here, I would also like to express my views on the above theme from a conceptual angle.

Empirically, the term social sector in this work relates to issues dealing with poverty alleviation, nutrition, health and education. These are areas in which governmental expenditures are involved. Expenditures on social sectors are deemed to reduce poverty and gender gaps, and improve nutritional status, health care services and the educational levels of a population. The three primary indicators of human development, are the improvement of life expectancy at birth, adult literacy rate (proportion of literate population above fifteen years of age), which should be reflected in the combined enrollment ratios in primary, secondary and tertiary spheres of education, and the GDP per capita on the basis of the international purchasing power parity of US dollars. Efforts have been made to readjust the indicators to provide for gender gaps. Different state governments in India and the Planning Commission itself have tried to look at the level of human development in terms of the above and enlarged set of indicators.

The primary postulate is that an improvement in the indicators connotes an improvement in the human development index. The objective of social sector expenditure policies is to improve the various indicators with reference to the states and the national economy. The concept of development is bifurcated between material development and human development. Actions in respect of commodity productions and their increase belong to the former realm. Actions related to improvements in life expectancy, education level and comparable per capita GDP belong to the realm of human development. Improvement in per capita GDP is considered to be an instrument in material development as well. There is therefore some overlap between material development and human development. Actually, in classical economics, labour is treated as a function of commodities of certain types and if there is surplus in production, portion of the surplus can be used for the development of human resources in the society. In the case of the latter, the inputs are almost all commodities. Thus, commodities, specially the surplus in commodity productions, produce both material development and human development. There is therefore an inherent tension between the use of surplus for further material development and enhancing the quality of life in terms of education, health, recreation etc., for human beings. As society advances, some elements of the latter also become crucial inputs in production.

The emergence of the human development approach is based on the idea that material development *per se* does not necessarily have a bearing on human development as such. Since, per capita GDP occurs in both, the implication is that the allocation of GDP has to be such as to promote the three and extended indicators of human development. Government expenditures related to social sectors mentioned above are supposed to lead to an improvement in the human development indicators.

The human development approach emerges as a critique as well as a supplement to mainstream economics concerning material development. Material development is achieved when commodities produce more and more commodities. Human development by contrast is achieved when commodities produce more commodities, but also result in improved life expectancy, education, health etc., It is believed that unless human development is induced as a special goal in development it will not occur automatically, or at least not for most human beings. A redirection along normative lines of surpluses is involved here. There are problems of choice in such redirections.

In welfare economics, if everyone's wellbeing improves or if some people's wellbeing improves without there being a decrease in the wellbeing of others then one can say that there has been an improvement in the general welfare. In mainstream economics, it is the consumption status of human beings that is crucial. If the consumption status of all increase or of some increase without a decline in those of others, then that indicates an improvement in the general welfare. Wellbeing is perceived in terms of consumption status. An improvement in productivity potential has no welfare significance unless related to similar improvement in the actual consumption status of all, or of some, without deterioration in the status of others. Let us now subject the human development concept to the above line of reasoning as in mainstream economics.

Take the first criterion. An improvement in life expectancy is supposed to increase human development. The concept of life expectancy itself is not examined in detail from a welfare angle. Let us assume that the improvement occurs at all age levels. Further, the well being significance of such improvement must be the same at all age levels. There will be a conceptual difficulty if there is a possibility of such improvement being higher in some age levels, and lower in others. We must assume that the marginal welfare significance of an improvement in life expectancy is the same at all age levels. Put in this manner, there is no support to the above assumption. Is the utility of an increment in life expectancy, the same for all irrespective of initial ages? Probably, one would think that this measure of utility is greater for persons at lower age levels than at the upper limits of the age level. We are also not clear as to whether the usefulness in better life expectancy is seen from the point of view of an individual or the society. What is the social utility of an increase in the life expectancy by one year of a person at say age 90? Is this social utility the same as that of a person at age 20? Old people might feel that an extension of life would be a burden. One might argue that living beyond an age without the necessary environment might not be an advantage. More provisions for old age homes may not contribute to an improvement in the wellbeing of old people. A model of overlapping generations where the generations live separately is not the same thing from the point of view of welfare as a model of overlapping generations in all families. I do not want to refer to the concept of euthanasia for old people. History tells us that only physically fit people were allowed to survive in Sparta. This might not be altogether untrue in a highly competitive, achievement oriented economy. I am afraid that the theory of human development has not been sufficiently refined to take into account issues like these. Mere survival for longer years is not necessarily an improvement in human development. Has the social environment changed to such an extent that an improvement in life expectancy brings the same measure of human satisfaction to all social classes in a society like India? Long ago, Myrdal drew attention to the differences in levels of living and opportunities between the white and the black. Without a change in the societal environment, the western criterion of an improvement in life expectancy is not class neutral even in the west and how can we say it is class neutral in a country like India?

Let me take the criterion of improvement in enrolment ratios. Is this improvement independent of the environment in which children are learning? The educational conditions of different classes and income groups are widely different in India and in other developing countries. Children from rich homes do not go to the same schools as the children who are poor. Even for minimum common learning, the facilities are markedly different. It is well known that the educational system perpetuates class distinctions. Can we assume that an improvement in enrollment ratios *per se* connotes the same level of increase in wellbeing or opportunities for all children irrespective of social class and income class backgrounds?

With respect to health and medical care, those who are financially better off go to nursing homes and star hospitals and the poor go to public hospitals. This means that the life expectancy of the rich has a better chance of going up whereas that of the poor does not. Apart from differences in the chance of survival there are differences in the chances of recovery of most ailments, given the fact that recoveries mean further opportunities for earning.

One criticism of human development approach is that the indicators are supposed to be best for advanced countries and the developing countries have to obtain such indicators through internal policies. In this context, it is important to stress that population growth in most advanced countries is close to zero or low. Other things being equal, their indicators will go up whereas in the case of countries like India, the population growth is so high that large extensions in social sector expenditures will not lead to improvements in human development indicators *pari passu*. This then leads to a situation where even with same aggregate social sector expenditure policies, reduction in population growth rates will move up the indicators of only some countries. What this implies is that all developing countries by just reducing population size can move up in the human development indicators. In other words, these indicators are not neutral in respect of demographic changes. As a result, some countries move up or move down in the rankings only because of demographic changes and not because of any social sector expenditures for improving indicators.

I have referred earlier, to the distribution aspects of different aggregate indicators. The distribution aspects can be understood from several angles depending upon the historical and environmental situations. Rawls tried to expand the concept of social justice by expanding the dimension of the minimum to encompass all societal levels in economics, politics, law, sociology etc. He visualised a holistic approach which is useful in working out different sets of indicators. Rawls introduced the notion of political liberalism as an element in a socially just society. Political liberalism is not the same thing as democracy. In the latter, it is the majority that counts, whereas in a liberal society, different constituent groups have an equal significance irrespective of numbers. Human development indicators as understood today completely ignore different types of societies in which people function. Politically illiberal and unfree societies may show big improvements and ranking may be high. But, the question is whether all the different groups in such societies are treated equally irrespective of numbers. Do all people have effective choices not simply from the individual's point of view, but also from that of the society.

The dimension of the social angle will bring in certain normative concepts of minimum with respect to each individual as a member of a society. This issue is not given much importance in developed countries which are mostly capitalistic and individualistic. We need to look at society as a network of relations between groups and individuals in a particular historical and environmental context. We cannot escape the notion of an optimal society in such an approach. An optimal society must have some minimum in respect of all. But, in defining such a minimum, we have to be neutral in respect of class backgrounds and the concept of class has to be wider than just that of income. Wellbeings are psychological states and a social sensitivity has to be at the background of any concept of wellbeing in countries like India.

Each human being is concerned with the development of his own individual personality and in several spheres, which should include the moral or ethical dimensions. There is no unidirectional relation between material and human development and ethical or spiritual development of human beings. Individuals want a society to conform to some ideals, and if it falls short of these, he might not consider the society to be developing, even if the indicators of material and human development are all positive. In the old days, the British Raj produced annual reports of the economy and polity under the title 'The Moral and Material Progress of India'. I am not clear that the moral aspects referred to here pertain necessarily to the human development components. It rather refers to individuals functioning in groups in which there are some implicit rules. These rules by habit or constitution are very important in determining moral dimension. For example, in Gandhiji's case, if the wellbeing of the lowest strata of a society, if improved continuously would reflect a higher moral state of that society. Such improvements might even imply a reduction in the narrowly conceived wellbeing states of the top strata. This criterion is the opposite of the Pareto criterion. Perhaps, the goal of social sector expenditures should be aimed at the Gandhian criterion. This means that even with a given level of indicators, a better state is one in which the lowest strata improves even at the cost of the highest or other strata.

I have mentioned above some limitations from a conceptual angle of the popular approaches to human development in relation to the social sectors. These are stray remarks. But, together, they point to the need for deepening the meaning of the indicators and their significance to welfare economics.

I am sure the collection of papers in this volume and the introduction by the editors will help to deepen the concept of human development and its relation to social sector goals.

Professor P.R. Brahamananda

Preface

The Department of Economics, University of Mumbai along with the Office of the UN Resident Co-ordinator in India and the National Bank for Agriculture and Rural Development, organised a symposium on 'Reforming India's Social Sectors: Strategies and Prospects', in order to consider the progress on four main themes: Poverty Alleviation Programmes, Nutrition, Health and Education. Each of the main themes were designed to analyse in depth, the issues and problems concerning each social sector and to provide suggestions toward the improvement of their functioning. This collection of essays has resulted from the symposium, with some augmentations of subsequent experience up to the completion of the volume in 2002.

The authors would like to express their heartfelt gratitude to the contributors for their co-operation and help. Special thanks are due to Dr Brenda McSweeney, UN Resident Co-ordinator and UNDP Resident Representative, Professor D.M. Nachane, former Director of the Department of Economics, University of Mumbai and Professor M.J.M. Rao, present Director, Department of Economics, University of Mumbai, for their unflinching support in the organisation of the symposium.

The authors would like to acknowledge Professor P.R. Brahmananda, scholar and teacher par excellence, for being a guiding force behind the theme of the symposium and for lending it conceptual rigour.

Thanks are also due to Sandhya V. Iyer, ICSSR Fellow, Department of Economics, University of Mumbai and Elena Borsatti, HDRC, UNDP, for cheerfully bearing the brunt of editing this present volume.

Views expressed by the editors are in their personal capacity and do not reflect the official position of the organizations to which they belong.

K. Seeta Prabhu and
R. Sudarshan

New Delhi
25 February 2002

Contributors

Datta, Ramesh, Professor, Department of Personnel Management and Industrial Relations, Tata Institute of Social Sciences, Mumbai.

De, Anuradha, member of Collective Research and Dissemination (CORD).

Dev, Mahendra S., Director, Centre for Economic and Social Studies, Hyderabad.

Deshpande, Lalit, Former Professor and Head, Department of Economics, University of Mumbai.

Deshpande, Sudha, Former Professor, Department of Economics, University of Mumbai.

Gumber, Anil, Senior Research Fellow, University of Warwick, United Kingdom and Senior Economist, National Council of Applied Economic Research, New Delhi (on lien).

Jesani, Amar, Programme Co-ordinator, Achutha Menon Centre (AMCSS), Sree Chitra Tirunal Institute of Medical Science and Technology, Thiruvananthapuram.

Jha, Shikha, Professor, Indira Gandhi Institute of Development Research (IGIDR), Mumbai.

Kamdar, Sangita, Research Associate, Economics for Education Unit, Department of Economics, University of Mumbai.

Karnik, Ajit, Professor and Head, Department of Economics, University of Mumbai.

Kothari, V.N., Former Head, Department of Economics, M.S. University, Baroda.

Kulkarni, B.N., General Manager, National Bank for Agriculture and Rural Development (NABARD), Mumbai.

Lalvani, Mala, Lecturer, Department of Economics, University of Mumbai.

Mungekar, B.L., Vice Chancellor, University of Mumbai and Professor, Department of Economics.

Noronha, Claire, member of Collaborative Research and Dissemination (CORD).

Prabhu, K. Seeta, Head, Human Development Resource Centre, United Nations Development Programme, New Delhi and Professor of Economics, University of Mumbai (on deputation).

Qadeer, Imrana, Professor, Centre of Social Medicine and Community Health, Jawaharlal Nehru University, New Delhi.

Shariff, Abusaleh, Principal Economist, National Council of Applied Economic Research, New Delhi.

Srinivasan, P.V., Professor, Indira Gandhi Institute of Development Research (IGIDR), Mumbai.

Sudarshan, R., is Adviser, Access to Justice, Oslo Governance Centre, Oslo.

Suryanarayana, M.H., Professor, Indira Gandhi Institute of Development Research (IGIDR), Mumbai.

Viswanathan, K.U., Assistant General Manager, NABARD, Mumbai.

Introduction

1. SOCIAL SECTORS: CONCEPT AND APPROACHES

The Concept

The connotation of the term social sectors varies depending on the user and the occasion on which it is used. Conventionally, the term is used to denote education, health and nutrition sectors, though in most countries with pervasive poverty, efforts to enhance social sector attainments rarely succeed without addressing the issue of poverty as well. However, most often in the appraisal of policies pertaining to social sectors, the success or otherwise of various poverty alleviation strategies is usually not included.[1]

Apart from the lack of a clear delimitation, social sectors are rarely considered an analytical category and most of the analysis is generally confined to identifying the determinants and problems related to individual components such as education, health and nutrition. Thus, a critical appraisal of the problems relating to social sectors as an integrated whole is often missing.

Thirdly, the theoretical underpinnings of the analysis on social sectors has not always been made clear. Consequently, the prescriptions to reform social sectors are often piece-meal in nature undermining the possibility for a coherent alternative social sector policy to emerge.

In what follows we critically examine alternative approaches to the analysis of social sectors and examine their implications for a social sector policy.

Approaches

Two distinct though related approaches, viz. the human capital approach and human development approach could be used to analyse social sectors (Prabhu, 1998).

The first approach emphasises investment in education, health and nutrition as a means of enhancing the quality of human capital which may be defined as 'stock of skills and productive knowledge embodied in people' (Rosen, 1989, p. 682). The human capital approach attracted attention during the 1960s when Schultz (1961) and Gary Becker (1962)[2] highlighted the viewpoint that education, health and nutrition cannot be considered merely as consumption goods.[3] Investment in these sectors is emphasised as a 'means' to higher productivity of labour force and justified on the basis of either financial rates of return (as in the case of education) or elasticity estimates emerging from production functions (as in the case of health).

The human capital approach has been very influential in focusing attention on the investment aspects of education, health and nutrition and has generated a large body of literature, particularly on the measurement of returns to such investment. Nonetheless, analysts since Blaug have been pointing out the limitations of this approach. Briefly, it has been noted that the human capital approach exaggerates the importance of returns to investment in schooling and ignores the importance of self-learning in enhancing the quality of human capital. Since the approach considers production in a mechanistic sense as being organised on an assembly line with individuals contributing to the production process, it fails to take cognisance of the contribution of individuals in evolving new technologies and practices (Blaug, 1976, Carnoy, 1995). Subsequent literature on endogenous growth theories incorporated the latter aspect with externalities accruing to society from investment in schooling as well as expenditure on research and development being given due importance (Romer, 1986, Lucas, 1988).

Despite this improvement, the basic orientation of the human capital approach continues to rely on private initiatives through individuals investing in themselves in terms of education, health and nutrition in expectation of higher financial returns from such investment in future. The role of the state is confined to investment in specific areas where high positive externalities to society or 'merit goods' considerations justify public investment. As issues of poverty and the consequent inability of individuals to invest in themselves do not directly enter the basic tenets of this approach, it seems to be of limited utility for the analysis of social sector policy in situations characterised by pervasive poverty.

The alternative approach, viz., the human development approach also known as the capabilities approach, views basic human attainments such as basic education, good health and nutrition as an 'end' in itself rather than as a 'means' to higher productivity and higher earnings. Social sector attainments are perceived as contributing to enhancement of the quality of life as well as to economic growth (Sen, 1994). Human development as a concept is defined as 'enlarging the range of people's choices' (UNDP, 1990) and encompasses the elements of empowerment, co-operation, equity in basic capabilities and opportunities, sustainability and security. As is evident, this approach has strong overtones of neo-Kantian philosophy.[4] The human development approach, while seemingly similar to the basic needs approach, is clearly distinguished from it by the fact that while the human development approach is concerned mainly with the 'state of existence of people—the lives they lead', the basic needs approach centres around assessing the extent of possession of detached objects (Anand and Ravallion, 1993, p. 135–36).

An important feature of the human development approach is that it considers the acquisition of minimum levels of education, health and nutrition as basic rights of the people and therefore assigns a key role to the state[5] in providing these rights. Thus, there is greater emphasis on the supply of public services as compared to the reliance placed on rise in general affluence to enhance basic capabilities. The state is not only a regulator but a provider of services as well. The focus of attention is not merely on workers who contribute to production but also the old and infirm who may not be in a position to make an economic contribution. Importantly, the approach needs no justification such as rates of return to investment to justify public expenditure on social sectors.

The human development approach is based on the premise that economic growth does not automatically lead to higher attainments and that the pattern of growth and social sector attainments. Income poverty, particularly, acts as an inhibiting factor in achieving desirable levels of social sector attainments. The role of the state, in this paradigm, extends from being a facilitator to that of investmenting directly in social services. This investment is sustained over decades in recognition of the long gestation period involved for reaping its benefits. More importantly, investment in social services is not a 'stand alone' policy measure. It is part of a redistributive ethos that permeates all policies, an essential tool for empowering the people and ensuring that the benefits of growth are equitably distributed. Specific measures to alleviate income poverty are seen as necessary interim measures to correct structural inequities.

Linkage between Approaches

It is obvious that the human development approach is more appropriate for developing countries like India which are characterised by structural inequalities and pervasive poverty. In fact, it is being increasingly realised that even for human capital to contribute to economic growth, it is essential to ensure a minimum level of social sector attainments. In recent literature, this has been stressed by reference to social capital.[6] In fact, the human development approach provides the preconditions for development of human capital in a region to contribute to economic growth.[7]

Human development could be enhanced through two routes of capability expansion, viz. growth-mediated security and public provision mediated security, both of which need to be combined judiciously for maximum impact. The former would include income generation through direct rural development and workfare programmes (popularly known as poverty alleviation measures) and the latter public provisioning of education, health and nutrition in a complementary and integrated manner.[8]

To recapitulate, three conditions need to be fulfilled for social sector policy to succeed; it needs to be (a) rooted in a redistributive ethos that permeates all public policies (b) recognise the long gestation period involved and sustain adequate investments over decades and (c) formulate and implement measures in a complementary and integrated manner so as to reap the benefits of the synergies thus generated (Prabhu, 1996).

2. SOCIAL SECTORS IN INDIA

Social sector policy in India in the light of the discussion above has been inadequate in addressing the challenges confronting the nation. Since the process of planning was initiated without altering initial structural inequities, the distribution of benefits of economic growth has not been egalitarian. Social sector policy, which could have acted as a redistributive measure, did not don this mantle. Further, the very approach of the state towards social sectors has been ambivalent. They have been considered either as constituting welfare, or as a means for enhancing human capital.

In a regime of fiscal stringency and competing demands, a welfare orientation towards social sectors has implied that the allocation of required amounts of resources to these sectors could be repeatedly diverted to 'productive sectors' which were seen as being more important. The adoption of the human capital approach, implies a focus on higher level facilities with not much attention being paid to the basic levels.[9] The results that this lack of vision about the role of social sectors in development strategy are reflected in the uneven progress that has been achieved, and the paradoxical situations that it has spawned.

The main challenge facing India's development is the high proportion of population that continues to be poor despite a high rate of growth of real per capita income (around 2 per cent per annum) being recorded between 1985–2001 (1980–1 prices). The fact that in 1999–2000 the official estimates of poverty indicate that over 260 million are below the poverty line (GOI, 2002) highlights the inadequacy of the development efforts. The high inequalities of income and the lack of a redistributive thrust is reflected in the paradox of a rising stock of over 58 million tonnes (as on 1 January, 2002 according to GOI, 2002) even as 26.1 per cent of the population live below the poverty line. This poverty explains the poor performance of the attainments in social sector.

The impressive improvements in the literacy rate from 18.33 per cent in 1951 and 52.21 per cent in 1991 to 65.38 per cent in 2001, and the resultant decline in the actual number of illiterates by 31.96 million between 1991 and 2001 (GOI, 2002) have been widely commended. While not undermining these gains, it needs to be mentioned that over one-third of the total population continues to be illiterate and our current achievements fall short of the 77 per cent literacy rate attained by the neighbouring country of Sri Lanka (UNDP, 2002) as far back as 1970. Though 'education for all' was to be achieved by the year 1990, and an allocation of 6 per cent of GDP as public investment in education (Kothari Commission, GOI,1966, Ramamoorthy Committee, GOI, 1991), was considered necessary for the purpose, public expenditure has hovered at best at 4.5 per cent of GDP.[10] The underinvestment has been compounded by misdirected priorities and inefficiencies in functioning of public schools.[11] While allocations for basic education have been inadequate, the generous subsidies to higher education in an milieu characterised by uneven access to such education owing to high inequalities in income has resulted in the paradox of the country being home in 2001 to the largest reservoir of illiterate children between 6–14 years of age (200 million, GOI 2001), even as it is lauded for the having one of the world's largest pools of highly trained technical and scientific personnel. The Approach Paper to the Tenth Plan candidly admits with respect to education that 'Our performance in education is one of the most disappointing aspects of our development strategy' (GOI, Planning Commission, 2002, para 3.57).

A similar dilemma is one of the incomplete epidemiological transition with the rising incidence of diseases such as tuberculosis even as lifestyle diseases claim much greater attention from the point of view of resource allocation-both human and financial. In terms of attainments, life expectancy at birth rose from a low of 37.2 years in 1951 to 60.4 years in 1997 (Government of India, 2002). This falls far short of the 65.1 years attained in Sri Lanka in 1970–75 (UNDP, 2002). Similarly, though India's infant mortality rate declined from 146 in 1951–61 to 70 in 1999 (GOI, 2002) it is higher than the 65.1 recorded by Sri Lanka in 1970–75 (UNDP, 2002). The allocations to the health sector have been much lower than those for education. Public expenditure on health, constitutes only 1.8 per cent of GDP. Inadequate facilities in the public sector and the poor functioning of even these facilities have led the households to rely on the private sector which accounts for three fourths of their expenditure on health and this is an important *cause* of poverty. The Planning Commission admits this in the Approach Paper to the Tenth Plan by stating that 'Data from NSSO indicate that the escalating health care costs is one of the reasons for indebtedness not only among the poor but also in the middle-income group' (GOI, Planning Commission, 2002, para 3.71).

What is indeed intriguing is that while India's social sector attainments fall far short of what countries such as Sri Lanka and China attained at least three decades ago, the current discourse on social sector expenditures continues to ignore this fundamental reality. In fact, the predominant opinion seems to be that since the current levels of public expenditure incurred on social sectors in India, 4.5 per cent of GDP on education and less than 2 per cent of GDP on health is similar to that of several East Asian economies, they are considered to be 'adequate'. This argument is fallacious as it is incorrect to compare the expenditure levels of countries at very different levels of attainment. Several official committees in India

(Kothari Commission 1966, Ramamoorthy Committee 1991 and ICSSR-ICMR Report 1981) have recommended that the expenditure on education and health be at least 6 per cent of GDP for each of these sectors. However, the current levels are far less than those stipulated as far back as the 1980s. Even these levels have been threatened since the initiation of economic reforms in India in 1991 (Prabhu, 1999). The dichotomy between public expenditure and resultant social outcomes becomes extremely pertinent in this context. Reforms undertaken in various social sectors across the states have further sought to advocate cost recovery and limited engagement of the government in the provision of social services. It is needless to say that the weakening of protective social security systems further aggravates the socio-economic security provided to the poorer sections of the population (Prabhu, 2001).

While inadequate resource allocation is a fundamental problem facing social sectors, there is much that can be accomplished even within the existing resources.

The first measure is to recognise the need for a more holistic conceptual framework in order to plan for social sectors in India. The second is to identify specific measures in each of the main areas constituting the social sectors and to recognise that there could be a need for conceptual and practical modifications in order to ensure that these well intentioned measures taken by the government yielded the desired results.

Poverty

India, as many other developing countries, is faced with the imperative of reducing the number of poor even while reining public spending. Targeting is often considered to be the answer to this predicament though it is not always easy to accomplish. In fact, errors associated with targeting have been the subject of much debate. In this scenario, self-selecting programmes, viz. rural public works programmes (RWPs), are recommended to avoid some of the direct and indirect costs of targeting schemes. The objectives of RWPs are to provide employment and create a rural infrastructure. The paper by Mahendra Dev, 'What have We Learnt from Rural Public Works', analyses the experience of RWPs, mainly the Employment Guarantee Scheme (EGS) in Maharashtra and the Jawahar Rojgar Yojana (JRY) at the national level.

The paper reiterates some well-known achievements of the scheme, including its notable impact on the intensity of poverty which has helped the ultra poor, especially women, and its indirect benefits, such as the creation of rural assets and the benefits accruing from the provision of employment which is high in the lean season and low in the peak season. The distinctive approach of considering employment as a legal entitlement, is seen as enabling the rural poor to improve their bargaining strength. The JRY has provided employment to the poorer sections of the society, although there is a significant variation in coverage across states. However, it did not reach out to women as effectively as the EGS in Maharashtra. In terms of targeting errors, an evaluation of the EGS with other poverty alleviation programmes like the IRDP and PDS, indicated better efficiency of targeting towards the poor. Further, secondary benefits from the EGS such as asset creation and provision of insurance benefits have considerably improved the living standards of the poor. The analysis also illustrates the difference in the scenario during drought and normal years.

Reforms suggested for improving the functioning of the EGS and ensuring that EGS works are not merely relief-oriented but contribute to the building of a rural infrastructure. These include enhancing the outlay for EGS, proper project selection and planning, speedy transfer of completed works to Zilla Parishads (district level panchayats) and allocation of adequate funds for maintenance. Another objective of the EGS works is ensuring the participation of people and voluntary organisations which contribute to the reduction in leakages and improve transparency in the scheme's operation. In the case of JRY, the use of buffer stocks of food for employment generation, involvement of panchayats and ensuring linkage with sectoral programmes have been stressed. In view of the poor employment scenario in India, it was decided that public works can be effective in combatting poverty.

The role of credit creation as an alternative strategy to the alleviation poverty is considered by Kulkarni and Viswanathan in the paper 'Innovative Rural Credit Delivery Systems for Poverty Alleviation—Some Experiences'. Despite the extensive rural financial infrastructure created by the initiatives of the Reserve Bank of India and the National Bank for Rural Development at various points, the formal credit structure has failed to adequately address the requirement of adequate and timely credit for the poor. Some of the models of alternative channel constituted by Non-Governmental Organisations (NGOs) and voluntary agencies and Self-Help Groups (SHGs), which are designed to reach the poor have been illustrated in this paper. The need for group commitment and minimal government intervention, limited to the provision of infrastructure, have been highlighted. The paper also emphasises the need for transparency in NGO funding and general support systems and exclusive provisions in the Banking Statutes.

It is necessary to recognise the rising importance of informal sector activities in the course of development in the country in order to be able to address issues of poverty reduction. The heterogeneity of the informal sector in India and the growing feminisation of labour are also important dimensions to be considered. The paper 'Gender and the Informal Sector: Implications for Poverty Alleviation' by Sudha Deshpande and Lalit Deshpande examines these issues using a sample of 200 women workers living in two slums pockets within Mumbai city. Several development programmes including income and employment generation programmes, housing programmes and vocational training programmes that are targeted towards working women as well as poor, downtrodden widows, destitute, and disabled women are analysed. The low allocations of public expenditure and the shortfall of allocated expenditure have been the main deterrants in ensuring the desired impact. Policies have been suggested in this paper which address the needs of home-based workers, and women who are in dead-end menial jobs. Stress is laid on training, both formal and informal, in the light of market demand and workers' needs. The need for creating a database for the formulation of appropriate policies has also been highlighted.

The definition of poverty and the linkages between income poverty and human poverty have been spelt out by Seeta Prabhu and Sangita Kamdar in the paper 'Human Poverty and Income Poverty: Linkages and Implications'. Measures proposed to quantify human poverty are considered in this paper and differences in the approaches used are highlighted. The Human Poverty Index (HPI) suggested by the UNDP and the Modified Human Poverty Index (HPIM) proposed by the authors are constructed for fifteen major Indian states. The HPIM attempts to address objections to the inclusion of both input and output indicators in the HPI. Both the computations indicate high deprivation in capabilities at the national level. The ranking of states with respect to per capita income, income poverty and human poverty is compared in order to understand the linkages between these variables. The analysis indicates that higher average levels of income do not necessarily imply lower levels of income poverty and human poverty. Political commitment in terms of government expenditures on social services is an important variable that explains variations in human poverty across states.

Nutrition

The relationship in India between foodgrains production, prices and rural poverty during the period from 1971–72 to 1991–92, has been spelt out by Mungekar in the paper 'Foodgrain Production, Prices and Rural Poverty in India'. An analytical framework is introduced to explain the determinants of poverty in India over two decades from 1971–72 to 1991–92. The explanatory variables of rural poverty are: (1) rural poverty (RPOV) (2) per capita availability of foodgrains (PUNAFD)—used as a proxy for foodgrains production (3) irrigation (IRGN) (4) real agricultural wages (RAWGS); (5) procurement of foodgrain as percentage of net availability (PROFD). Real agricultural wages emerged as the most important factor explaining the decline in rural poverty. Irrigation had a strong negative impact on rural poverty. The increased use of irrigation raised cropping intensity of Indian agriculture which in turn resulted in an increase in the demand of labour and a lowering of prices. Procurement of foodgrains had also a negative effect. Foodgrain production represented by per capita net availability had a negative impact on poverty, although its impact was minimal as compared to that of other variables. It has been pointed out in this paper that an inegalitarian agrarian structure, along with social and cultural inequalities, reduces the impact of increase in foodgrains production which could otherwise reduce rural poverty.

Shikha Jha and P.V. Srinivasan assess the efficacy of distribution of foodgrains through the public distribution system (PDS) in the paper on 'Targeting Food Subsidies'. The analysis indicates that despite some improvement in the functioning of the existing Public Distribution System (PDS) from the mid-1990s, and its much higher pro-poor bias than other public services, the PDS seems to have failed to transfer grains from surplus to deficit states. Inter-regional biases in distribution of PDS supplies persist. In order to limit subsidies to the poor, the Targeted Public Distribution Scheme (TPDS) was introduced in 1997. Difficulties in identifying the population below the poverty line, those without a residential address have reduced the effectiveness of this scheme. Experiences of other countries, which highlight the possibilities of either incorporating self-selection measures or incentive effects of public transfer suggest the desirability of introducing a link between PDS and employment based programmes.

Reforms relating to PDS should concentrate on improving the self-targeting feature of the universal system. Targeting through the identification of group characteristics could minimise errors of exclusion. Further, it has been suggested that government costs can be reduced by increasing the operational efficiency of the Food Corporation of India (FCI) and limiting its role to only price stabilisation.

Nutrition security is also an important element to be considered and addressed if people's choices have to be enlarged. Suryanarayana in his paper 'Nutrition Security in India: Issues and Policies' attempts to examine and quantify the degree of nutrition security (particularly with reference to cereal consumption and calorie intake) across states and at the all-India level. During the decade 1983–84 to 1993–94, poverty declined across Indian states, with the exception of Assam and Haryana where rural poverty levels increased. However, contrary to expectations, average calorie intake declined in both rural and urban sectors in the majority of the states. Analysis indicates that this was due to an increase in cost of cereals as a result of the changes in production conditions, cropping patterns, exchange entitlements of the rural poor, and consumption preferences. From this perspective, policy instruments such as the PDS have a major role to play in ensuring adequate cereal availability and calorie intake, particularly in calorie deficient states. These facts also indicate that poverty alleviation programmes alone may not ensure nutrition security. Policies have to ensure the availability of cereals and additional efforts are necessary to put the consumer education programmes in place, in order to guide consumer choices.

Health

The next set of papers deal with the health sector. The need to give priority to preventive care, and to regulate the health care delivery sector in general and the private sector in health in particular are the two main themes considered by Amar Jesani in 'Social Objectives of Health Care Services: Need and Strategy for Regulating the Private Sector'. The specific social objective of medical care is making available basic health services, such as curative, preventive and promotive, to all who need it. The distribution of health care services in India is characterised by dominance of the private sector and de-ruralised in terms of availability of health infrastructure as well health care personnel. The relatively unregulated functioning of the private sector has made health a commodity. The large size of the health sector and private sector dominance has created a social force that needs to be taken into account in planning for public health and in achieving the social objective of making health care universally accessible. The basic reorganisation of medical care would create greater space for both public health as well as community health services.

In the paper on 'Primary Health Care: From Adjustment to Reforms' Imrana Qadeer discusses the transformation of primary health care system in India. The concept of primary health care includes along with the provision of basic health services, the provision of various developmental inputs, secondary and tertiary care. Evolving health care services according to the needs affordability and participation of the people is extremely important. The Alma Ata Declaration recognised the importance of 'political will' but did not spell out the consequent prerequisite for primary health, which and led to the dilution of the term to basic health care. During economic reforms there were cutbacks in the public sector, fiscal restraints on welfare measures and growth in emphasis of the market mechanism. Thus, while measures to strengthen primary health care were explored, its role was truncated to imply primary level health care. For effective primary health care provisioning, there is a need to invest in the welfare sector, so that the most vulnerable sections of the society are covered and the quality of care standardised. Decentralisation is considered to be effective in making primary health care more community oriented. The role of NGOs, in providing specific services and keeping a vigil over local institutions, and medical education is also important. Monitoring the co-ordination with the private sector, in the provision of primary health care, should also be introduced.

Ajit Karnik and Mala Lawani discuss the 'political' dimension of the alleviation of poverty and ensuring availability of basic facilities in 'Building Coalitions: Moving from Subsidies for Interest Groups to Social Sector Spending'. In order to re-orient government spending towards genuine welfare activities and away from subsidies to interest groups, it is necessary to emphasise that a potential loss of political support from interest groups could be compensated by a gain in support from beneficiaries of welfare oriented spending. This process must involve a change in the configuration of interest groups through the coalitions of beneficiaries of welfare spending. Estimates indicate that a mere 1 percentage point hike in recovery rates would yield enough resources to provide health benefits to approximately 10 million persons. Even if some of these beneficiaries are non-voting, such numbers could compensate the loss of political support arising out of curtailment of subsidies. It is therefore suggested that, even within the existing framework of political economy, it is possible to transcend the status quo and improve the quality of government interventions.

The health sector in India is beset with many problems. Despite substantial public investment in health infrastructure in India, access and use of services varies considerably across population groups, regions and different settlements. These variations are the result of not only differences in health-seeking behaviour of the people concerned, but also due to the types of policies, programmes and investments across states. Abusaleh Shariff and Anil Gumber in 'Health Care Services in Rural India: Implications for Reproductive Health' examine the use of health care services and treatment facilities for women and men according to socio-economic status in different population settings. A scrutiny of the pattern of health expenditures across various states indicated wide inter-state disparities in government health expenditure, high out of pocket expenditures as well as under utilisation of existing facilities. Among various factors considered, the availability of health care facilities and female literacy are the most important factors in influencing the utilisation of reproductive health care facilities as well as child immunisation. It is suggested that an expanded definition of primary health care (not associated only with immunisation and maternal and child health services), including basic curative, preventive and promotive services be adopted. The paper recommends a new approach to set up an organised public-private mix to attain universal coverage of health care.

Education

The last set of papers attempts to analyse various aspects pertaining to the education sector. Anuradha De and Claire Noronha discuss the results of a field survey conducted in 1996 in 188 villages of Uttar Pradesh, Bihar, Rajasthan and Madhya Pradesh, which found that parental indifference towards the importance of educating their children is only a myth. The interplay between high parental motivation and low quality of government schools, which often results in the rapid spread of private schools even in rural areas, is spelt out in their paper 'Parental Motivation and Private Schooling'. Demand for education is not homogeneous, and has a strong gender bias, which influences educational attainments of the children belonging to the same household. It was also found that demand for education does not often translate into demand for schooling, mainly because of high cost involved. These factors lead to investment on education of few children and deprivation for other children in the same household. Incentives such as food rations, mid-day meals and free text books have attracted children to school. Despite high parental motivation towards education, poor quality of education coupled with lack of sufficient infrastructure in government schools have led to poor education attainments. These factors have contributed partly, towards a growing reliance on private schooling. While high parental motivation presents immense scope for achieving universal elementary education, unless the decay in government schools is reversed, the achievement of this goal will not be possible.

The education sector faces a severe resource crisis, which could be tackled by introducing higher fees. Kothari in the paper 'Should Higher Education in India be Self-Financing?' identifies practical consequences of a fee structure, and spells out the rationale for public expenditure on higher education. The higher education sector would shrink in size if a self-financing approach is introduced, as enrolment of girls, students from rural areas, and from disadvantaged classes of population would decline as enrolment based on merit would be replaced to a significant extent by a system that is ordered on financial ability. If higher education became self-financing, a larger quantum of resources would become available to ensure universal enrolment of children. An attempt is made to indicate the resources that could then be freed in terms of total budgeted revenue expenditure on higher education by the education departments of the state and central governments, as well as other departments. The role of public expenditure on higher education is emphasised as a means to maintain adequate supply of educated manpower and to facilitate social integration across the deprived population. A possible fee structure could be introduced so that the majority of the students are able to pay fees, and for others who are not in a position to pay, mechanisms could be introduced so that fees are waived or some financial aid is provided.

According to the human capital theory, skills acquired in school are directly related to the characteristics that labour needs, and results in improved economic performance. Productivity is an intervening variable in the connection between education and earnings. The role played by formal education at the level of a firm is analysed by Ramesh Datta in the paper 'Human Capital, Performance and Earning: A Firm Level Study'. This study includes performance rating as an intervening variable, although it attempts to incorporate the effects of other variables as well (viz. motivation, regularity, etc.). Empirical estimation conducted using a recursive model while supporting the human capital approach to earnings determination, shows that traditional simple human capital variables (e.g. years of formal education and experience on the job) do not necessarily determine performance variations on the job. It also emphasises the importance of in-firm and off-the-job training to upgrade the workers' skills. The paper draws attention to the fact that in the present era of competition, where the gap between skills required to work with new technologies and the existing ones is constantly growing, new human capital in the form of continuous in-firm and off-the-job training to upgrade workers' skills is therefore imperative.

CONCLUSION

The papers, taken collectively, address aspects of the social sectors that recognise the importance of including structural inequities as an integral part of the analysis. Very little work has been done in this area. The book has put forth a common point of view that stresses empowerment, participation of people and voluntary organisations, and greater government responsibility in ensuring the enhancement of capabilities of the masses. The collection, while covering a vast canvas, does not pay sufficient attention to issues of gender equity and decentralisation, though they are touched upon by several authors. Also missing is an analysis of financing for human development. The omission of these issues is more due to constraints of time and space rather than being unaware of their importance in the current context. We hope that despite some limitations, including the inevitable time gap between the preparation of the papers and their final publication, the volume will serve as a useful compendium to articulate the human development paradigm and focus attention on various reforms in India's social sectors that require urgent attention from academics, civil society and policy makers.

END NOTES

1. It is only recently that the Government of India has acknowledged the importance of providing an annual review of the measures undertaken in social sectors. Consequently, a chapter on social sectors has been included in the Economic Survey that precedes the presentation of the Union Budget. Significantly, poverty alleviation programmes are included

in this chapter along with a discussion on measures to enhance the education, health and nutrition levels.

2. Schultz (1961) perceived a country's human capital at any given date as an important factor in analysing its production possibilities and stated '... investment in human capital accounts for most of the impressive rise in real earnings per worker' (Schultz, 1961, p. 1). Gary Becker (1962) added another dimension of on-the-job training to the formation of human capital and influenced the analysis of firm-specific investment in training, labour relations and contracts.
3. The expenditure on schooling, health, on-the-job training, searching for information about job opportunities and migration, constitutes investment that people make in themselves.
4. The basic proposition of Kant was that '... all rational beings come under the *law* that each of them must treat itself and all others *never merely as means*, but in every case *at the same time as ends in themselves* (Kant, 1785, p. 58, emphasis as in original).
5. Dreze and Sen (1995, p. 17) have defined the state as encompassing governance, legislative and the political system prevailing in a region.
6. Social capital has been defined by Abromovitz (1995, p. 45) as 'a set of attitudinal and institutional characteristics'. Krishna and Uphoff (1999, p. 8) use the term to refer to both *social networks* as well as *shared norms, values, attitudes and beliefs*.
7. The linkage between the two approaches can be illustrated in terms of the East Asian economies that emphasised universalisation of primary education along with complementary provisioning of higher levels of education, even as they pursued higher levels of investment and growth, which enabled these countries to achieve growth with equity.
8. Dasgupta (1993) has emphasised complementary public provisioning of services to enable investments in human capital to yield higher rates of return and proposes a social contract that pre-commits the access to commodities such as nutrition, housing, primary and secondary education, basic health care and legal services.
9. Of the allocations for education, less than 50 per cent is allocated for elementary education (Tilak, 2001).
10. The Ramamoorthy Committee (1991) recommended that 6 per cent of GDP should be invested in education. This has been accepted by the Government of India and is expected to be implemented from the Tenth Plan period.
11. The PROBE report covering a sample of 1376 households, in 234 randomly—selected villages of Bihar, Madhya Pradesh, Rajasthan, Uttar Pradesh and Himachal Pradesh reported that of all the school buildings '... only 58 per cent had at least two *pucca* rooms and nearly two-thirds have a leaking roof, which disrupted the classroom activity for weeks during monsoon.' The Report also indicated that due to single teachers

handling large number of students, the effective teaching time amounted to less than one minute of individual teaching attention per pupil per day over the whole year. (PROBE, 1998, p. 45)

REFERENCES

Abromovitz, M. 1995. 'The Elements of Social Capability' in *Social Capability and Long—Term Economic—Growth*. Eds. Koo B.H. and D.H. Perkins. New York, St. Martin's Press.

Anand and Ravallion, 1993. 'Human Development in Poor Countries: On Role of Private Income and Public Services', *Journal of Economic Perspectives*, 7(1):130–50, Winter.

Becker, G., 1962. 'Investment in Human Capital: A Theoretical Analysis,' *Journal of Political Economy*, Vol. LXX(5): 9–49.

Blaug, M., 1976. 'The Empirical Status of Human Capital Theory: A Slightly Jaundiced Survey,' *Journal of Economic Literature*, 14: 827–55.

Carnoy, M., 1995. 'The Economics of Education: Then and Now' in *International Encyclopaedia of Economics of Education*, Cambridge, Cambridge University Press.

Dasgupta, P., 1993. *An Inquiry into Well-being and Destitution*, Oxford, Clarendon Press.

Dreze, J. and Amartya Sen, 1995. *India: Economic Development and Social Opportunity*, Oxford, Oxford University Press.

Government of India, 1966. Report of the Education (Kothari) Commission, 1964–66 New Delhi.

———, 1991. Committee for Review of National Policy on Education, 1986 (Ramamoorthy Committee), New Delhi.

———, 2002. *Economic Survey*, Ministry of Finance, GOI, New Delhi.

Indian Council of Social Science Research (ICSSR) and Indian Council of Medical Research (ICMR), 1981. *'Health for All: An Alternative Strategy'*, Indian Institute of Education, Pune.

Kant, I., 1785. *Fundamental Principles of the Metaphysic of Morals*, Illinois, Henry Regnery Company Chicago.

Krishna, A. and Uphoff, N. 1999. 'Mapping and Measuring Social Capital: A Conceptual and Empirical Study of Collective Action for Conserving and Developing Watersheds in Rajasthan, India' (Cornell University, *http://www.ids.sussex.ac.uk/*) p. 8.

Lucas, R.E. 1988. 'On The Mechanics of Economic Development', *Journal of Monetary Economics*, 22(1): pp. 3–42.

Planning Commission, 2001, *Approach Paper to The Tenth Five Year Plan, 2002–2007*. Government of India, New Delhi.

Prabhu, K. Seeta, 1998. 'Social Sectors in Economic Development', *Journal of Social and Economic Development*, 1(2), pp. 268–87.

______, 1999. 'Social Sectors During Economic Reforms: The Indian Experience', *Oxford Development Studies*, 27(2), pp. 187–210.

PROBE, 1999. *Public Report on Basic Education In India*, New Delhi, Oxford University Press

Romer, P.M. 1986. 'Increasing Returns and Long Run Growth', *Journal of Political Economy*, 94(5), pp. 1002–37

Rosen, S., 1989. 'Human Capital' in J. Eatwell, M. Milgate and P. Newman (eds), *The New Palgrave Dictionary of Economics*, Vol. 2. London, Macmillan Press

Schultz, T.W., 1961. 'Investment in Human Capital', *American Economic Review*, 51(1): 1–17

Tilak, J.B.G., 2001. 'Public Subsidies in the Education Sector in India', Paper presented at a Conference on Fiscal Policies to Accelerate Economic Growth, organised by the World Bank, 21–22 May 2001, New Delhi.

United Nations Development Programme (UNDP) 1990, 2002. *Human Development Report*, Oxford University Press.

part one

Poverty

chapter 1

Rural Public Works

• *S. Mahendra Dev*

1. INTRODUCTION

Targeting is regarded as an attractive method of intervention to alleviate poverty in many developing countries that face the necessity both of reducing the number of poor and limiting the extent of public spending. The rationale for targeting is that the benefits are higher for the population at the lower end of the income distribution than at the upper end. However, targeting schemes have many direct and indirect costs. To avoid some of these problems, particularly high administrative costs, programmes that are self-selecting in character are recommended for poverty alleviation. Rural public works programmes (RWPs) have become important instruments for alleviating poverty and hunger in many developing countries. The case for RWPs lies in the self-targeting nature of these schemes. There is a growing theoretical and empirical literature on the impact of public works programmes (or 'workfare') on poverty alleviation (Dreze and Sen, 1989; Ravallion, 1991; Besley and Coate, 1992; Besley and Kanbur, 1993; Sen, 1995). 'Workfare' is supposed to enable a social planner to separate the non-poor from the poor by connecting income transfers to participation in public works. Public works also fit into the ideas of Ragnar Nurkse (1957), who regarded surplus labour in low-income countries useful for capital formation. The objectives of RWPs are to provide employment and to generate 'public goods' such as physical infrastructure. It may, however, be noted that while public works are supported by the public sector, it is possible that implementation may sometimes rest on private sector and community level initiatives. On the other hand, certain public works, such as land development, may be publicly sponsored and executed but may generate private benefits.

India has been experimenting with labour intensive public works since long. After attaining independence in 1947, many schemes were sponsored by the central government, beginning with the Rural Manpower programme in 1960.[1] The Employment Guarantee Scheme (EGS) implemented in the state of Maharashtra received acclaim from several sources. It is a particularly interesting example because of its unprecedented feature of guaranteed rural employment, which makes it a model for other states in India and in the developing world.[2] At the national level, the Jawahar Rojgar Yojana (JRY) and Employment Assurance Scheme (EAS) are important programmes implemented in rural areas. The JRY was restructured in 1999 and renamed Jawahar Gram Samridhi Yojana (JGSY). In terms of person days of employment created, India's rural public works programmes are the largest in the world. The JRY reached around one billion person days in recent years. The share of JRY expenditure in government expenditure on social sectors is quite high; around Rs 200 billion was spent on wage employment programmes during the Eighth Five-Year Plan (1992–7). It is necessary, therefore, to assess the working of these programmes.

The main objective of this paper is to analyse the experience of rural public works programmes in India in order to learn some lessons regarding poverty alleviation. The problems encountered and the lessons learnt in the functioning of these schemes would be useful for suggesting reforms in India's wage employment programmes. In this study, we restrict ourselves to two major schemes, one at the state level (EGS) and the other at the national level (JRY). Apart from these experiences, it is also important to be clear about the conceptual issues relating to public works.

Thus, the specific objectives of the paper are to: (a) provide an overview of conceptual issues (Section 2); (b) analyse India's experience in public works (Section 3); (c) discuss lessons from India's wage employment programme (Section 4); and (d) suggest reforms for better working of public works in order to reach the poor more effectively (Section 5).

2. CONCEPTUAL ISSUES

Several earlier studies have discussed the theoretical and empirical issues on public works programmes.[3] In this section we provide a brief overview of the conceptual issues for better understanding the working of RWPs.

2.1 Costs of Targeting and the Case for Self-targeting Schemes

Targeting costs can be classified into four types. They are administrative, incentive (dead-weight), disutility and stigma, and political.[4] The administrative and political economy costs are more serious as compared to other costs but can be minimised in the case of self-targeted public works.

(a) Administrative Costs

The administrative costs mainly relate to costs borne to identify the poor, which can be particularly high if targeting is based on income-based means tests. Exclusion errors (failure to include all the poor) can also be quite high if there is a shift from universal to targeted schemes.[5] It has also been shown that attempts to achieve 'more for the poor' through the use of indicator targeting may in fact mean less for the poor (Gelbach and Pritchett, 1995). However, exclusion errors can be minimised with self-targeted schemes like rural public works.

(b) Incentive Costs

One negative incentive effect often mentioned about targeted subsidies is distortions in labour-leisure choice. According to a study of the effect of receipt of a rice ration on labour supply in both rural and urban areas (Sahn and Alderman, 1995), there has been substantial reduction in the level of work effort in response to receiving the rice ration. In other words, workers increased their leisure time due to the rice scheme. This, however, cannot be called as dead-weight loss. In a strict welfare sense, the worker's overall utility (in terms of work and leisure) might be higher now as compared to the period before the introduction of food subsidies.

The disincentive to work is a problem associated with programmes targeted according to income-based means tests. The beneficiaries may change their behaviour by altering their labour supply and hence their income.[6] The workers may be better off by remaining poor in order to be eligible for the benefits under the means test based scheme. The beneficiary may not lose anything from the programme but society as a whole would lose their output.

(c) Stigma and Disutility Costs

It is argued that stigma and disutility are possible negative consequences of means-tested government transfer programmes. The recipients may lose their self-esteem because they have to rely on public support and the non-recipients may treat the recipients differently due to targeting. Moreover, universalisation itself is some kind of a targeting objective because the aim is to cover more numbers of the poor. Public works programmes do not carry the stigma attached to charity handouts.

(d) Political Economy Costs

Any anti-poverty programme needs political support. It has been argued that while politicians and governments generally support programmes with wide or universal coverage, finely targeted programmes may not have political support. However, self-targeted programmes may have wider support as compared to income-based means-tested programmes. For example, the Employment Guarantee Scheme has considerable political support in Maharashtra.

The effectiveness of the programme depends on factors such as costs, benefits (direct and indirect), wage rates and the source of financing.

2.2 Direct Transfer Benefits due to Rural Public Works Programmes

Direct benefit, also called transfer benefit, is the income (wages times number of days employed) a labourer gets which depends on factors such as the share of wages in the total expenditure, costs of participation (e.g., transport costs) and the income forgone from alternative employment (see Table 1). In some countries, the poor who participate in public works may have to pay part of their wages to officials, contractors, or politicians which may potentially reduce programme benefits. A hypothetical example is given in Table 1. In this example, out of government expenditure of Rs 100 on public works, the net direct transfer benefit to the poor is only Rs 18. In this example, we assumed 50 per cent as share of wages, 2 per cent of wage cost as cost of transportation and other transaction costs, 30 per cent of wages as foregone incomes, and 20 per cent of wages as leakages.

Thus, if the share of wages is high, transfer benefits will be higher. Similarly, if the cost of participation (such as transportation), forgone income and leakages are low, the net transfer benefits will be larger.[7] Targeting efficiency depends on the design of the programme with respect to wage rates, mode of payment etc.

2.3 Indirect Benefits

Theoretical literature has concentrated more on the targeting aspect and issues like mode of payment (e.g., cash vs food), rather than

TABLE 1. TRANSFER BENEFITS TO THE WORKERS: HYPOTHETICAL EXAMPLE

	(Rs)
Total Budget	100
Share of wages (proportion)	0.50
Gross Transfer Benefit	*50*
Cost of participation*	2
Foregone incomes	15
Leakages (corruption)	10
Net transfer benefits to workers	*23*
Targeting Efficiency (coverage of the poor)	80 per cent
Net Transfer to the Poor	*18*

Note: *Transportation and other transaction costs.

on the 'general equilibrium' or indirect benefits in public works programmes. The case for RWPs as compared to other poverty programmes lies more in the indirect benefits that they bestow.

(a) Stabilisation Benefits

One of the most important aspects of RWPs is the seasonally stabilising effect on the incomes of the poor. If the timing of the programmes synchronises with the agricultural slack season, when the demand for labour is low, labourers are most likely to gain from the resulting income stabilisation and consumption smoothing. Reducing fluctuations in income can be as important to the poor as raising average incomes. It can prevent acute distress and avoid the need for costly forms of adjustment, such as selling productive assets. In other words, even if the increase in employment and income is not very large as compared to aggregate needs, the existence of a form of income or employment insurance can be quite significant. The value of the insurance function of public works will depend on other factors such as the ease with which employment is actually obtainable and the costs of alternative mechanisms, e.g., credit.

(b) Asset Creation and Impact on Agricultural Growth

The second round effect of public works is the contribution to the creation of rural assets. The projects mainly relate to soil conservation, land development, irrigation and rural roads. They can have substantial impact on agricultural growth. There are two issues regarding asset creation. First, the assets created have to be productive in order to have an impact on rural growth. For example, the RWPs should not build roads that get washed away in the next monsoon. The second issue is that even if the assets are productive, the benefits of the created assets can go to the non-poor. The poor, however, can get continuing benefits in the form of employment from rural asset creation like land improvements.

(c) Upward Pressure on Agricultural Wages

The RWPs exert an upward pressure on agricultural wages. They increase the bargaining power of unskilled labourers during negotiations with an employer or the landlord. Thus, RWPs can curb the oligopsonistic power of large landlords (Gaiha, 1996). However, if wages are too high, demand for labour in agriculture may be reduced and large farmers may resort to labour-displacing mechanisation.

2.4 Workfare Schemes vs Uniform Untargeted Transfers

If indirect benefits like creation of productive assets and upward pressure on rural wages are not substantial, it is possible to argue that workfare schemes are no better than uniform untargeted transfers. As mentioned by Ravallion and Datt (1995), 'the direct impact on poverty incidence arising from employment on public works schemes was no greater than could have been achieved with a uniform (untargeted) allocation of the same gross budget across all households'. This is because in public works there is loss to the poor associated with forgone incomes, administration, supervision, and other non-wage costs generated by the public works. Thus, indirect effects seem to be crucial in order to argue the case for public works. It may be noted, however, that the mechanism of uniform, untargeted allocation of the budget across all households is a hypothetical scenario.

2.5 Wage Rate Determination and Targeting

Wage rate determination in public works is the most critical policy decision. Two considerations come into play in wage determination. First, labour market characteristics and labour/capital price ratios, both of which determine choice of technology in public works programmes in a specific setting and season of implementation, and second, reservation wage rates for the poor (including self-employed or subsistence farmers) who participate in the labour market. These two considerations suggest, on the one hand, a concern that wage rates should not be too low to reach the desired skill and productivity levels and so as not to overextend labour intensity and, on the other hand, a concern that wage rates should not be too high to render the maintenance of the self-targeting feature of public works programmes under fiscal constraints difficult (Braun,1995).

The general argument is that wage rates should be at a subsistence level so that the poor may participate in such programmes through self-selection. It tends to be tempting to set wage rates in public works at levels too high (for instance at public sector minimum wage rates) which then results in employment rationing under prevailing fiscal constraints. This in turn usually excludes more of the relatively poorest segments of interested employees. There is some merit in the low wage argument if one wants to concentrate on reducing the intensity or severity of poverty. However, if the aim is to take the poor up to the so-called poverty line, obviously higher wages are needed.

2.6 Cash vs Kind

The mode of payment of wages—cash or in kind (food)—is an important design feature that influences participation decisions. Payment in kind may attract more women than men to worksites. Whether wages in public works should be in the form of cash or kind depends on local circumstances relating to the risk of market failure.[8] Cash is preferred to food in well-developed markets while food is preferred to cash in case of market failure. When increased demand for food is induced through a large public works scheme, food must be forthcoming locally or it may induce inflationary pressures. Inflation may also hurt non-participating households if food supply is not increased in the local market.[9] Giving cash as wages may provide more freedom to labourers to purchase goods of their choice. However, food is preferred to cash if the aim is to attract more women and improve the nutrition level of the households. Food for work is also preferable if governments have surplus buffer stocks of food at their disposal.

2.7 Social Opportunity Cost of Funds

Are there better alternative programmes that can reduce poverty as compared to labour intensive public works? Would they have had an effect, that are different in the short and long term, if the same resources were put for alternative uses (e.g., investment on irrigation, education, health) by the government? This is an empirical question. To some extent, computable general equilibrium models can capture the impact of alternative policies on the poor.[10]

(a) Source of Financing

The related issue is the mode of financing, which can influence the sustainability of the programme and impact on the poor. If employment were expanded entirely through an aid-financed scheme, the transfer benefits to workers would be straightforward. If public works are funded from specific taxes, the government has a choice: tax non-target groups or tax the whole population. For instance, an urban employment tax in Maharashtra is used to partially finance an employment guarantee programme. In this case the resources are being redistributed from the relatively rich to the poor. On the other hand, if the programme is financed out of general tax revenues, the implications for the poor could be different. If the costs are high, it may require deficit financing and the ensuing inflationary pressures may hurt the poor disproportionately.

2.8 Opportunity Cost for the Individuals

As mentioned previously, participation in public works involves some costs to workers. Opportunity costs are defined here as the expected wage forgone by participating in public works when that person works on his or her farm or on his or her household or chooses leisure. From society's point of view, however, there may not be loss of output because others may take up the jobs left by public works employees. Similarly, even for the public works employees, the opportunity cost is much less if employment is provided during the slack season, when the choice for the labourer is between leisure and work under public works.

2.9 Conflicts between the Objectives of Relief Employment and Development

There is generally a conflict between the short-term objective of providing relief employment and the long-term aim of asset creation. If the wage share were very high in the projects, the funds available for materials and other non-wage costs would be low. On the other hand, the long-term development type projects have a somewhat lower labour share in total cost due to higher planning and capital costs. The issue of the employment-asset creation trade-off arises most sharply when public works programmes are utilised as time-limited, crisis mitigating instruments. Excessive emphasis on short-term employment effects for the target group may, however, result in programmes lacking technical and economic viability ('digging holes' programmes). On the other hand, disregarding the short-term self-targeting feature of public works programmes overlooks the key potential for poverty reduction with this instrument.

3. THE INDIAN EXPERIENCE: IMPACT ON THE POOR

3.1 Employment Guarantee Scheme

The Employment Guarantee Scheme (EGS) introduced in Maharashtra in the early 1970s is an innovative anti-poverty intervention. The EGS provides a guarantee of employment to all adults above 18 years of age who are willing to do unskilled manual work on a piece rate basis. The scheme is self-targeting in nature and is totally financed by the state government. The main objectives of the EGS are to improve household welfare in the short run (through provision of employment) and to contribute to the development of the rural economy in the long run through strengthening rural infrastructure.[11] Here we examine the costs and benefits due to EGS.

(a) Details on Costs of the EGS

From a modest beginning of only Rs 19 million in 1972–3, the scheme's expenditure expanded to Rs 578 crores in 2000–01 (Table 2). During the 1970s and 80s, the EGS consistently claimed between 10 to 14 per cent of the total plan expenditure of the Maharashtra government. During the Eighth Plan period, however, the share of EGS in the plan expenditure declined to around 8 per cent.

The cost per person day (in current prices) increased from about Rs 4 in the first year to around Rs 31 in 1989. The real cost per person day increased mainly in the 1980s and was particularly high in 1989–90. The real cost has not risen in the 1990s. The average real wage per person day (at 1971 prices) rose from Rs 1.7 in 1977 to Rs 3.3 in 1983, then fluctuated until 1988. Since 1988, real wages have been about Rs 4 because of the rise in minimum wages (Table 2).

From 1977 to 1984, the share of EGS expenditure on wages ranged between 74 to 82 per cent. There has been a significant decline in this share since 1985. The main reason is that capital costs have been rising much faster than wage rates. As a result, the share of wages in total

TABLE 2. QUANTITATIVE DIMENSIONS OF THE EGS: 1972–73 TO 1995–96

Year	*Total Exp. (Rs million)*	*Per cent of Wage Exp.*	*Employment gene. (Person days in million)*	*Nominal Cost per day (Rs)*	*Nominal Wage per day (Rs)*	*Real Cost per day (Rs)*	*Real Wage per day (Rs)*
1	*2*	*3*	*4*	*5*	*6*	*7*	*8*
1973	18.8	N.A.	4.5	4.18	N.A.	3.64	N.A.
1974	18.9	N.A.	5.1	3.71	N.A.	2.73	N.A.
1975	137.2	N.A.	48.1	2.85	N.A.	1.73	N.A.
1976	346.1	90.95	109.5	3.16	N.A.	2.00	N.A.
1977	511	75.04	136.5	3.74	2.81	2.23	1.75
1978	515.4	73.98	117.3	4.39	3.25	2.53	1.95
1979	741.7	79.58	163.5	4.49	3.61	2.50	2.19
1980	1092.3	81.89	205.4	5.32	4.36	2.63	2.31
1981	1221.2	75.90	171.5	7.12	5.40	3.04	2.56
1982	1261.7	77.74	156	8.09	6.28	3.23	2.63
1983	1309.3	76.20	128	10.23	7.80	3.90	3.29
1984	1849.8	75.34	164.5	11.24	8.41	3.88	3.17
1985	2320.4	63.68	178	13.04	8.30	4.15	3.06
1986	2722.4	66.85	189.5	14.37	9.60	4.23	3.39
1987	2434.3	63.47	187.6	12.98	8.23	3.56	2.72
1988	2883.1	53.19	133.2	19.06	9.11	4.92	2.76

(Table 2 contd...)

1989	2542.3	50.00	81.3	31.27	15.02	7.52	4.09
1990	2392.8	53.30	78	30.68	15.53	6.93	3.97
1991	2389.2	57.37	89.8	26.16	15.02	5.28	3.77
1992	3085.4	65.79	119.4	25.84	16.91	4.51	3.28
1993	4210	60.30	143	30.59	18.45	4.92	3.01
1994	3100	—	97.4	—	—	—	—
1995	4131.5	—	94.1	—	—	—	—
1996	4437.5	—	97	—	—	—	—
1997	3667.5	9.01					
1998	3530	9.00					
1999	4566.6	9.19					
2000	4939.7	9.49					
2001	5780	11.12					

Notes: 1. In Col. 1, year 1973 refers to 1972–3 and so on.
2. Consumer price indices for agricultural labourers are used for obtaining real wages.
3. Implicit price deflators for State Domestic Product of Maharashtra are used to obtain real cost per day.

Sources: 1. Cols. 1 to 7, Planning Dept. of Maharashtra (1997): 'Employment Guarantee Scheme,' Planning Department, Government of Maharashtra (GOM), Mumbai, mimeo.
2. Col. 8 calculated by the author.

expenditure declined over time. Based on recent share of wage costs, we can say that around Rs 1.66 are needed to transfer Re 1 to EGS employees. Further, if we assume that 90 per cent of them are poor, Rs 1.84 are needed to transfer Re 1 to poor EGS workers.

(b) Benefits due to EGS

(i) *EGS and Targeting.* There has been a debate about the effectiveness of the EGS in covering the target group. Using landless labourers as the criterion for target group, the PEO study (1980) reveals that only 40 per cent belonged to the target group under the EGS. Ravallion (1991) questioned this criterion and stated that 'it is the *poor* whom we are trying to reach, not the landless *per se*'. According to him, a better test would be to compare the income distribution among participants with that of the rural population as a whole. Using results of micro studies, he demonstrated that the EGS was well targeted towards the poor. For example, Dandekar's study (1983) indicated that almost 90 per cent of EGS workers belonged to the poorer sections.

Using the International Crop Research Institute for the Semi-Arid Tropics (ICRISAT) Village Level Studies' data, a number of studies have examined the targeting performance of the EGS. Most of these studies concentrated on Shirapur and Kanzara villages of Maharashtra. Walker and Ryan (1990) found that wealth in the form of total assets was strongly and inversely related to participation in the EGS. The results also revealed that the size of that relationship was larger for women as compared to men in both the villages. Between the two villages, the inverse relationship was much stronger in Kanzara, where the opportunity cost was higher because of abundant availability of agricultural employment opportunities.

Deolalikar and Gaiha (1993) also examined targeting performance in these two villages. With respect to female participation, this study indicated that the scheme was well targeted towards young female agricultural labourers with low levels of schooling who were household heads and who came from low-income and low-asset households. A study by Datt and Ravallion (1992) on these two villages revealed that in general, participants with relatively lower wealth and other assets tended to participate in this programme. However, according to this study, there were signs that social stigma and work disabilities diluted targeting performance somewhat. In other words, the possibility of participation for low-wealth high-caste persons and persons with physical disabilities was lower.

However, recent studies by Gaiha (1997) revealed that the EGS was mistargeted, contrary to the conclusions of former researchers. According to these studies, a little over 48 per cent of the EGS participants in 1979 were poor. In 1989, the share of the poor among EGS participants was a little over 27 per cent. Thus, the proportion of non-poor rose more than moderately. Gaiha's conclusions were based on data sets for two villages in Maharashtra (viz., Shirapur and Kanzara). First, this evidence may not be true for entire Maharashtra. Second, the poverty lines used by the author appear to be much lower than official poverty lines. Most of the other evidence shows that EGS is well targeted to the poor.

(ii) *Mitigation of Underemployment and Unemployment at the Aggregate Level.* Based on the estimates at the aggregate level, it can be concluded that the contribution of the EGS to total employment/underemployment in the state varied from less than 10 per cent to 30 per cent. However, the equivalent of 10 to 30 per cent of full-time employment has an impact on a much larger part of that group because EGS employment is considered only as supplementary or part-time employment.

Average labour attendance under the EGS was approximately 0.50 million in the year 1993–4. In the same year, the NSS 50th Round data revealed that there were 23.2 million workers (self-employed as well as wage employed) above 15 years. Thus, the share of EGS workers in the total rural workers was only 2.2 per cent in the state. In the absence of the EGS, at least theoretically, unemployment among rural workers would have been up by 2.2 per cent.

This is reflected in the trends in unemployment rates for Maharashtra (Table 3). The incidence of unemployment declined much faster in Maharashtra as compared to All-India. The decline was particularly significant between 1983 and 1987–8. However, unemployment for both males and females increased in Maharashtra between 1987–8 and 1993–4 and between 1993–4 and 1999–2000. During the same period, the level of female unemployment at the All-India level declined. Reasons for the increasing person day unemployment in Maharashtra in the 1990s are yet to be explored.

(iii) *Transfer Benefits of EGS.* At the aggregate level, we can estimate transfer benefits to the workers under EGS. Assuming that the available funds are Rs 100, the gross transfer benefits to unskilled workers would be Rs 60 (i.e. share of wage costs). Assuming 30 per cent of wages as forgone income and targeting efficiency of 90 per cent, the net transfer benefit would be Rs 35 to Rs 40 out of Rs 100. By assuming 27 per cent transfer efficiency as per Gaiha, the amount reaching the poor is

TABLE 3. INCIDENCE OF PERSON-DAY UNEMPLOYMENT IN RURAL MAHARASHTRA AND RURAL INDIA

(In Percentages)

Year	Maharashtra		All India	
	Male	Female	Male	Female
1972–3	7.7	11.7	6.8	11.2
1977–8	5.9	9.3	7.1	9.2
1983	6.3	7.2	7.5	9.0
1987–8	2.9	3.5	4.6	6.7
1993–4	4.6	4.0	5.6	5.6
1999–2000	6.3	6.9	7.2	7.0

Note: Incidence of person-day unemployment is defined as a ratio of unemployment days to labour force person-days.

Sources: (i) Sarvekshana (1982), Vol. V, Nos. 1–2; (ii) Sarvekshana (1988) Vol. XI, No. 4; (iii) NSSO (1990), Key results of Employment and Unemployment Survey, All India Part 1–I, NSS 43rd Round, July 1987–June 1988, National Sample Survey Organisation, Dept. of Statistics, Government of India, New Delhi; (iv) NSSO (1997) Employment and Unemployment in India, 1993–4, Fifth Quinquennial Survey, NSS Fiftieth Round (July 1993–June 1994), NSSO, Dept. of Statistics, Government of India.

only Rs 11 out of Rs 100. However, a study of two villages from Maharashtra (Shirapur and Kanzara) by Ravallion and Datt (1995) indicated that half of the gross budget disbursement directly reached the participants, most of whom were poor. This study found that the foregone income from employment on public works schemes was quite low—around one quarter of gross wage earnings; most of the time displaced was in domestic labour, leisure and unemployment. This indicates that workers have not been losing much by participating in the EGS at least in the study villages.

(iv) *Impact on Poverty.* The problem of poverty is much wider than the coverage of EGS, which alone cannot alleviate poverty. Despite the scheme's existence, poverty in Maharashtra has not declined more rapidly than that experienced in the country on an average. As some calculations indicate, even if workers work full time on the EGS, they cannot earn enough to cross the poverty line. The importance of EGS lies in both direct and indirect benefits. Although EGS may not have a significant impact on poverty in terms of head count ratio, it has had an impact on the intensity of poverty and has helped the ultra-poor. The gap between the ultra-poor and the poor has been narrowing in recent times (Table 4). This picture could be even better for districts where EGS is concentrated. The anti-poverty record of EGS is better understood by looking at district or region level data, since the macro-level poverty ratios do not fully capture the impact of EGS on the poor. This is due to the fact that EGS is concentrated in a few districts: almost two-thirds of all EGS employment is concentrated in one-third of the districts.

TABLE 4. POOR AND ULTRA-POOR FOR RURAL MAHARASHTRA: 1977–78 TO 1993–94

Year	*HCR (Head Count Ratio) 1*	*HCR (Head Count Ratio) 2*	*(HCR2 /HCR1) *100*
1977–8	63.97	54.10	84.60
1983	45.23	34.70	76.70
1987–8	40.78	28.10	68.90
1993–4	37.93	24.60	64.86

Sources: 1. HCR1 from Government of India (1993): 'Report of the Expert Group on Estimation of Proportion and Number of Poor', Perspective Planning Division, Planning Commission, Government of India, New Delhi.
2. HCR2 estimated by the author.

(v) *Wage Debate.* The dilemma to be resolved is whether the wage should be below or equal to market wage rate or legally fixed minimum wages (generally market wages are below minimum level). Initially, EGS wages were below the market agricultural wages. In 1988, with the doubling of the statutory minimum wage rate, EGS piece rates were also doubled. A study by Ravallion *et al.* (1993) reveals that higher wages have led to rationing the guarantee of employment. They argued that lower wages should be maintained in order to have wider coverage, which would help the poor better as compared to rationing due to higher wages. This issue should be resolved before replicating the EGS to other states. There is some merit in the low wage argument if one wants to concentrate on reducing the intensity of poverty. However, if the aim is to take the poor up to the so-called poverty line, obviously higher wages are needed. In recent years, workers seem to have been shifting from EGS to JRY in Maharashtra because of the higher wages (Prabhu, 1996). Therefore, one has to verify whether the reduction in EGS employment has been due to increase in wage rates or shifting of workers to JRY.

(vi) *Indirect or Secondary Benefits.* The case for EGS relies more heavily on indirect (or secondary) and stabilisation benefits, rather than on direct benefits. One of the second round effects of EGS is its contribution to the creation of rural assets. The EGS projects mainly relate to soil conservation, land development, percolation tanks and roads. They can have substantial impact on agricultural growth (Sathe, 1991). The EGS has been criticised for neglecting the creation of durable assets and paying more attention to employment generation. There is some merit in this argument but it may not be true for all EGS assets. A related criticism is that agricultural growth in Maharashtra was very low during the 1980s inspite of the EGS[12]. Here too one has to look at the disaggregate data, i.e. trends in agricultural growth at the district level.

Second, EGS exerts upward pressure on agricultural wages.[13] The guarantee part of EGS increases the bargaining strength of unskilled labourers during negotiations with an employer or landlord. There is evidence that the EGS wage rate has influenced agricultural wage rate in Maharashtra (Acharya, 1990). Third, one of the important aspects of the EGS is its insurance function. In the absence of unemployment insurance in India, EGS can act as insurance for rural workers. The existence of a form of income/employment insurance could be quite significant although the increase in employment and income is not very large as compared to the needs at the aggregate level.

The EGS also has a stabilisation benefit in the sense that the employment under the scheme is high in the lean season (April to July) and low in the peak season (October to January). The fourth aspect that needs to be noted is that in rural Maharashtra, EGS is known as a 'programme of women'. Various micro studies have shown that women constitute 40 to 50 per cent of the EGS workers. These large percentages could be due to the predominance of female labour in casual unskilled work in rural areas. The fifth point is that EGS makes employment an entitlement and thus enables the rural poor to undertake collective political action, improve their bargaining strength and promote the realisation of common interests. A number of organisations have come up to help the EGS workers.[14]

(vii) *Opportunity Cost to Workers and Society.* Participation in EGS involves some costs that need to borne by the workers. However, since most of the employment under EGS is created during the lean season, the opportunity cost of workers could be low. Social costs could be very low because EGS employment is a net addition to society.

(c) Targeting Errors: EGS as compared to other Anti-poverty Programmes

The success of the EGS needs to be judged against alternative anti-poverty programmes or policies. Many evaluation studies have shown that the performance of EGS is much better as compared to programmes like IRDP. None of the other programmes have sustained large scale operations for a lengthy period or dealt with corruption and other administrative problems as effectively as the EGS.

In recent years, there have been comparisons between the EGS and the Public Distribution System (PDS), although official information is not readily available for comparing the two. For illustrative purposes, we give here the comparison of cost-effectiveness as provided by Guhan (1994) (Table 5). It shows that although transfer efficiency is higher under PDS than in EGS, the benefit cost-ratio in the PDS may be only half of that in employment programmes, because of better targeting in the latter programmes. However, the coverage is much wider for the PDS (S. Mahendra Dev, 1996a).

Cornia and Stewart (1995) divide the errors of 'target' government expenditures on the poor into two: 'E' mistakes in which benefits are provided to the non-poor as well as the poor, and 'F' mistakes in which some of the poor fall outside the scope of the programme. In employment programmes, which are generally self-targeted, the 'E' mistakes would be lower than 'F' mistakes. In the untargeted programme like PDS, the 'E' mistakes (coverage of non-poor) are expected to be larger than in targeted programmes.

TABLE 5. COMPARISON OF COST-EFFECTIVENESS IN THE EMPLOYMENT GUARANTEE SCHEMES (EGS) AND PUBLIC DISTRIBUTION SYSTEMS (PDS) IN INDIA

	EGS	*PDS*
1. Budgetary cost	100[1]	100[2]
2. Overheads	50[3]	37[4]
3. Leakage	10[5]	35[6]
4. Gross benefit (1–2–3)	40	28
5. Participation Cost	16[7]	Neg[8]
6. Net Benefit (4–5) i.e. transfer efficiency	24	28
7. Targeting efficiency (coverage of poor)	0.9	0.4
8. Final Transfer to poor (benefit-cost ratio)	21.6	11.2

Notes: [1]Aggregate cost for creating one person day of employment. [2]Cost of food subsidy. [3]Administrative overheads and non-labour expenditures. [4]Distribution overheads such as freight, storage, costs, interest, etc. being 57 per cent of 65 per cent reaching consumers. [5]Under payment of wages. [6]In transit and at point of sale. [7]Foregone earnings. [8]Neg: Negligible, assuming that foregone earnings due to waiting time and transport costs to retail shops are not significant.

Source: Adopted from Guhan (1994).

(i) *'E' and 'F' mistakes for EGS.* In the case of employment programmes, 'E' mistakes are expected to be lower and 'F' mistakes are expected to be higher as compared to those of the PDS. According to a survey conducted in the year 1979–80, an estimated 90 per cent of the workers employed in the Employment Guarantee Scheme were poor (Dandekar, 1983). In contrast, the 'F' mistakes were high in employment programmes because of the non-coverage of many poor persons. Another point is that the EGS is considered superior to the PDS even if it does not create any assets (Parikh, 1994). EGS scores much more over other poverty alleviation programmes if secondary benefits such as asset creation, increase in agricultural wages, insurance benefits etc. are considered. Once these benefits are considered, the impact of the EGS on the poor could be much higher than that of the PDS.

To sum up, given some of the limitations in the design and implementation of the EGS, many studies, particularly at the micro level, have shown that the EGS has made a positive impact on the levels of living of the poor in Maharashtra. The unemployment rate declined considerably and incomes of the poor have increased over time.

3.2 Jawahar Rojgar Yojana (JRY) and Employment Assurance Scheme (EAS)

Two massive centrally sponsored wage employment programmes in operation at present are the Jawahar Rojgar Yojana (JRY) and Employment Assurance Scheme (EAS). The objectives of these schemes are (a) to generate gainful employment for the unemployed and underemployed and (b) to create sustained employment by strengthening rural economic infrastructure and community assets.

The JRY, a centrally sponsored scheme implemented by the state governments, was created in 1989 with a substantial funding and has been implemented in all villages in the country. The expenditure under the programme is to be shared between the centre and states on an 80:20 basis. During the Eighth Plan (1992–7), that was the largest single anti-poverty programme.[15]

The implementation of the EAS started on 2 October 1993 in the rural areas of 1,778 blocks of 261 districts, in which the Revamped Public Distribution System (RPDS) was in operation. The scheme aimed at providing assured employment of 100 days of unskilled manual labour to the rural poor who need and seek employment. The assurance of 100 days was extended to all men and women over 18 years and below 60 years of age and normally residing in the villages of the blocks covered by EAS. A maximum of two adults per family were to be provided employment under the scheme. The total number of blocks covered under EAS was 3,197 as on March 1996. The expenditure under EAS was shared between the centre and the states on an 80:20 basis. More than 20 million people registered themselves under the EAS till March 1996. The EAS is a demand driven programme and no physical targets are fixed under it.

(a) Costs of JRY and EAS

In the Union budget, the Central Plan outlay on JRY and EAS together increased from around Rs 20.01 billion in 1990–1 to Rs 47.71 billion in 1995–6 and declined in the following two years. It may be noted that the expenditure at constant prices increased in 1993–4 and 1994–5, unlike the trend in current prices which declined in 1995–6 (Table 6). The central plan outlay on JRY and EAS as per cent of GDP declined from 0.54 in 1993–4 to 0.35 in recent years. However, the share of wage employment programmes in the social sector showed a significant increase in the 1990s (except in 1991–2) at the expense of programmes like IRDP.

(i) *Cost per day.* In 1995–6, Rs 43,911.2 million was spent on JRY to create 885.2 million person days. Similarly, Rs 17,206.1 million was spent on EAS to create 346.5 million person days of employment in the same year (GOI, 1997). The cost per person day in JRY and

TABLE 6. CENTRAL PLAN OUTLAY ON WAGE EMPLOYMENT PROGRAMMES (IN RS BILLION)

Year	*Outlay (RE)*					
	JRY	*EAS*	*Total (Current Prices)*	*Total (1990–1 Constant Prices)**	*Per cent of GDP*	*Per cent share of social sector*
1990–1	20.01	—	20.01	20.01	0.42	49.6
1991–2	18.25	—	18.25	15.91	0.33	42.5
1992–3	25.46	—	25.46	20.47	0.40	51.5
1993–4	33.06	4.38	37.44	27.51	0.53	53.1
1994–5	35.35	11.4	46.75	31.4	0.54	58.1
1995–6	29.55	18.16	47.71	29.88	0.48	56.9
1996–7	16.55	18.4	34.95	—	0.33	—
1997–8	20.77	19.7	40.47	—	0.35	—

Note: *Implicit GDP deflator is used for prices. RE is revised expenditures.
Sources: Computed from the Budget data; last column taken from Guhan (1995)—'Social Expenditure in the Union Budget', *Economic and Political Weekly*, 30 (18 and 19).

EAS was about Rs 50 in 1995–6, while the cost per person day in the Maharashtra EGS was around Rs 30.

(b) Benefits of JRY and EAS

(i) *Employment at Macro Level.* About Rs 230.33 million has been spent on JRY since its inception up to March 1996, leading to the creation of employment to the tune of 6,203.6 million person days. The wage employment programmes (JRY, EAS etc.) generated 1,073 million person days of employment during 1993–4 and 1,225 million person days during 1994–5. The extent of underemployment sought to be covered by a JRY/EAS type of wage employment programme was estimated to be around 3,000 million person days. If employment generated both under JRY and EAS in 1994–5 were included, it is likely that underemployment would be reduced by about 40 to 45 per cent (Nayyar, 1996). This estimate for 1995–6 is likely to be around 50 per cent.

(ii) *Contribution of RWPs to Casual Labour Days: Independent Evidence.* National Sample Surveys on Employment and Unemployment provide independent evidence on employment under public works. The contribution of public works to the total rural casual labour days was only around 2 per cent in 1993–4, while that of wage employment programmes which were thinly spread throughout the country, was much higher at around 5.5 per cent in a drought year like 1987–8 (Table 7). If rùral non-agricultural person days are also considered,

TABLE 7. CONTRIBUTION OF PUBLIC WORKS TO CASUAL LABOUR DAYS (PER CENT): 1987–88 AND 1993–94

Year	*Male*	*Female*	*Total*
Per cent of Public Works in Total Rural Casual Labour Days			
1987–8	4.8	5.5	5.0
1993–4	1.4	2.6	1.8
Per cent of Public Works in Casual Labour in Rural Non-Agriculture			
1987–8	18.0	26.7	22.2
1993–4	6.2	20.0	9.1

Sources: i) NSSO (1990), 'Key Results of Employment and Unemployment in India, All India Part 1–I, NSS 43rd Round, July 1987–June 1988, National Sample Survey Organisation, Dept. of Statistics, Government of India, New Delhi; ii) NSSO (1997), Employment and Unemployment in India, 1993–4, Fifth Quinquennial Survey, NSS Fiftieth Round, (July 1993–June 1994), NSSO Dept. of Statistics, Government of India, New Delhi.

the contribution of public works varied from 9 per cent in a normal year (1993–4) to 22 per cent in a drought year (1987–8). It is worth noting that the contribution of public works to female employment has been higher than that for males.

(iii) *Employment and Income Benefits: Concurrent Evaluation of JRY.* The forgoing aggregate magnitudes do not show the extent of employment generated per person, which would be a better indicator of the success of schemes as a means of raising incomes. To have a correct assessment of the JRY, the Government of India (GOI) undertook a concurrent evaluation of the JRY. The concurrent evaluation of JRY for 1993–4 (June–May) indicated that a JRY worker obtained on an average, 11.06 days of employment (or 133 days per year) from panchayat JRY works during the reference period of 30 days preceding the date of survey. State-wise variations (Table 8), however, indicated that in some poorer states like Madhya Pradesh and Orissa, JRY workers secured less than 10 days of work per month.

TABLE 8. AVERAGE PERSON DAYS OF EMPLOYMENT GENERATED DURING THE LAST 30 DAYS PRECEDING THE DATE OF SURVEY: MAJOR STATES, 1993–94

State	*By Self Under JRY*	*State*	*By Self Under JRY*
Andhra Pradesh	12.53	Madhya Pradesh	9.34
Assam	17.94	Maharashtra	11.80
Bihar	10.13	Orissa	8.58
Gujarat	10.67	Punjab	30.00
Haryana	11.84	Rajasthan	11.02
Himachal Pradesh	15.00	Tamil Nadu	12.30
Jammu & Kashmir	9.65	Uttar Pradesh	12.22
Karnataka	12.89	West Bengal	8.52
Kerala	11.59	All India	11.06

Source: GOI (1997a), 'Concurrent Evaluation of Jawahar Rojgar Yojana, 1993–4', Planning Commission, Government of India.

According to the concurrent evaluation study, the average daily wage rate was Rs 33.36 (Rs 30.54 cash + Rs 2.82 value of foodgrains). On an average, a JRY worker at the All-India level earned Rs 369 during the 30 days preceding the date of survey. The poverty line income per month per family is around Rs 917 (GOI, 1997a).[16] In other words, a JRY worker earned on an average 40 per cent of the poverty line threshold. Thus, JRY seems to be contributing substantial income to the families working under the scheme.

(iv) *Targeting Under JRY*. The concurrent evaluation for the year 1993–4 shows that 82 per cent of the workers had an annual family income of less than Rs 11,000 which is the revised cut-off point for the poverty line (GOI, 1997a) (Table 9). Therefore, largely, workers who were provided with employment belonged to the poorer sections.[17] There is significant variation in the coverage of the poor under JRY across states. In Andhra Pradesh, 52 per cent of JRY workers were non-poor. This percentage was quite high also for Bihar, Karnataka and Uttar Pradesh. On the other hand, it was less than 10 per cent for Assam, Gujarat, Orissa, Rajasthan, Tamil Nadu and West Bengal.

TABLE 9. PERCENTAGE OF NON-POOR COVERED BY JRY (WORKERS WITH ANNUAL INCOME OF RS 11,000 AND ABOVE: MAJOR STATES, 1993–94

State	*Per cent of Non-poor Under JRY*	*State*	*Per cent of Non-poor Under JRY*
Andhra Pradesh	51.73	Madhya Pradesh	13.67
Assam	4.02	Maharashtra	20.62
Bihar	22.13	Orissa	3.38
Gujarat	5.62	Punjab	56.00
Haryana	19.5	Rajasthan	3.40
Himachal Pradesh	9.33	Tamil Nadu	3.17
Jammu & Kashmir	0.00	Uttar Pradesh	30.19
Karnataka	34.10	West Bengal	8.90
Kerala	30.36	All India	18.06

Source: GOI (1997a), 'Concurrent Evaluation of Jawahar Rojgar Yojana, 1993–4', Planning Commission, Government of India.

According to the concurrent evaluation, the share for women in JRY employment was only around 17 per cent despite the earmarking of 30 per cent for them in JRY works. Thus, the contribution of JRY to women's employment has been much less than that of EGS in Maharashtra.

(v) *Cost and Transfer Benefits*. As per the concurrent evaluation, the wage component of JRY expenditure in 1993–4 was, on an average, 53 per cent and Rs 1.87 were required to transfer one rupee of income to a household in rural areas. The evaluation also indicated that 18 per cent of JRY workers were non-poor and that an additional expenditure of Rs 2.28 would be required to transfer one rupee of income to the poor rural households. These numbers, however, vary from state to state.

The gross transfer benefit to the employees was 53 per cent (share of wage costs) under JRY. If we assume forgone income for the individual is 30 per cent of the gross wages and 82 per cent targeting efficiency (as given by concurrent evaluation) out of every Rs 100, the poor obtained benefits to the tune of Rs 30 under JRY.

(vi) *Cost per One Rupee Transfer to the Poor: Comparison of RWPs with Other Programmes.* Employment programmes fare better than food transfer programmes in terms of cost effectiveness, though the Integrated Child Development Scheme (ICDS) appears to transfer income to the poor at lower cost (Radhakrishna *et al.* (1997), GOI (1997a), GOM, 1993–4). Our estimates show that the costs of employment programmes are lower than those provided by Radhakrishna *et al.* (Table 10). For instance, our estimates for JRY, based on recent concurrent evaluation, indicated that Rs 2.28 is required to transfer one rupee to the poor. In general, employment programmes are most cost effective in reaching the poor.

(vii) *Asset Creation.* Regarding asset creation, a large number of public works have been taken up at the village level. Major assets created during the period 1993–4 include rural link roads (26.96 per

TABLE 10. COST PER RE 1 OF INCOME TRANSFERRED BY VARIOUS PROGRAMMES

Schemes	*Radhakrishna* et al. *in Rs (1989–90)*	*Our estimates in Rs (1993–4)*
PDS	5.37	—
Andhra Rice Scheme	6.35	—
JRY	4.35	2.28
Maharashtra EGS	3.10	1.85
ICDS	1.80	—

Notes: 1. Our Assumptions on JRY: Share of wages 52 per cent and only 18 per cent of workers belonged to non-poor sections.
2. Assumptions on EGS: Share of wages 60 per cent and only 10 per cent of workers are non-poor.

Sources: (i) Radhakrishna *et al.* (1997).
(ii) Our Estimates 1993–4: (a) JRY-GOI (1997a), 'Concurrent Evaluation of Jawahar Rojgar Yojana, 1993–4', Planning Commission, Government of India; (b) Employment Guarantee Scheme (EGS), Planning Division, Government of Maharashtra.

cent), buildings for schools, Panchayat Ghars, Anganwadis, etc. (10.37 per cent), drainage and anti water-logging works (8.96 per cent), work benefiting SC/ST (7.25 per cent), construction or renovation of community irrigation wells or village tanks (4.58 per cent) (GOI, 1997a). It may be noted that village panchayats in various states accorded the highest priority to construction of rural link roads and construction of buildings for welfare of the community and therefore JRY contributed to the strengthening of rural infrastructure.

(viii) *Strategies for Women during Drought and Normal Years.* What do the women who are working in public works programmes in drought years do in normal years? Unni (1996) has examined this question using survey data on Gujarat villages and has compared a drought year 1987–8 when a large proportion of women were engaged in relief works programmes and a normal year 1993–4.

Some of the findings of this study are summarised as follows:

(i) Women who were outside the labour force in a normal year usually entered the visible work force in a drought year. This is reflected in higher worker population ratios for females in the drought year as compared to the normal year whereas for males these ratios were more or less the same. Further, the worker-population ratios for females were higher for scarcity households as compared to all households. The percentage of workers with a subsidiary activity in the drought year for both males and females was higher as compared to the normal year.

(ii) In the drought year 1987–8, 84 per cent of the female scarcity workers were casual labourers whereas in the normal year, the percentage of casual labourers was only 34 per cent (Table 11a). Many of the workers shifted to self-employment in a normal year.

(iii) The industrial distribution of scarcity workers differs from drought year to normal year. In the drought year, while 83.5 per cent of women worked in the construction sector and only 16.5 per cent

TABLE 11a. DISTRIBUTIONAL ACTIVITY STATUS OF SCARCITY WORKERS: FEMALES, 1987–88 AND 1993–94

	1987–8		*1993–4*	
	Scarcity HH	*All HH*	*Scarcity HH*	*All HH*
Self-employed	15.6	57.7	64.8	76.6
Casual Wage labour	84.4	40.0	33.8	22.6
Regular employment	—	2.3	1.3	0.8

Source: Unni (1996).

worked in agriculture, 95.6 per cent worked in agriculture and less than one per cent worked in construction during a normal year (Table 11b).

TABLE 11b. INDUSTRIAL DISTRIBUTION OF FEMALE SCARCITY WORKERS IN SIX VILLAGES OF MEHSANA DISTRICT OF GUJARAT, 1987–88 AND 1993–94

Sectors	*1987–8*	*1993–4*
Agriculture	16.5	95.6
Household Industry	—	0.9
Other Industry	—	0.4
Construction	83.5	0.7
Relief and Wholesale Trade	—	0.7
Community, Social and Personal Services	—	1.6
Total	100.0	100.0

Source: Unni (1996).

(iv) The study indicated that one-third of the poor households were engaged in scarcity relief works in the drought year and used it clearly as an insurance against shock. The rest were found to be engaged in productive activities in the normal year though the intensity of employment and returns to it left much to be desired.

Rightly, the study argues that employment created should be more productive and that public works programmes should be used for development of productive activities.

4. LESSONS FROM INDIA'S WAGE EMPLOYMENT PROGRAMME

4.1 Lessons from EGS

(a) Employment on a large scale

The EGS has shown that Rural Public works can be designed and administered on a large scale.

(b) Urban-rural transfer of resources

Taxing the urban middle and upper (or the rich) class for the EGS funds indicates that it is also a means for urban-rural transfers of resources.

(c) Fixing of Wage Rate

Another important lesson that can be learnt from the EGS is regarding the wage rate to be adopted in rural public works programmes. Initially,

EGS wages were below the market agricultural wages. In 1988, with the doubling of the statutory minimum wage rate, EGS piece rates were doubled. The EGS is now required to pay wages at the statutory minimum rates, which are higher than market wage rates. 'This requirement implies substantial budgetary outlays and potentially high social costs in lost output from alternative employment' (World Bank, 1990). Ravallion *et al.* (1993) have argued that lower wages should be maintained in order to have wider coverage that would help the poor better as compared to the rationing due to higher wages. They have also shown that an increase in EGS wages in 1988 did not have an impact on agricultural wages. Rationing of the EGS has, however, dampened the expected second round income effects arising through the agricultural labour market and the insurance effect.

Recent experience, however, suggests that there is a need for increase in EGS wages because these wages are lower as compared to those given in programmes like the JRY.

(d) Sustainability of the Programme

The urban population provides half the resources for the EGS budget. Government officials say that finance has not been a problem. There has been widespread support for the EGS because it offers something for everybody and is one of the state's most popular programmes. These factors have been responsible for sustainability of the programme.

(e) Maintenance and Utilisation of Assets under EGS

Maintenance and utilisation of assets created under EGS have been observed to be far from satisfactory. Some evaluation reports on this aspect (Acharya, 1990), show that utilisation of assets has not been uniformly satisfactory in all the districts. However, in some other areas, the assets created under the EGS have led to positive developments for agriculture and rural non-agricultural activities. Other RWPs can learn lessons from the EGS regarding its successes and failures with respect to maintenance and utilisation of assets.

(f) Voluntary Organisations

There are many lessons to be learnt from the role of voluntary organisations, which help in delivering EGS benefits to the workers. For example, the Lal Nishan Party is active in helping the poor in Pune, Dhule and Ahmednagar districts. A study on Jawahar Taluka of Thane district (Deshpande, 1988) shows that the existence of a receiving mechanism in the form of a labour organisation, namely the Bhoomi Sena, helped in improving the delivery of EGS benefits.

(g) Famine Prevention

As shown by Dreze (1990), public works programmes helped in preventing famine during the drought of 1970–3 in Maharashtra in spite of the low and declining per capita availability of foodgrains in the state. African countries can learn a great deal from the experiences of Maharashtra in the prevention of famines.

In addition, EGS offers lessons on how to reach the poor in an effective manner, reducing gender inequities, responsiveness to crisis, responsiveness to seasonal fluctuations and spatial differences in poverty and generating many indirect benefits.

4.2 Lessons from JRY

(a) JRY and EAS have also shown that India can organise large-scale wage employment programmes and generate more than a billion person days of such employment.

(b) JRY has managed to keep a high level of targeting efficiency as shown by the concurrent evaluation.

(c) Employment programmes seem to be more useful during drought years. The incidence of poverty has not increased in India in a drought year like 1987–8 mainly because of the purchasing power created by the massive employment programmes in the drought affected states.

(d) Another lesson is that local level governments like panchayats are directly involved in implementing JRY projects. There are still some problems at the panchayat level but over time, the efficiency of projects is likely to increase.

(e) Because of the relatively high wage rate, as revealed by the concurrent evaluation study, JRY is able to contribute substantially to the incomes of the poorer households.

(f) Employment programmes sometimes make use of the surplus buffer stocks of foodgrains. This is important because giving food as wages may improve the nutrition of the households.

5. REFORMS NEEDED FOR RURAL PUBLIC WORKS

The main criticism against public works has been that these programmes are relief oriented and do not create durable assets. Around 40 to 50 per cent of total funds under public works have been used for non-wage purposes. What is happening to these funds? How productively are these funds being used? The major issue is how to generate productive assets without diluting the primary objective of employment guarantee and poverty alleviation.

5.1 Reforms under EGS

The EGS has been in existence for a long period (twenty-five years so far). There is need for some changes, which would enable the EGS to be more effective in helping the poor without altering the basic structure of EGS. Some of them are the following:

(a) Wage Rate

The workers under EGS in Maharashtra seem to be shifting from EGS to JRY because of the higher wage rates in the latter. The data for 1995–6 shows that around 91.2 million person days were created under JRY. This number is almost equal to that created under the EGS. It is necessary to have some parity between these two schemes. The wage rate must be raised in such a way that a person working for 300 days a year can lift himself or herself and his or her dependants above the poverty line.

(b) Resources under EGS

The government may resort to employment rationing if the hike in EGS wages is not accompanied by a matching increase in the outlay. This seems to have happened in the late 1980s. In real terms, there has not been much increase in the outlay under EGS in recent years. The resources have to be increased if the government is serious about increasing wage rates under the scheme.

(c) Asset Creation and Organisational Aspects

Some organisational aspects have to be sorted out in the EGS. Improper planning, inadequate project selection and design, lack of technical and organisational supervision, and finally long delays in implementation have affected the productive quality of capital constructed. The EGS has been criticised for neglecting the creation of durable assets by paying more attention to employment generation. The initial emphasis on creation of durable assets got watered down due to public pressure for starting road works. One major weakness of the EGS is the lack of adequate planning for assets. It may be noted that a volatile demand from the workers also creates problems for projects. Droughts, natural calamities or even seasonal changes cause dramatic shifts in demand. Because of sudden increase in demand, new projects have to be undertaken which may be of little productive value (Dantwala, 1978).

(d) Maintenance of Assets

Maintenance and utilisation of assets are observed to be far from satisfactory. The problems in ensuring adequate maintenance are two-fold. First, there has been considerable delay in handing over completed works to the Zila Parishads for maintenance. Second, even where the works have been handed over, the local bodies did not allocate resources for the maintenance of EGS assets. Consequently, maintenance of assets has been neglected. There is a need to allocate some part of the EGS funds for maintenance of assets.

(e) People's Participation

Some evaluations have shown that without people's participation, the bureaucracy dominates EGS plans and implementation. People's participation in selection and management would improve the productivity and sustainability of the assets.

(f) More Importance to Watershed Development

Water management is crucial for increasing agricultural production and productivity in Maharashtra. It may be noted that even after utilising the ultimate irrigation potential, over 60 per cent of the cultivated area may have to depend on uncertain rainfall. Therefore, EGS projects should concentrate more on water conservation. Similarly, emphasis has to be given to the promotion of horticulture.[18] There are already models like Pani Panchayats, Ralegaon Siddhi etc. that provide suitable guidelines.

(g) Involvement of Voluntary Organisations for Effective Implementation of EGS

Along with local people's participation, involvement of voluntary organisations would improve the working of EGS. Corruption and leakages in the EGS has been a point of major concern. A number of cases of corruption have been cited in the reports of the legislature committee on the EGS from time to time.[19] Involvement of NGOs and local people can reduce such corruption.

5.2 Reforms under JRY:

(a) Are the Resources Enough for Wage Employment Programmes?

It has been noted previously that the person days under public works contribute only 3 to 5 per cent to the total casual labour days in rural areas.[20] This indicates that All-India programmes are thinly spread and are unlikely to have a significant impact in any given state.[21] This can be interpreted in two ways. One view is that these funds should be diverted for investment purposes since they do not have much impact on poverty, particularly in normal years. On the other hand, it can be argued that funds should be increased under wage employment programmes in order to have a significant impact on poverty. For example, Parikh (1998) argues that a nationwide EGS with increased wage and easy access to all can provide individual food security against both chronic and transient hunger to the employable hungry. This can be done at a cost of about Rs 147.75 billion per year to cover both rural and urban areas. It has been assumed that other programmes like PDS are not necessary for employable persons.[22] Obviously we need more resources for public works in order to have a significant impact on poverty.

(b) Minimum Wage Rate

Higher wages in public works may be important from the point of view of income guarantee. The use of minimum wage rates for JRY work, however, raises several issues. Where the minimum daily wage is above the market wage, as may be the case in poorer localities, there is a danger that persons with other market based work opportunities will be attracted to JRY, which detracts from targeting and inflates demand for JRY employment, possibly necessitating rationing. On the other hand, in some places the minimum wage rate appears to be well below the market wage, in which case no one would be attracted to engage in JRY work unless higher wages are paid in a disguised manner (violating JRY guidelines). The question that naturally arises is whether JRY is needed at all localities where the market wage far exceeds the minimum wage. If there is no demand for JRY employment at the minimum wage rate, the programme could simply be dispensed with in that locality, leaving more resources available where they are truly needed in poorer localities. Attraction of some of the non-poor to JRY mentioned earlier could also be due to higher wages under this programme.

(c) Using Excess Bufferstock for Public Works

Sometimes governments have excess bufferstock as happened in 1995, when it reached a peak of 37 million tonnes in May. The government has several options to dispose of this excess stock. These are: (a) exporting the grains, (b) selling in the open market, (c) increasing the demand for PDS by reducing the issue price, and (d) using these stocks for public works programmes. Among these options, the last option of linking foodgrains with public works programmes, like JRY, seems to be the most effective strategy for buffer stock reduction. Similar views were expressed by Ghosh *et al.* (1996, p. 1,235). According to them, existence of food stocks 'provides a tremendous opportunity in terms of a substantial non-inflationary expansion in public works and other infrastructure development and maintenance which can be organised through food-for-work and similar schemes'.

(d) Public Works can be used for Targeting PDS

Various options are being discussed regarding targeting of PDS to the poor. There is, however, some sort of consensus that PDS should be linked with public works programmes because of their excellent self-targeting characteristics. Giving food coupons as part of the wages to the workers in public works can be experimented with.

(e) Involvement of Institutions

It is the general impression that the effectiveness of employment programmes on the lives of the people is lower as compared to the funds spent on such schemes. The major criticism of the government based anti-poverty programmes relates to lack of people's participation. The approach seems to be more technocratic and top-down while implementing these programmes. There is a need for involving panchayats and NGOs, self-help groups, and community based organisations for strengthening government employment programmes.

(i) *More Involvement of Panchayats*: With the 73rd and 74th Constitutional Amendments, people at the village level are now empowered through participation in local government to exercise their rights and manage their own developmental activities. It opens up space for potentially meaningful, and creative, local development efforts with inbuilt pressures for accountability. Thus, people's participation through panchayats would strengthen government activities. There are, however, apprehensions that given the highly stratified and unequal socio-economic structure of Indian villages, the dominant land-owning caste elites would effectively control power and are unlikely to be concerned about the welfare of the poor and women. However, over time the poorer sections are likely to participate in the panchayat system.

JRY is implemented through panchayats. However, as mentioned in the concurrent evaluation, only 43 per cent of the heads of elected panchayats were imparted training for implementation of JRY works. Therefore, there is a need for more orientation of heads of village panchayats through training programmes. In general, panchayats are working better in West Bengal and Kerala.

(ii) *Voluntary Organisations (NGOs, CBOs)*: Wherever voluntary organisations have shown interest, the effectiveness of government programmes has improved. Non-Governmental Organisations (NGOs) and Community Based Organisations (CBOs) thus play a vital role in strengthening the hands of the government. Voluntary organisations also make the panchayats accountable. For accountability two instruments are needed. They are: (a) The right to information and access to information (b) social mobilisation. The activities of the government at the local levels have to be transparent and the people should have the right to information regarding funding and other activities. The NGOs and CBOs can also facilitate social mobilisation of people and, in particular, of women. Also, some of the special employment programmes like DWCRA can be given to self-help groups for implementation.

(f) Leakages under the Programmes

There are many stories throughout India on leakages under JRY. There is no accountability either of officials or of panchayats. The right to information and involvement of voluntary organisations can reduce such leakages.

(g) Better in Drought Years?

An interesting dimension of the rural works programmes is that they seem to work remarkably well during drought years as relief programmes. There is evidence that the poor have better access to food during periods of scarcity as compared to normal years.[23] It is worth examining why the bureaucracy that works efficiently during drought years fails in normal years.

(h) Need for Linkages with Sectoral Programmes for Productive Employment

The special employment programmes may have to be continued in the short run until the growth process generates the required employment. However, it is necessary to recast the employment programmes with a view to making them more effective in meeting not only the short term objective of providing temporary work, but also in building up the productive capacity of individuals or areas which in turn, would make greater employment on a more sustainable basis feasible (Nayyar, 1995). For example, public works programmes should create assets, which can provide sustainable productive employment in future. They should not be relief programmes. The case for using rural public works as a development activity and for providing productive employment has been argued by Hirway and Terhal (1994).

The most glaring weakness of the expenditures made every year in public works is that they are not conceived in the framework of overall development plans (Rao, 1992). Action plans of JRY are nothing more than lists of schemes having hardly any interconnections between them. Again, there is hardly any integration between JRY programmes and the schemes of various line departments. The potential of JRY type programmes can be fully utilised if the projects of these schemes are identified in the framework of planned development of an area. Some novel experiments can also be tried for effective utilisation of these programmes at the local level. For instance, one can try Zimbabwe-type public works in which the government provides only the casual wage cost and requires the community to mobilise its own resources for non-wage expenses.

6. CONCLUSION

This paper shows that India needs public works as one of the mechanisms for poverty alleviation. Public works are often criticised, with some justification, for creating unproductive (low productive) assets. It is also argued that these programmes provide only short-term relief and supplementary income (current benefits) and are not useful for long term benefits.[24] As Dantwala (1978) mentions, 'the public works approach to unemployment would make sense if it is so organised that there will be progressively less and less reliance on it, so that ultimately it becomes redundant'. It may be noted that they are not meant to function as a permanent escape route from poverty. One has to recognise the insurance or stabilisation function of these schemes. Further, the primary objective of most of these schemes is guaranteeing employment and poverty alleviation. Moreover, as mentioned earlier, the success of a public works programme needs to be judged against alternative poverty alleviation programmes. In other words, one has to examine whether there are any other programmes that can reach the poor cost effectively as compared to public works.

However, a case can be made for creating productive assets under wage employment programmes without diluting the primary objective of poverty alleviation. Effective involvement of panchayats, planning of projects at the local level using local priorities, involvement of voluntary organisations, right to information at the panchayat level, social mobilisation etc. can contribute towards the creation of high productive assets and better maintenance of the created assets. Also, in order to ensure effectiveness of the programmes, it is important that projects of these schemes are identified within a framework of planned development of an area.

Finally, special wage employment programmes are not a substitute for a sustained and broad based growth process. However, in a country like India, which has surplus labour and poor infrastructure, public works can be a useful component of poverty alleviation strategies.

ENDNOTES

1. From the 4th century BC when the ancient Indian political economist, Kautilya, wrote his *Arthasastra*, there has been emphasis on public relief works, particularly at times of famine.
2. The EGS is commended by the Human Development Report (UNDP, 1993) as one of the largest public works programmes in the developing world.
3. For example, see several papers in Van de Walle and Nead (eds., 1995) and Lipton and Van de Gaag (eds., 1993). Also see an excellent review on South Asia by Ravallion (1991).
4. For a useful discussion on costs of targeting, see Sen (1995). Dreze and Sen (1989) say that there are broadly three ranges of options for targeting, depending on the programme. They are: administrative selection, market selection and self-selection.
5. Cornia and Stewart (1995) use the term 'F' mistakes for exclusion of the poor.
6. See Kanbur *et al.* (1995) for assessing changes in labour supply.
7. For more on transfer benefits see Ravallion (1991), Datt and Ravallion (1992).
8. For a discussion on cash vs food in public works programmes see Dreze and Sen (1989).
9. On the impact of public works on non-participating households see Basu (1996), Mahendra Dev and Ranade (1997).
10. For example, see Parikh and Srinivasan (1995).
11. For more details on EGS, see Mahendra Dev (1995, 1996).
12. Suresh Tendulkar, Delhi School of Economics (personal communication).

13. There is also casual evidence of a labour shortage in Maharashtra, along with significant seasonal unemployment.
14. Also see Echeverri-Gent (1988), Subbarao (1992), Hirway and Terhal (1994) on the benefits of EGS.
15. Preference is given to the Scheduled Castes, the Scheduled Tribes and freed bonded labourers. At least 30 per cent of the employment is to be provided to women under the Yojana.
16. Annual family income of Rs 11,000 is considered as poverty line.
17. The concurrent evaluation for the year 1992, however, shows that around 56 per cent of the JRY workers were non-poor in 1992. This result could be due to the low poverty line (Rs 6,400 per annum) used in this evaluation.
18. There is already one scheme on horticulture under EGS.
19. It may be noted, however, compared to other anti-poverty programmes in India, corruption may be lower in the EGS. The decisions of the officers responsible for planning and implementing the EGS are more open to outside scrutiny.
20. On the other hand, Nayyar (1996), Papola and Sharma (1996) show that JRY and EAS jointly take care of 40 to 50 per cent of the underemployment in the country.
21. This point is due to Suresh Tendulkar, Delhi School of Economics (personal communication).
22. Parikh says along with EGS, a PDS to reach the old and the infirm who cannot work on EGS would be required. The EGS with supplementary PDS for 5 per cent of the poor requires around Rs 167 billion for both rural and urban areas.
23. Regarding this, it is worth quoting here R.K. Laxman's cartoon in the Times of India (3 December 1996). A villager goes to see a minister. The minister's P.A. conveys the villager's observation to the minister as follows. 'He is grateful for rushing food during the recent drought. He is asking what to eat when there is no drought, sir'. Also see Sainath (1996) for interesting stories on droughts.
24. Another valid criticism of public works is that they do not increase the skills of workers. Also, in future, skill based workers are going to get much higher wages and the wage employed will continue to get lower wages (Dantwala, 1996). The gap between unskilled and skilled would widen further particularly after the introduction of economic reforms in the country.

REFERENCES

Acharya, S., 1990. 'Maharashtra Employment Guarantee Scheme: A Study of Labour Market Intervention', ILO-ARTEP, New Delhi.

Basu, K., 1996. 'Relief Programmes: When it may be Better to give Food instead of Cash', *World Development*, 24(1): 91–6

Besley, T. and S. Coate, 1992. 'Workfare vs Welfare: Incentive Arguments for Work Requirements in Poverty Alleviation Programmes', *American Economic Review*, 82:249–61.

______, and R. Kanbur, 1993. 'Principles of Targeting', Chapter 3 in Lipton, M. and J. van der Gaag (eds.), pp. 67–90.

Braun, J. von. (ed.), 1995. 'Employment for Poverty Reduction and Food Security', International Food Policy Research Institute, Washington, D.C.

Cornia, G.A. and F. Stewart, 1995. 'Two Errors of Targeting', Chapter 13 in van de Walle and Nead (eds.), pp. 350–86.

Dandekar, K., 1983. 'Employment Guarantee Scheme—An Employment Opportunity for Women', Gokhale Institute of Politics and Economics, Pune.

Dantwala, M.L., 1978. 'Some Neglected Issues in Employment Planning', *Economic and Political Weekly*, 23(6&7): 291–94.

______, 1996. 'Employment Guarantee Scheme', *Economic and Political Weekly*, 31(9): 563, 2 March.

Datt, Gaurav and Martin Ravallion, 1992. 'Impacts on Time Allocation and Poverty of Public Works in Two Maharashtra Villages', Welfare and Human Resources Division, World Bank, Washington, D.C.

Deolalikar, A. and Raghav Gaiha, 1993. 'Targeting of Rural Public Works: Are Women Less Likely to Participate?' Discussion Paper Series No. 93–105, Institute for Economic Research, University of Washington, Seattle.

Deshpande, S.K., 1988. 'Local Level Management of a Rural Anti-Poverty Programme: A Case Study of the Employment Guarantee Scheme in Maharashtra', A dissertation submitted on partial fulfilment of the requirements of the Fellow Programme in Management, Indian Institute of Management, Bangalore (February 1988).

Dreze, Jean, 1990. 'Famine Prevention in India' in Jean Dreze and A. Sen (eds.), *The Political Economy of Hunger*, Vol. 2, Clarendon Press, Oxford, pp. 13–122.

______, and Amartya Sen, 1989. 'Hunger and Public Action', Clarendon Press, Oxford.

Echeverri-Gent, John, 1988. 'Guaranteed Employment in an Indian State: The Maharashtra Experience', *Asian Survey*, 28:1294–310.

Gelbach, J.B. and L.H. Pritchett, 1995. 'Does More for the Poor Mean Less for the Poor?' Policy Research Working Paper 1523, World Bank, Washington D.C.

Gaiha, R., 1996. 'Impoverishment, Wages and Oligopsony in Rural India', mimeo, Faculty of Management Studies, University of Delhi.

______, 1997. 'Do Rural Public Works Influence Agricultural Wages? The Case of the Employment Guarantee Scheme in India', *Oxford Development Studies*, 25(3): 301–14.

Ghosh, Jayati, Abhijit Sen and C.P. Chandrasekhar, 1996. 'Using Foodstocks Productively', *Economic and Political Weekly*, 31(21):1235–7.

Government of India (GOI), 1997. 'Annual Report of the Ministry of Rural Development 1997', Government of India, New Delhi.

______, 1997a. 'Concurrent Evaluation of Jawahar Rojgar Yojana, 1993–4', Planning Commission, Government of India.

Guhan, S., 1994. 'Social Security Options for Developing Countries', *International Labour Review*, 133(1):35–54.

______, 1995. 'Social Expenditure in the Union Budget' *Economic and Political Weekly*, 30(18 and 19).

Hirway, I. and P. Terhal, 1994. 'Towards Employment Guarantee in India', Sage Publications, New Delhi.

Lipton, M. and J. van der Gaag (eds.), 1993. 'Including the Poor', Johns Hopkins University for the World Bank, Washington, D.C.

Kanbur, R. Michael Keen, and Matti Tuomala, 1995. 'Labour Supply and Targeting in Poverty Alleviation Programmes', Chapter 5 in van de Walle and Nead (eds.).

Mahendra Dev, S., 1995. 'Alleviating Poverty, Maharashtra Employment Guarantee Scheme', *Economic and Political Weekly*, 30(41 and 42):2663–76.

______, 1996. 'Experience of India's (Maharashtra) Employment Guarantee Scheme: Lessons for Development Policy', *Development Policy Review*, 14(3): 227–53.

______, 1996a. 'Food Security: PDS vs EGS: A Tale of Two States', *Economic and Political Weekly*, 31(27): 1752–64.

______, and Ajit Ranade. 1997. 'Cash vs Food in Public Works Programmes', Indira Gandhi Institute of Development Research, Mumbai (mimeo).

Nayyar, Rohini, 1996. 'New Initiatives for Poverty Alleviation in Rural India,' in Rao, C.H. and Hans Linnemann (eds.), *Economic Reforms and Poverty Alleviation in India*, Sage Publications, New Delhi, pp. 171–98.

Nurkse, Ragnar, 1957. 'Problems of Capital Formation in Underdeveloped Countries', Basil Blackwell, Oxford

Papola, T.S. and A.N. Sharma, 1996. 'Structural Adjustment, Poverty, Employment and Safety Nets: The Indian Experience', *Indian Journal of Labour Economics*, 39(3): 591–624.

Parikh, K.S., 1994. 'Who Gets How Much from PDS: How Effectively Does It Reach the Poor?' *Sarvekshana*, 17(3): 1–39, Jan–March.

______, 1998. 'Food Security: Individual and National', Chapter 11 in Ahluwalia, I.J. and I.M.D. Little (eds.), *India's Economic Reforms and Development: Essays in Honour of Manmohan Singh*, Oxford University Press, New Delhi, pp. 253–79.

______, and T.N. Srinivasan, 1993. 'Poverty Alleviation Policies in India', Chapter 17 in Lipton, M. and J. van der Gaag (eds.), *Including the Poor*, Johns Hopkins University for the World Bank, Washington, D.C., pp. 392–410.

Programme Evaluation Organisation (PEO), 1980. 'Joint Evaluation Report on Employment Guarantee Scheme in Maharashtra', PEO, Planning Commission, New Delhi.

Prabhu, Seeta K., 1996. 'Promotional and Protective Social Security During Economic Reform: A Study of Two Indian States', *Review of Development and Change*, 2(1).

Radhakrishna, R. and K. Subbarao with S. Indrakant and C. Ravi, 1997. 'India's Public Distribution System: A National and International Perspective', World Bank Discussion Paper No. 380, The World Bank, Washington D.C.

Rao, C.H. Hanumantha, 1992. 'Integrating Poverty Alleviation Programmes with Development Strategies: The Indian Experience', *Economic and Political Weekly*, 27(48): 2603–7.

Ravallion, Martin, 1991. 'Reaching the Rural Poor through Public Employment: Arguments, Evidence, and Lessons from South Asia', *The World Bank Research Observer*, 6(2): 153–75.

______, and Gaurav Datt, 1995. 'Is Targeting through a Work Requirement Efficient? Some Evidence for Rural India', chapter 15 in van de Walle and Nead (eds.), pp. 413–44.

______, Gaurav Dutt and S. Chaudhuri, 1993. 'Does Maharashtra's Employment Guarantee Scheme Guarantee Employment? Effects of the 1988 Wage Increase', *Economic Development and Cultural Change*, 42(2): 251–76.

Sainath, P., 1996. 'Everybody Loves a Good Drought: Stories from India's Poorest Districts', Penguin Books, New Delhi.

Sahn, D.E. and H. Alderman, 1995. 'Incentive Effects on Labour Supply of Sri Lanka's Rice Subsidy', Chapter 14 in van de Walle and Nead (eds.), pp. 388–410.

Sathe, M.D., 1991. 'Rural Employment and Employment Guarantee Scheme in Maharashtra', Development Group, Vijayanagar, Pune, Maharashtra.

Sen, A., 1995. 'The Political Economy of Targeting', Chapter 2 in van de Walle and Nead (eds.), pp. 11–24.

Subbarao, K., 1992. 'Interventions to Fill Nutrition Gaps at the Household Level: A Review of India's Experience', in Harriss, B., S. Guhan, R.H. Cassen (eds.), *Poverty in India: Research and Policy*, Oxford University Press, New Delhi, pp. 231–58.

Unni, Jeemol, 1996. 'Employment Security: Relief Work Programmes vs Productive Employment', *Indian Journal of Labour Economics*, 39(2): 353–64.

United Nations Development Programme (UNDP), 1993. *Human Development Report 1993*, Clarendon Press, Oxford.

Van de Walle, D. and K. Nead, 1995. 'Public Spending and the Poor: Theory and Evidence', Johns Hopkins University Press and World Bank, Baltimore.

Walker, T.S. and James G. Ryan, 1990. 'Village and Household Economies in India's Semi-Arid Tropics', Johns Hopkins University Press, Baltimore.

World Bank, 1990. 'World Development Report 1990', Oxford University Press, New York.

chapter 2

Innovative Rural Credit Delivery Systems for Poverty Alleviation

• *B.N. Kulkarni and K.U. Viswanathan*

1. INTRODUCTION

The approach to rural development in India's first four Five-Year Plans was unique in that it integrated the objective of eradication of poverty with agricultural development. The concept of social justice was considered to be inherent in agricultural development, implying that the overall growth of the agricultural sector would lead to equitable distribution of gains through generation of additional employment. However, this expectation could not be fulfilled, as agricultural growth on its own could not substantially reduce the incidence of poverty even in regions that experienced remarkable growth. This was mainly because of the fact that the poor were out of the purview of the costly seed-fertiliser-irrigation technology which implied that the trickle-down effect of the technology was weak. Second, the emphasis on maximisation of yield led to input intensification in developed areas leaving a large part of the country, particularly the dry land areas, devoid of new technology. This consequently gave rise to inter-regional disparities in income and incidence of poverty.

The target group programmes viz., Small Farmers Development Agency (SFDA), Marginal Farmers and Agricultural Labourers (MFAL), and Area Development Programmes for fragile resource regions like drought prone, tribal, hill and desert areas were designed and implemented during the Fourth and Fifth Five-Year Plans. This marked a shift in the approach from mere growth to growth with distributive justice. The dichotomy between agricultural growth oriented programmes and poverty alleviation programmes became distinctly clear at the beginning of the Sixth, Seventh and Eighth Five-Year Plans, wherein the strategy of direct attack on poverty was adopted through beneficiary oriented programmes i.e., the Integrated Rural Development Programme (IRDP), National Rural Employment Programme (NREP), Rural Landless and Employment Guarantee Programme (RLEGP), Jawahar Rojgar Yojana (JRY), etc. It was widely believed, and rightly so, that the vicious circle of low income, low saving and low investment prevailing among the majority of agriculturists pursuing subsistence farming and the lack of access to capital assets were the major constraints to overall agricultural growth. Credit was, therefore, considered to be a facilitator in augmenting production and income.

Providing credit as a component of poverty alleviation strategy was widely adopted with the initiation of the IRDP. The World Summit held in 1997 in Washington also endorsed the provision of micro credit as an effective means to achieve reduction in the incidence of poverty.[1] However, despite having a multiplicity of institutions and a wide network of rural branches, institutional credit fell short of reaching a section of the rural poor. The co-operatives, in which mutual help and thrift were watchwords, could not succeed in helping the poor in any significant way because of their structural and financial shortcomings. Rural co-operatives in developing areas brought little benefit to the masses of poorer inhabitants and could not generally be regarded as agents of change and development for such groups. It was the better-off rural inhabitants who mainly took advantage of the services and facilities such as government supported credit and technical assistance channelled through co-operatives (UNRISD, 1975). Though the subsequent induction of the commercial banks and Rural Regional Banks (RRBs) into rural credit helped in creating a wide financial infrastructure across rural areas, these institutions faced a large number of problems, which endangered their viability. It is against this background that the involvement of non-governmental organisations (NGOs), voluntary agencies and Self-Help Groups (SHGs) was thought of as an alternative channel to reach the poor, including women, at minimal cost in an effort to help them cross the notional poverty line.

In what follows, some of the early initiatives in credit assisted poverty alleviation in India and the constraints experienced in those initiatives have been examined (Section 2). Further, a description of the recent innovative credit delivery systems evolved and implemented by the National Bank for Agriculture and Rural Development (NABARD) from time to time (Section 3) has been provided with a view of suggesting possible areas for reforming the rural credit delivery system (Section 4).

2. EARLY INITIATIVES OF INSTITUTIONAL CREDIT IN POVERTY ALLEVIATION

Various policies of the Reserve Bank of India (RBI) and Government of India (GOI) in expanding the rural network of institutional credit agencies and in dispensation of credit to the economically weaker sections of society have aimed at income redistribution and reduction in income inequality. The number of institutional rural credit outlets in the country have expanded such that one outlet was available for 3.95 villages and for every 5,000 rural population by the end of 1996. The RBI/ NABARD had maintained from the beginning that small and marginal farmers were essentially producers of foodgrains and any effort to ameliorate the conditions of the poor would require bringing them within the fold of institutional credit. With this end in view, small and marginal farmers were given preference in the provision of short-term credit for crop production by earmarking a share of about 20 per cent in the total amount of disbursement by banks. Concessional rates of interest, lower down payments, longer loan maturities, etc., were some other protective measures adopted. The small and marginal farmers were also given, and have continued to be given, precedence over other farmers with regard to the provision of term loans.

The credit system has an in-built mechanism of providing relief to the farmers in the event of crop failures due to natural calamities like drought, floods, etc.[2] Some provision for consumption loans was also made an integral part of the production loan for marginal and small farmers to help them meet part of their consumption needs. Further, consumption requirements were adequately taken care of while fixing the debt-service liability of borrowers of term loans by allowing 50 per cent of the incremental income for consumption purposes. The banking sector has also played an important role in the distribution of food, which proved crucial for poverty alleviation programmes. Bank credit has been extended for the purpose of financing the procurement of foodgrains and supporting the public distribution system. As of 31 March 1995, food credit accounted for 6.2 per cent of the gross bank credit amounting to Rs 122.75 billion.

2.1 Integrated Rural Development Programme (IRDP)

Small and marginal farmers have not been the only vulnerable sections of the rural society. Landless labourers, rural artisans, etc. also constitute a distinct group belonging to the weaker sections. Some of them do not possess land but have enough entrepreneurial skill and production potential. Unless their income level and purchasing power is raised they would continue to be vulnerable sections of the society. The vicious circle of low income, low savings, and low investments and thereby low income in subsequent periods in which the poor have been trapped, is well known. Recognising the important cause of poverty to be their low asset base and limited access to institutional credit, the IRDP was conceived as a poverty alleviation programme. The Government of India has, since 1978, launched the Integrated Rural Development Programme (IRDP) wherein identified poor beneficiaries have been provided finance by the banking system for the purchase of income-generating assets in occupations like dairy, poultry, piggery, goatery, small business and retail trade, and professional and self employment. The 'Antyodaya Programme' in which a few of the poorest of the poor families within each village were chosen for upliftment, was an extreme case of the strategy of direct attack on poverty.

Notwithstanding the criticism and differences of opinion with respect to the efficiency of its implementation, there are no two opinions about the programme's success in reducing poverty in India. Under the programme, Rs 117.52 billion and Rs 67.49 billion, respectively, were provided as credit by the financial institutions such as commercial banks, co-operative banks and RRBs and subsidy by the central and state governments to 27.9 million families living below the poverty line during the Seventh and Eighth Five-Year Plans. National Bank for Agriculture and Rural Development (NABARD) had extended refinance to the extent of Rs 71.94 billion. The programme covered both farm and rural non-farm sector activities.

The varied success[3] achieved under the IRDP in reducing the proportion of the population living below the poverty line has been attributed to some of the weak features of the programme and leakages in its implementation. It is obvious that the gap between what poor people need and what the banking system provides would not be uniform in all regions or spaces, sectors or seasons. In irrigated regions with high population density and strong market forces, there would be a concentration of bank branches competing with each other to reach the people. In the process, the ability of the bank to reach the poor in such regions would be considerably enhanced through better information and institutional environment (Dixit *et al.*, 1989).[4]

2.2 Coverage of the Poor in other Lending

Even after massive rural branch expansion, mass lending programmes, provision of protection to the poor and their access to formal credit institutions remained limited. For instance, about 68 per cent of the term credit from commercial banks was extended to farmers holding above 2 hectares (5 acres) of land (Table 1).

TABLE 1. SHARE OF SMALL AND MARGINAL FARMERS IN THE CREDIT, 1993–94

	Upto 5 Acres		*5 Acres and above*		*Total*	
	No.	*Amt.*	*No.*	*Amt.*	*No.*	*Amt.*
Short-term loans						
CBs	78.06	66.75	21.93	33.25	100.00	100.00
PACs	49.88	34.97	27.00	49.92	100.00@	100.00@
Term-loans						
CBs	72.60	32.35	27.90	68.24	100.00	100.00
PACs	56.99	46.62	43.01	53.37	100.00	100.00

Note: @Figures do not add up to 100 as distribution for some loans is not available.
Source: Reserve Bank of India: Report on Currency and Finance, Vol. II.

In the case of short-term credit from co-operatives, nearly 50 per cent was extended to farmers holding above 2 hectares (5 acres). The restricted access of small farmers to co-operative credit is further highlighted by the fact that only 30 per cent of the farmers holding less than 1 hectare were members of Primary Agricultural Credit Societies (PACS) whereas almost all the farmers holding above 4 hectares were members of PACS (Rath, 1989). The reality as perceived from field level studies from different parts of the country seems to suggest an even more restricted access of small and marginal farmers to institutional credit than these data reveal.

The limited access of small farmers to credit has been well documented. Haque and Verma (1988) reported that the households with a low asset base (below Rs 10,000) depended on non-institutional sources for their credit needs and the dependence on institutional sources increased with rising asset base. The credit institutions could not, perhaps, cover a sizeable segment of the rural poor due to the high cost of administering such a large number of small loans and also due to perceived lending risks in the absence of any collateral, unionisation of staff and poor recovery of loans. Though it was observed that the share of small farmers in loans has been higher as compared to their share in the operated area (Gadgil, 1986), this need not be construed as a favourable development for small farmers as the impact of credit on small farms has not been satisfactory (RBI, 1989). The evidence from field studies reveals that marginal and small farmers continue to be dependent on non-institutional sources for as much as half of their credit needs (Singh and Mrutyunjaya, 1992).

2.3 Constraints on Credit to the Poor

Despite the implementation of target-oriented and special area programmes, the outreach of the financial institutions in backward areas and accessibility of the rural poor to formal credit appears to have remained highly restricted. These can be attributed to a variety of reasons such as the high cost of credit supply, an inadequate branch network, rigidity in fixing the time and size of the loan, intra-organisational features, which either prevent proper appreciation of the problems of the poor or result in insufficient response. Therefore, a wide gap between the needs of the poor and the services provided by the banking system continues to exist. This gap is not uniform across regions and spaces, sectors or seasons. For instance, in the irrigated regions with high population density and strong market forces, it is inevitable that there would be a concentration of bank branches competing with each other to reach the people. In unirrigated areas with mainly cottage industries, rainfed crops, forest based activities, etc., may not attract as much credit or as easily as minor irrigation, mechanisation or cash crop cultivation. In high-risk environments or backward regions like drought prone areas, flood prone regions and hill areas, the gap between the needs of the poor and the supply system is likely to be much higher. This is because a majority of the marginal producers in high-risk regions have a deficit in their household budgets.

In the areas where market forces are weak, voluntarism in the form of people's participation and formation of groups has taken a lead. Social organisations like non-governmental organisations (NGOs) have been considered as an important, if not essential, instrument for the rural poor to mobilise their own resources and in self-help actions (Milton, 1978; Hollnsteiner, 1979). A series of case studies from Asia, on experiences in the rural development effort through NGOs that seek to encourage rural people in their own advancement through group formation and effectiveness of collective action have demonstrated the effectiveness of the participative approach (Korten, 1980; Janvry *et al.*, 1993). One of the most successful and largest poverty alleviation programmes anywhere has been the Grameen Bank of Bangladesh, which started on account of the efforts of a single person and has now become a large national project with government support covering more than a million families. It has been replicated in several other countries in Asia, for example, Swarinar and Bangladesh Rural Advancement Committee (BRAC) in Bangladesh, Self Employed Women's Association (SEWA) and Bharatiya Agro Industries Foundation (BAIF) in India, Agha Khan Rural Support Programme (AKRSP) in Pakistan and Project Amanath IKHTAR in Malaysia.

Linking Self-Help Groups (SHGs) with commercial financial institutions through NGOs has been encouraged to provide the poor access to credit. Assisting the rural poor for pursuing income generating activities in the formal sector is viewed to be an effective way to achieve financial deepening and mobilisation of domestic capital resources from a sector which otherwise falls out of the purview of the formal credit system. The available literature on the subject has indicated a few distinct advantages in the formation of SHGs and linkage of formal and informal sectors. They include (i) macro-economic objective of economic growth could be pursued more effectively, (ii) economies of scale from mobilising savings or meeting capital requirements of micro-enterprises could be overcome successfully, (iii) it not only tends to reduce the transaction cost of dealing with the poor but also provides in terms of security, an alternative to the conventional collateral and helps to improve the efficiency of the domestic financial market, (iv) it enables to focus attention on the development of women, (v) since the SHGs have been managed by the beneficiaries themselves, unlike IRDP, the needs of the local people get adequate attention while preparing action plans, (vi) as NGOs function as the intermediaries between the financial institutions and the poor, leakages due to interference of several layers of intermediaries can be minimised, (vii) the formation and financing of SHGs have been found effective in significantly reducing 'adverse selection' of the beneficiaries and default rates, and (viii) there has been substantial reduction in transaction costs at the borrower level as well on account of elimination of cumbersome and time-consuming documentation procedures, costs incurred on repeated visits to the banks, etc. (Puhazhendhi, 1995; Llanto and Chua, 1996).

3. INNOVATIVE APPROACHES

Some measures have been undertaken to revamp the rural credit system in order to improve, among other things, the access of the poor to credit. Among them a few noteworthy measures initiated by NABARD have been the execution of the memorandum of understanding (MOUs) with co-operatives and RRBs based on the Development Action Plan (DAP) and supplementary credit delivery system/mechanism (1991–2). The role of NGOs, VAs and SHGs in the rural credit scene, by way of organising the poor into informal groups for mutual help and benefit, was pursued in this context. Amidst the shortcomings of the formal financial system in catering to the rural poor, an informal segment, particularly those comprising small, indigenous SHGs that have been engaged in mobilising savings and lending activities for mutual help on a very micro scale, are being linked to the formal credit system. NGOs play a vital role in bridging the gap between the rural poor, who are unable to reach the formal system, and the banks by helping the poor form groups and further nurturing, stabilising and guiding the SHGs into a cohesive and dynamic group inculcating the habits of thrift and credit management. Many of these groups have been provided credit support through credit institutions.

Based on the merits of linking SHGs with formal financial institutions through NGOs, as seen earlier, and out of the quest to reach 'the unreached poor' with financial services or support, NABARD has initiated a number of credit linkage projects across the country. The endeavour has been to replicate some of the successful models from countries like Bangladesh, Indonesia, Malaysia and Thailand.[5] Among the various credit linkage projects initiated by NABARD, the following few models have demonstrated success. They are (i) the SHG-Bank Linkage Programme (ii) bulk lending support to NGOs (iii) the tribal development project in Gujarat (iv) the Maharashtra Rural Credit Project (v) Community Development Societies in Kerala, and (vi) the Indo-German Watershed Development Programme.

3.1 Self Help Groups Bank Linkage Programme

The fifth general assembly of the Asian and Pacific Regional Agricultural Credit Association (APRACA) held at Bangkok in December 1984 exhorted the agricultural and rural development finance institutions in the Asia and Pacific region to mobilise savings from rural areas with the object of providing loanable funds for agriculture and rural development. It was also noted at the conference that the framework adopted in many countries was such that it made mobilisation of rural savings less attractive for financial institutions for on-lending for agriculture and rural development. The experience in some of the member countries of operating informal SHGs of rural people that prompted savings among members, which in turn were used for meeting the credit needs of their members, were considered to be useful innovations that merited greater study and support. In pursuance of a recommendation made by the APRACA, NABARD in collaboration with some other member institutions of the APRACA, undertook field studies of selected SHGs and experiments for the benefit of the poor. The study revealed that the SHGs were formed with an emphasis on self-help and with a view to promoting objectives like freedom from exploitation, economic improvement and raising resources for development. By and large, the SHGs were of 'target group' people consisting of small and marginal farmers, agricultural labourers, artisans, scheduled tribes and women. The SHGs represented a variety of groups like savings and credit groups, joint farming groups, irrigation groups, sericulture farming groups, social forestry groups, trade groups and non-farm activity groups (NABARD, 1989).

The SHG-Bank linkage programme was started by NABARD in 1992. It provides 100 per cent refinance support to the banks and gives policy guidance, technical and promotional support mainly for capacity building of NGOs and SHGs, and exposure training to banks and NGOs having potential and interested in promoting SHGs. Under the programme, different models have emerged. In one such model, the banks are directly linked to the SHGs without the intervention of the NGOs. Under the second model, banks have been providing credit to SHGs and NGOs to act as SHG Promotion Institutions. In the third model, the NGOs act as both promotion institutions and financial intermediaries for channelling the credit from banks to SHGs. The progress of the SHG-Bank linkage programme has been encouraging and by March 1998, over 13,804 SHGs have been linked with the banks. Group savings under the linkage programme aggregated over Rs 80 million while bank credit and refinance from NABARD was to the tune of Rs 220 million and Rs 200 million, respectively. The coverage of the programme was more than .17 million poor families, of which 76 per cent were women. Some results of the SHG-Bank Linkage programme are set out in Table 2.

TABLE 2. SELF HELP GROUPS: BANK LINKAGE PROGRAMME ACHIEVEMENTS AS ON 31 MARCH 1997

1. Number of SHGs linked	13,804*
2. Number of states & UTs covered	18 + 2
3. Bank loans disbursed	Rs 220* million
4. Number of commercial banks linked	29
5. Number of RRBs linked	79
6. Number of co-operative banks linked	12
7. Number of poor families covered	1,50,000
8. NGOs that received Revolving Fund Assistance from NABARD	12
9. Revolving Fund Assistance by NABARD	Rs 320 million
Working results as on 31 March 1996	
1. Average Membership per SHG	21
2. Average savings per SHG	Rs 4,645
3. Average loan per SHG (by NGOs)	Rs 2,587
4. Average loan per SHG (by bank)	Rs 5,520
5. Average bank loan outstanding	Rs 4,662
6. Average savings per member	Rs 219
7. Average bank loan per member	Rs 260

Note: *figures relate to 31 March 1998.

The efforts made by different agencies in documenting the performance of SHGs bring out the positive impacts of the project such as increase in loan volume of SHGs, definite shift in the loaning pattern from consumption to production activities, nearly 100 per cent repayment performance, significant reduction in transaction costs of lending and gradual increase in the income levels of the SHG members.

3.2 Bulk Lending Support to NGOs

Besides the linkage programme, NABARD introduced a scheme of bulk lending to NGOs for on-lending to rural micro and household enterprises, with a view to providing credit support to individuals and small groups who have for one reason or the other not formed themselves into SHGs. According to this scheme, select NGOs that would act as financial intermediaries are provided with a 'revolving fund' for on-lending to individuals and groups. Besides, refinance support has been made available to banks for providing credit support to such NGOs for the purpose. Till March 1997, NABARD had sanctioned a cumulative sum of Rs 123.5 million under the Bulk Lending Scheme to fifteen NGOs and VAs through the Revolving Fund Assistance and Corpus Fund Support.[6] It had the twin objectives of providing credit on special terms and building/strengthening a new set of strong financial intermediaries capable of lending micro-credit on a sustainable basis. These NGOs have been organising micro-credit institutions and have established co-operative societies, co-operative urban banking systems, and non-banking financial services, replicated the Grameen Bank model and formed thrift and credit groups. Since the present licensing policy does not provide scope for recognising these specialised institutions as banks (except SEWA), the scope of their operations continues to remain restricted.

3.3 Tribal Development Project (the Wadi Project) in Gujarat

The NABARD has supported, since 1995, an innovative tribal development programme in the Dharampur taluk of Valsad district in Gujarat. Besides alleviating poverty of the tribal community, this programme has multi-pronged objectives that include restoration of forest lands, checking seasonal migration, community hygiene and inculcating self-help among the tribals. This programme is funded by Kreditanstalt für Weideraufbau (KFW), the German Development Bank, through NABARD and implemented by Bharatiya Agro Industries Foundation (BAIF), an NGO based in Pune. It involves the development of 8,000 tribal families in eighty-nine villages for over eleven years through the provision of resources, materials, skills and guidance to develop 4,000 hectares of marginal land in their immediate surroundings. Each family is expected to prepare a 'wadi' (orchard) of approximately 0.5 to 1.5 acres, and grow horticultural crops like mango, cashew and some forest species on the fence. Besides financial assistance, the beneficiaries of this programme are paid wages when they do this work on their own land. Further, it includes certain measures for improving their health. The programme also has a separate component of assisting 2,000 landless tribal women who would raise nurseries and kitchen gardens.

A quick evaluation of the programme has shown encouraging results in the form of transformation of marginal land belonging to tribals into developed horticultural lands. Nearly 4,000 families have developed about 1,400 hectares of marginal land in the first two years. As on 31 March 1998, the project covered 6,424 families and an area of 5,888 hectares. The programme has demonstrated that tribals can remain in their territory and do what they know best—forestry, horticulture—and yet improve their lot on a sustainable basis.

3.4 Maharashtra Rural Credit Project (MRCP)

The MRCP has been implemented from the year 1995 in the first phase in 400 villages belonging to four districts of Maharashtra viz. Chandrapur, Nanded, Yeotmal and Pune. The programme mainly focuses on people's participation in credit planning and credit administration for the poor and non-poor, developing saving habits and a credit culture among the ultra poor through the medium of SHGs, procuring support/social services from various agencies and thereby ensuring socio-economic development of the villages. The project thus aims at improving the delivery of financial services to the rural poor and making a majority of them bankable clients. It has been jointly implemented by NABARD, Government of Maharashtra, Maharashtra Arthik Vikas Mahamandal (MAVIM), Maharashtra Industrial and Technical Consultancy Organisation (MITCON), Maharashtra Centre for Entrepreneurship Development (MCED), National Institute of Bank Management (NIBM) and NGOs. The NGOs have to promote and support SHGs, with active support from banks in the area, to provide training and technical expertise in the project areas. The project has been funded by the International Fund for Agricultural Development (IFAD) through NABARD. Project implementation involves participation of banks that disburse credit through improved credit delivery mechanisms.

The Government of Maharashtra, through its Rural Development Departments (DRDAs) and district line agencies, provides infrastructural and support services, organises participant training and administers capital grant assistance under the Government of India's poverty alleviation programmes. The MAVIM mobilises women, promotes women's SHGs for informal savings and credit, assists women to gain access to credit and imparts training for income-generating activities. The NGOs promote and support SHGs and provide training and technical expertise to project villages. MITCON trains the district level consultants and establishes a market intelligence service and MECD trains the entrepreneurs and trainers. NIBM acts as technical adviser to the project, guiding the overall design of the village outreach approach and providing training to senior and middle level bank executives.

The innovations brought into the project include (a) ensuring people's participation through Village Development Assemblies, (b) preparation of People's Action Plan including credit and non-credit inputs and (c) emphasis on skill development and self-help approach. The ground level disbursement of financial assistance under this project reached a level of Rs 300 million (December 1997) while the number of SHGs formed was 747 and number of beneficiaries trained was 4,175 (March 1997). Within a period of two years this innovative and complex project has made significant progress in terms of social as well as economic development through proper selection of economic activities and borrowers for micro and other credit, aftercare, support, training and repayment discipline. Apart from developing regular thrift habits and proper credit culture among members, SHGs have taken up economic activities individually and on a group basis. Bank loan repayment rates have improved significantly, particularly in the case of loans to the poor (from 30 per cent to about 75 per cent). Similarly, the loan utilisation rate, particularly with respect to the poor, has gone up to 90 per cent from 40 per cent.

(i) Gender Development through Credit

The NABARD has also taken upon itself the task of redesigning credit policies in order to aid the empowerment of women. It has been observed in several studies that female members of rural households lack access to formal credit, which prohibits them from utilising their knowledge and skills in a productive manner. The experiments conducted by Amul Dairy in Anand and the Aga Khan Foundation (AKRSP) in Junagadh district of Gujarat have amply demonstrated that female members of poor households are better managers of the credit provided to them to undertake income generating activities. NABARD has also taken the initiative to establish informal/unregistered groups under Development of Women and Children in Rural Areas (DWCRA), a sub-scheme of IRDP, formed on the basis of guidelines issued by the Government of India. The NABARD has also introduced an exclusive scheme for the development of rural women, viz. Assistance to Rural Women in Non-Farm Development (ARWIND) which is a single-window scheme to take care of the credit and promotional needs of groups of rural women in non-farm development. Under ARWIND, up to the end of Mach 1997, forty schemes have been sanctioned with grant-cum-revolving fund assistance of Rs 11.7 million fourteen states and involving activities such as the Rural Entrepreneurship Development Programme, skill upgradation, Mother Units/Common Service Centres for activities like handloom, handicrafts, coir, SSI (leather, readymade garments, hosiery and electronics), etc. Besides, in order to strengthen the institutional capabilities of co-operative banks and RRBs to deal with gender related issues in credit and support services effectively, NABARD has been providing grant assistance for establishing Women's Development Cells (WDC).

3.5 Community Development Society, Alappuzha, Kerala

State governments in the country have been playing an important role in promoting micro-credit projects for women, especially in the state of Kerala. A unique approach to poverty alleviation of rural women called the 'Community Development Society' (CDS) experiment is under implementation in Alappuzha and Mallapuram districts of Kerala. Under this, formal agencies like the Government of Kerala, NABARD, United Nations Children's Fund (UNICEF) and banks have joined together to create a participatory structure to help women to prioritise their expenditures, identify income-generating activities and implement their own programmes. A three-tier integrated model has been devised for implementing the programme.

Under this programme, one woman each from twenty to forty identified poor families is chosen to be a representative in the base level body known as Neighbourhood Group (NHG). Each NHG selects a president called the Resident Community Volunteer (RCV), and has a five-member committee consisting of the RCV and four other representatives of identified poor families. At the ward level, Area Development Societies (ADSs) have been constituted comprising of eight to ten NHGs representing about 200 poor families. The ADSs are federated at the top level in the Community Development Society (CDS). The governing body of the CDS consists of chairpersons, vice chairpersons and secretaries of all ADS and a few government functionaries co-opted as non-voting members. The CDS that is present at the panchayat level is registered under the Travancore-Cochin Literacy and Charitable Societies Act, 1955. The responsibility for the preparation of an action plan and its implementation is vested with the respective NHG. The ADS and NHGs work like branches of CDS in all the financial matters related to groups. The NHGs also function as thrift societies collecting small savings from their members and depositing them through the ADSs in the banks. The corpus that is collected is used to provide loans to members for household needs like medical expenses as well as income-generating activities like coir units, mat making, umbrella making, fish vending, etc. The CDS also receives financial assistance from UNICEF and state governments, which is being used as a revolving fund.

Two commercial banks lend to the CDS for income generating activities at the NHG member's level with refinance from NABARD. The notable feature of this experiment is that poor women are held together as thrift groups having a common need for some economic activity 'to earn a little more'. The priorities with regard to utilisation of funds collected and/or of savings are decided by the women themselves and there is no intervention of any outside agency like government or voluntary agencies with interest on capital subsidy. Experience shows that the loans granted have been utilised properly by group members and loans have been serviced within the stipulated time period with no overdues. Every proposal received is scrutinised by the group and every member of the group is aware of the activity undertaken by other group members. In extraordinary situations, members of other groups come to the rescue of the borrowers in repaying the loans. Thus, this proposal turns out to the best example of supervised credit.

While there is a revolving fund with money from UNICEF and the Government of Kerala, there is no subsidy either in the form of capital or interest for any purpose from the outside agency. The rates of interest for all the purposes are generally fixed by the members themselves and is approximately 25 per cent per annum. The size of the biggest individual loan does not exceed Rs 3,000 at a time while smaller loans of the size of Rs 200–300 are more numerous. The biggest loans are to be repaid in ten months while the small loans are to be repaid in two to three months. The banks do not assess individual loan proposals but accept the assessment by CDS and its local level bodies. Thus in the management of NHGs, there is no cheap credit nor is there any subsidy as long as the members know that the funds managed by them are their own hard earned savings. This ensures proper usage of the funds and repayment of the money. By the end of September 1996, 62 per cent of the total outstanding loans was from member's savings while 38 per cent was from the banks and the revolving fund.

The success of the programme has clearly demonstrated that women can prove better credit managers if a proper environment is created by the support system, including the government. The experiment has been conferred with the UN community award.

3.6 Indo-German Watershed Development Programme

The dryland areas in the country, which account for nearly 70 per cent of the net sown area, are too economically fragile to support sustainable agriculture. A sizeable proportion of the rural population is affected because of typical characteristics of these dryland areas such as resource degradation, poor vegetative cover, high run-off, severe soil erosion, etc., leading to out-migration of the poor from rural areas and overcrowding of urban centres. The severe drought conditions in Maharashtra in 1972 gave an impetus to the efforts for conservation of water resources by undertaking a programme of construction of new dugwells, and construction of percolation tanks and KT weirs on the streams as effective drought-proofing measures. Watershed development also emerged as a major device in effectively cutting down the wasteful run off of rain water, erosion of soil and instability in agricultural yield. While steps were taken at the government level, a few NGOs like Ralegaon Siddhi by then had demonstrated that if the technology of water conservation is efficiently implemented, it can successfully control drought conditions. The Indo-German Watershed Development Programme is one such programme, which has been adopted to develop dryland areas for sustainable agriculture and help the rural poor in economically fragile areas.

The IGWDP has been implemented jointly by the Government of Maharashtra, Government of India, NABARD and KFW through intermediation of NGOs. This programme aims at:

(i) developing micro-watershed in a comprehensive manner to provide sustainable livelihood to the inhabitants of the area; (ii) to encourage them to form village groups by mobilising their degraded land through participatory self-help initiatives. The message to inhabitants of the area through this programme is that poverty can be alleviated and eradicated through harnessing their production potential, by coming together and deciding to help themselves by forming SHGs. The actual implementation rests with the watershed community. The local NGO acts as a catalyst and support organisation for the promotion of SHGs. The Government of India, Government of Maharashtra and external donors play an important role in funding and evolving the participatory process. Technological components of the programme include treatment of non-arable lands, treatment of arable lands, treatment of drainage lines, preparation and adoption of a scientific cropping plan, economic practices, timely and adequate provision of inputs to the farmers and availability of scientific manpower.

Certain necessary preconditions have been laid down for any watershed to qualify for selection for implementation of IGWDP programme. These include close engagement of stake holders, all support including political at different levels, creation of confluence of interest, creation of local watershed planning bodies which can technically defend their proposal to the funding agencies, local level collaboration of NGOs, creation of a mechanism which channels funds to the local organisation, four days of 'shramdan' by the community equivalent to 16 per cent of the unskilled labour cost, commitment by the community to reduce the biotech pressure on land, restrictions on water intensive crops and the constitution of a watershed committee representing different sections and geographic regions within the project area with specific representation of women and the landless. For effective implementation, a special institutional structure is created which includes a project-sanctioning committee, programme co-ordinator, village watershed committees, the establishment of support organisations and participatory planning procedure, etc.

The programme co-ordinator has a key role in the overall programme strategy as well as implementation. The programme co-ordinator is essentially to be a representative of NGOs who has the responsibility of liasioning between NGOs, government agencies and NABARD for all programme-related activities and undertakings, monitoring and evaluation of on-going projects, etc. The ultimate responsibility of planning and implementation of the watershed project rests with the village level organisation viz. the village watershed committee (VWC). It is at this level that the village watershed community participates effectively in the project. Project grants are transferred to the account of the VWC, which has financial control over the project. However, the VWC has been entitled to withdraw money from the account with the consent of the supporting NGO, which is a co-signatory for withdrawal. The NGOs initially were expected to provide technical guidance to the VWC. With the expansion of activities in the project area, a separate technical NGO called the Watershed Organisation Trust (WOTR) has been established to provide technical support. The entire capacity building activity and most of the new project preparation work for smaller NGOs is done with the assistance of the WOTR.

The programme initially began as a financial cupertino involving only the KFW and NABARD. Bilateral aid from the Federal Republic of Germany was routed through the KFW to NABARD for the mainline phase and from the GTZ to the WOTR for the capacity building phase. The programme covered 92,000 hectares of private and other land in twenty districts in Maharashtra. The results that have emerged from the project area have been encouraging. It has been reported that most villages have recorded an improvement in drinking water availability, reduction in off-season migration, increase in milk production in villages which were once water scarce, etc. (Nanda, 1997). As on 31 March 1998, 35 NGOs have been working in fifty-five watersheds, covering an area of 61,322 hectares under implementation and 15,749 hectares in the pipeline.

4. ISSUES IN CREDIT-LINKED POVERTY ALLEVIATION

The role of credit in sustainable poverty alleviation strategy need not be overemphasised. Past attempts to reach the poor fell short of both needs and expectations. A qualitative difference in the approach was felt necessary and it was realised that credit support would yield better results when there is group commitment. The success of various alternative models of linking SHGs with banks and participatory development programmes has been indicative of this. However, some issues need to be resolved for making this alternative channel effective. The creation of an environment that would be conducive to such policy through measures by the state government is a pre-requisite for establishing the link between informal groups and the formal credit system. While the government would have to provide all types of support including creation of required infrastructure, it should abstain from intervening in the day-to-day management of the SHGs. The government should also take sufficient care not to introduce subsidy oriented programmes in the areas of SHGs as it is likely to disturb and destroy the self-help institutions created by the poor which are willing to work on a commercial basis. Therefore, government intervention has to be minimal and restrict itself to provision of infrastructure. The government could possibly create a Trust or a Society (as in the case of Rashtriya Mahila Kosh) and give a corpus fund for the Trust to discharge its responsibilities with respect to effectively reaching the poor through innovative delivery mechanisms.

The NGOs have been promoting SHGs of the poor. They have been playing a credit plus role by meeting training needs of the poor, supplying inputs and providing necessary assistance in marketing. For a sustainable linkage between SHGs and the formal banking system, the NGOs should be autonomous and have their own funding arrangements. For funds, as far as possible, NGOs should depend on formal credit institutions and not on the government as flow of government funds may lead to an increase in government interference in the working of the NGOs. For ensuring this, there should be transparency in NGO funding. The transaction cost of NGOs should also be minimised since it would ensure a minimum margin in the interest rate. Further, the existing provisions in the banking statutes are not adequate and conducive for growth of micro-credit institutions. The recognition of NGOs as purveyors of credit and their linkages with SHGs, promotion of micro-credit institutions by NGOs or promotion of specialised institutions for the purpose of micro-credit would require general support systems and exclusive provisions in the banking statutes.

ENDNOTES

1. The latest world poverty estimates indicate that 1.3 billion people had incomes below the poverty line in 1993 (World Bank, 1996a, p. 4). If trends continue, the number is expected to rise to more than 1.4 billion by the year 2000. About 80 per cent of the poor live in rural areas in developing countries, half of them in less favoured rural areas (World Bank, 1996b). Numerically, the most important sub-groups of the 'rural poor' are small hold farmers and the landless. It is estimated that 70 per cent of the world's poor are women.
2. The rationale of such a relief system lies in the fact that the farmers' income levels tend to shrink due to crop failures and therefore, they should be provided relief by way of postponement of repayment of the bank loan so that their access to food does not get jeopardised.
3. The micro level evaluation studies conducted by NABARD across states have revealed a wide variation in the impact of the IRDP in raising the poor above the poverty line. For instance, in Sagar district of Madhya Pradesh, only 13 per cent of the sample families could cross over the

poverty line with financial assistance under IRDP while the percentage of families crossing the poverty line in Valsad district of Gujarat state was as high as 58 per cent of the selected households (NABARD, 1994 & 1995).

4. As per the Planning Commission estimates, the incidence of poverty was 37.4 per cent in 1983–4, which declined to 29.9 per cent in 1987–8. The Expert Group on Estimation of Proportion and Number of Poor estimated the incidence of poverty in 1983 at 44.8 per cent and in 1987–8 at 39.3 per cent. For the period between 1987–8 to 1993–4, the population below the poverty line declined marginally by 2.89 percentage points. A recent study conducted by the Indian Statistical Institute, Delhi, estimated the decline in poverty ratio at 6.25 percentage points. Both estimates were based on the methodology recommended by the Expert Group and are indicative of a not very comfortable achievement under poverty alleviation in the country. As per the Human Development Report (UNDP, 1997), India ranked 47th in the world in terms of the Human Poverty Index.
5. The NABARD–APRACA International Seminar on Credit Delivery to the Rural Poor through the SHGs, Bangalore, India, 28–31 May 1995 has brought out several successful models of linkage from various countries like Bangladesh, Indonesia, Malaysia, Thailand, etc.
6. The Small Industries Development Bank of India (SIDBI) also launched in 1994 a scheme for micro-credit under which financial support to well-managed NGOs for on-lending to rural poor with emphasis on women for setting up micro-enterprises is envisaged. Cumulative assistance under the scheme was Rs 830 million to seventy-two NGOs with a membership of 48,000 poor.

REFERENCES

Dixit, M.R., Anil K.Gupta, T.V. Rao, S.P. Seetharaman and P.M. Shingi, 1989. 'Banking the 'Non Bankable' Poor: Bridges, Brokers, Banias or Bankers', Final Report of NABARD-sponsored study on 'Poverty Control through Self Help', Indian Institute of Management, Ahmedabad.

Gadgil, M.V., 1986. 'Agricultural Credit in India: A Review of Performance and Policies, *Indian Journal of Agricultural Economics*, 41(3), July-Sept.

Haque, T. and Sunita Verma, 1988. 'Regional and Class Disparities in the Flow of Agricultural Credit in India', *Indian Journal of Agricultural Economics*, 43(3), July–Sept.

Hollnsteiner, Mary Racelis, 1979. 'Mobilising the Rural Poor through Community Organisation', *Philippine Studies*, Vol. 27, July-September; pp. 387–416.

Janvry De Alian, Elisabeth Sadoulet and Erik Thorbecke, 1993. 'World Development', Vol. 24, pp. 565–75.

Korten C. David, 1980. 'Community Organisation and Rural Development:

A Learning Process Approach', *Public Administration Review*; September-October, pp. 480–511.

Llanto G.M. and R.T. Chua, 1996. 'Transaction Costs of Lending to the Poor: A Case Study of Two Philippine Non-governmental Organisations', Foundation for Development Cupertino, Brisbane, Australia.

Milton J. Esman, 1978. 'Development Administration and Constituency Organisation', *Public Administration Review*, March–April, pp. 166–72.

NABARD, 1989. 'Studies on the Self-Help Groups of the Rural Poor', NABARD, Mumbai.

______, 1994. 'Investments financed under IRDP in Valsad District', Gujarat state. *Evaluation Study Series No. 5*, Regional office, Ahmedabad.

______, 1995. 'Ex-post Evaluation Study of Integrated Rural Development Programme in Alwar District (Rajasthan state)' *Evaluation Study Series No. 5*, Regional Office, Jaipur.

______, 1997. 'Annual Report, 1996–7', Mumbai.

Nanda, Y.C., 1997. 'Delivery System in Participatory Poverty Alleviation: A Case Study of the Indo-German Watershed Development Programme', *Grameeya*, Vol. III (1&2), July-Jan.

Puhazhendhi V., 1995. 'Transaction Costs of Lending to the Rural Poor: Non-governmental Organisations and Self-help Groups of the Poor as Intermediaries for Banks in India', Foundation for Development Cupertino, Brisbane, Australia.

Reserve Bank of India, 1989. 'A Review of the Agricultural Credit System in India', *Report of the Agricultural Credit Review Committee*, Bombay (Chairman: A.M. Khusroo).

Rath, N., 1989. 'Institutional Credit for Agriculture in India', *Journal of Indian School of Political Economy*, 1(2): July–December.

Singh, S.P. and Mrutyunjaya, 1992. 'Impact of Short-Term Credit on Income and Employment of Marginal and Small Farmers', *Agricultural Economics Research Review*, 5(1), January-June.

United Nations Research Institute for Social Development (UNRISD), 1975. 'Rural Co-operatives as Agents of Change: A Research Report and a Debate', Geneva.

World Bank, 1996a. 'Poverty Reduction and the World Bank Progress and Challenges in the 1990s', Washington, D.C.

______, 1996b. 'Rural Development: Putting the Pieces Together' Washington, D.C.

chapter 3

Gender and the Informal Sector: Implications for Poverty Alleviation

• *Sudha Deshpande and Lalit Deshpande*

1. INTRODUCTION

The failure of the United Nation's First Development Decade was essentially a failure of the productive sectors in the Less Developed Countries (LDCs) to grow fast enough to reduce poverty and unemployment. Unemployment was not only more visible but also politically more explosive because of its concentration in the cities. In an effort to answer two questions—how did people survive when they were unemployed for so long, and why did they migrate to the cities despite high urban unemployment—two researchers discovered the importance of what soon came to be called the urban informal sector. Hart (1973), one of the two researchers, coined the term and highlighted the sector's positive contribution to development in alleviating poverty and unemployment on the one hand and encouraging saving, investment and skill formation on the other. Todaro (1969), who addressed the second puzzle, saw it as a vestibule in which fresh migrants, lured to the cities by the high formal sector wage, waited till they were admitted to the formal sector. For much the same reasons as in the First Development Decade, the informal sector grew absolutely and relatively in the Second Development Decade. And now, liberalisation and globalisation, aided and abetted by new information technology, are expected to lead to informalisation and feminisation of formal employment and thereby increase the share of an urban population dependent on the informal sector for its livelihood even faster.

Growing feminisation of the labour force can be interpreted in two ways. It could either be due to rise in demand for cheaper female labour relative to male labour or due to economic distress resulting from loss of employment of male members of the household. Women, particularly from poor households, seek informal sector employment, mainly to enhance family income.

The present study discusses the efficacy of the policy measures that are meant for the betterment of women engaged in informal sector activities in urban India. Four of every five women workers in urban India in 1993–4 were employed in the informal sector. We do not know how many of them were poor. Though not all workers in informal employment would be poor and not all persons living in slums would be employed in the informal sector, it would not be too unrealistic to assume that a large majority of the workers, particularly women workers living in slums and engaged in informal activities, would be poor. Thanks to Shramashakti (Government of India [GOI], 1980) we know relatively more about self-employed women workers though we know very little about the wage employed.

Since we want to base our policy recommendations on facts, which, though statistically inadequate, illustrate the enormous heterogeneity of the informal sector and women's employment, we draw partly on a recent study of a sample of 200 women workers living in two slum pockets within Mumbai done by one of the co-authors of this paper. The older slum that is located close to the textile industry in the Island City is named Slum 1 in further discussions. The other relatively new slum, Slum 2, is located in the western suburbs near the Santacruz Electronic Export Promotion Zone (SEEPZ).

The paper is outlined as follows: Section 2 brings out the heterogeneity referred to earlier, Section 3 offers a few comments on the policies in operation and Section 4 provides suggestions for a set of appropriate policies to address the diversity that characterises the world of working women in urban India.

2. HETEROGENEITY OF CONCEPTS: INFORMAL SECTOR, GENDER AND TRAINING

The two concepts, gender and informal sector, are very heterogeneous. Women can be divided into many demographic, social and economic groups. A common policy prescription for a working girl child and an adult woman worker is likely to fall between two stools. Nor can we address a uniform policy to the self-employed and wage workers though both may be women. The heterogeneity in the informal sector is enormous. Some of the goods and services produced in this sector are consumed by the rich, others by the poor; some are exported, others domestically consumed; some are sold directly to the final consumers, others to intermediaries. The diversity of arrangements under which goods and services are produced and marketed is enormous too. Hence, care has to be taken to see that the policies formulated and implemented in a specific location are based on the knowledge of the profile of women workers in the informal sector and their felt needs in that place.

In what follows, we discuss the personal characteristics of the respondents, their economic profile, perceptions about the nature of employment and the kind of training presently undertaken in most informal sector activities. This is followed by a perusal of the nature and issues related to female employees in each category of the informal sector.

2.1 Personal Characteristics

In Mumbai, the personal characteristics of women workers, their industrial and occupational affiliation differed between old and newly settled slums. Nearly one half of the sampled workers were illiterate and the other half had six years of formal education. Hence, the set of policies to be addressed to the two groups has to be different. The overall personal characteristics of the respondents in Slum 1 and Slum 2 are presented in Table 1. The average age of most respondents was thirty-six. Of the total respondents, 70 per cent were married. Only

TABLE 1. PERSONAL CHARACTERISTICS OF RESPONDENTS

Characteristics	*Slum 1*	*Slum 2*	*All Slums*
No. of respondents	100	100	200
Average age in years	38.3	33.2	35.8
Percentage currently married	59.0	79.0	69.0
Percentage that never went to school	46.0	55.0	50.5
Average number of years of schooling	5.4	6.6	6.0
Scheduled Caste (SC)	36.0	31.9	34.0
Other Backward Classes	22.0	7.7	14.9
Non-Scheduled Caste/Tribe	41.0	43.9	42.5

Source: Field Survey.

one half of the respondents were literate and the other half had only six years of formal schooling.

Poor literacy rates coupled with high poverty have reduced choices available to these workers in seeking occupations with better wages. In fact, girls were often channelled into courses that were essentially an extension of their household and reproductive tasks—sewing, food processing, nutrition, home economics and so on. As a result they are limited, at an early age, to occupations in the service sector and trade or marginal areas of production.

2.2 Economic Profile

The economic profile of the respondents (Table 2) provides details about the nature of occupations, the average income of a woman worker and her contribution to the household income.

To most illiterate women, home-based work offered the first point of entry into the workforce.[1] Many reported working in factories as temporary or casual employees. Surprisingly, not many took up construction or trade as their first occupation. One out of every five women workers started her working career as a domestic and almost as many started as self-employed. A quarter were casual wage employees and just about 12 per cent were contract workers in their first employment in Mumbai. Obviously, fresh entrants to the workforce were concentrated at the lower end of the income ladder.

TABLE 2. ECONOMIC PROFILE: FIRST AND CURRENT JOBS

Job Characteristics	*Slum 1*	*Slum 2*	*All Slums*
Age of entry into labour market	24.7	21.7	23.2
First Job			
Major occupation (per cent)			
Domestic work	27.0	9.0	18.0
Factory work	7.0	32.0	19.5
Home-based work	32.0	15.0	23.5
Employment Status			
Permanent workers	1.0	2.0	1.5
Temporary workers	16.0	29.0	22.5
Casual workers	3.0	16.0	9.5

(Table 2 contd...)

(Table 2 continued)

Job Characteristics	*Slum 1*	*Slum 2*	*All Slums*
Contract workers (at establishments)	9.0	11.0	10.0
Self-employed	18.0	24.0	21.0
Home-based workers (put-out work)	20.0	7.0	13.5
Unpaid family workers	8.0	2.0	5.0
Part-time workers	25.0	9.0	17.0
Total	100.0	100.0	100.0
Average income (in Rs)	235.36	295.27	265.32
Current Job			
Major occupation (per cent)			
Domestic work	28.0	6.0	17.0
Factory work	5.0	38.0	21.5
Home-based work	26.0	11.0	18.5
Employment Status			
Permanent workers	9.0	11.0	10.0
Temporary workers	0.0	31.0	15.5
Casual workers	15.0	7.0	11.0
Contract workers (at establishments)	0.0	10.0	5.0
Self employed	25.0	26.0	25.5
Home-based workers (put-out work)	17.0	8.0	12.5
Unpaid family workers	5.0	1.0	3.0
Part-time workers	29.0	6.0	17.5
Total	100.00	100.00	100.00
Average income (in Rs)	830.5	728.0	779.25
Average income per household (in Rs)	2,240.41	2,390.40	2,315.41
Percentage current income of household income	37.1	30.5	33.7

Source: Field Survey.

About one-fourth of the respondents in our study were employed as home-based workers (Table 2). Slum 1, located close to the textile industry, had a greater proportion of home-based and domestic workers, 32 and 27 per cent respectively. About 32 per cent of the respondents in Slum 2 were employed mainly as casual workers in factories. This trend was exhibited while considering the first and current employment of the respondents.[2]

The fresh female entrant is mostly employed as a temporary worker or as a self-employed home-based worker or is employed in the putting-out system. With a change in employment, most respondents shifted towards permanent employment, casual wage employment and part-time employment. On an average, the percentage contribution of female workers was over one-third of the total household income.[3]

For a little less than half of the working women, the job they were doing was merely an extension of their housework and required no special training; 37 per cent learned skills on the job while barely 10 per cent reported having attended short training courses. Most women worked close to their homes and walked to their workplace. A woman earned Rs 728 per month on an average but this amount differed between municipal wards.

2.3 Perceptions of Work

About a third of the workers were dissatisfied with low pay, uncertainty of work and income and the exploitation involved in getting work through middlemen. Nearly 25 per cent of dissatisfied workers wanted home-based work from manufacturing units, 17 per cent were prepared to travel to distant places for work if they were given a higher pay, while 13 per cent would have liked to be in the food processing business. Not many wanted to do tailoring or cared for secure work.

We requested women to identify for us the most important problem they faced in their occupation. Many reported low income, intense competition in the trade they were engaged in from others living in the same slum and low piece rates paid by contractors on whom they depended for work as the most important problems they faced. Despite these problems, many women continued in the occupation because they had no skills to do any other kind of work. Presence of children at home restricted their mobility. Surprisingly, non-availability of funds did not figure in the list of the most urgent problems faced by those who wished to start their own business. Probably, given their poor background, very few could even think of starting some activity on their own to earn a livelihood.

Almost a third of the women workers felt that the government or an NGO could help them get work at home and thereby eliminate middlemen. A little more than a fifth wanted training programmes to help them acquire skills, while barely 12 per cent wanted credit at low rates of interest to start their own businesses. Age, education and experience determined the income levels of women workers.[4]

2.4 Training

It is not always clear what people mean when they speak of training. In fact, training may mean many things to many people. It is not certainly confined to what takes place in recognised institutions for two or three years to prepare relatively few school-leavers without a job history for a limited number of standard occupations. The term applies broadly to any transfer of knowledge, skills, or attitudes, which is organised to prepare people for productive activities or to change their working behaviour. Training may therefore concern first time learners, and people who have worked all their lives; it covers in and out-of-school efforts; it encompasses vocational, technical, managerial, entrepreneurial, societal and other useful skills; it need not even be called training, as in the case of business advisory services (Fluitman, 1989). Defined this way, it could be said that all workers need training of one type or the other throughout their working life to enhance their earnings and for making their own lives more liveable.

Needless to say, training needs of women in the informal sector are varied and have been recognised by policy makers the world over. It is necessary also to review how effective training and education have been in meeting the needs of women in the informal sector. Women all over the world, and in India in particular, do not have as much access to education as men do. This was true of women we interviewed in the slums of Mumbai as well. But it is not always obvious who should be trained and how it should be done. It often goes unrecognised that many women in the informal sector have been able to acquire certain skills without external help—a fact which should be kept in mind while designing training programmes. Training that is properly conceived can help change the lives of a lot of women who currently lack the skills required to make a decent living. A list of such women would include among others, illiterate women, school drop-outs or those who could not continue education, and women solely responsible for feeding their families but who were never trained because men were supposed to be the bread winners.

It is necessary also to review how effective training and education have been in meeting the needs of women in the informal sector. Women all over the world and in India in particular do not have as much access to education as men do. This is true of women we interviewed in the slums of Mumbai as well. Parents' perceptions mattered in educating girls.

This does not mean however that women entering the informal

sector have no skills. They do possess some skills but these are learnt traditionally within the family. Some of them relate to production and others to marketing but both are rather rudimentary, limited in their scope and economic viability. While the skills that girls acquire within the family or community could form a basis for future employment, they do not lead to high-income opportunities or self-employment. Additional training is usually required to break out of the narrow range of economic activities having low levels of skills, productivity and earnings (Goodale, 1989).

Experience shows that even the formal training programmes for girls have been viewed differently not only by those who frame them but also by those who teach them. Vocational and technical training imparted to women was often limited in scope. This could be attributed to the inability to get trained staff to teach the courses or simply lack of awareness of other alternative courses which could be offered. More often than not, training was imparted without finding out the scope it offered to the trainees in the labour market. Course content was so devised that girls rarely have access to the managerial and entrepreneurial skills needed for the creation or expansion of small businesses.

There was a need to change women's perceptions regarding the kind of training they prefer. Self and Girling (1983) in their study carried out in India reported that women in their survey population were keen to acquire income-earning skills of their own, but their perception of their employment potential was exceedingly narrow due to their lack of awareness about alternatives to typically female occupations such as knitting, sewing and lace making. Information about training and alternative employment opportunities should be made available to women.

2.5 *Type of Activity*

(a) Home-based workers: Putting-out system and Self-employment

So far, we have used terms such as home-based work, for instance, without pointing out the heterogeneity they hide. Workers who work without leaving their homes are called home-based workers. Very often even in official documents home-based work has been described as 'the production of a good or the provision of a service for an employer or contractor under an arrangement whereby the work is carried out at a place of the worker's own choosing, often the worker's own home, where there is no direct supervision by the employer or contractor' (International Labour Office (ILO), 1992). Alternative terms used to refer to home-based workers are 'out-workers' or 'piece-rate workers'. This definition applies to only one type of home workers, those on the putting-out system, which is carried out as a part of a manufacturing process or industrial work. The other type of home-based workers are the self-employed who work individually or in groups and provide goods or services directly to consumers.

(i) *Putting-Out System.* Women working in slums on the putting-out system carried out work for manufacturing industries like food products, textiles, garments, paper, leather, plastics and even chemicals. Most were contacted by contractors either through sub-contractors or traders. They learnt most of the skills required while doing the specific work. They hardly ever came in contact with the principal employer who owned the industry. The chain of middlemen between the worker and the principal employer could be long or short. Wage that a worker earned was inversely related to the length of the chain of middlemen between the principal employer and the out-worker. These home workers, though they lived in the same slum, could never hope to organise themselves into trade unions; they were neither aware of who their employer was nor who their fellow workers were. They were entirely at the mercy of the middlemen for work and were forced to accept whatever wage or piece-rate they were offered. More often than not, most women received abysmally low wages, worked for long hours to finish the work and perpetually faced uncertainty of work and income. These were the main problems that confronted home-based workers on the putting-out system.

(ii) *Self-Employed.* Self-employed home-based workers were mostly in traditional trades like cooking, food processing, sewing, tailoring and embroidery, activities generally done by all women. There were some, especially the young, who had acquired specific skills by attending special courses in assembly work, beautician's training, computer data feeding, screen printing etc. Such women formed a minority among self-employed home workers. These workers faced two types of problems. First, inadequacy of funds to invest in better equipment and expand their trade.[5] The second problem faced was that of locating the market for the goods they made. For the slightly better qualified, say those with skills in screen-printing or computer data feeding, the question was of locating clients who needed their skills.

(iii) *Economic Status.* Women, both self-employed home workers and those engaged in the putting-out system were generally in a weak and disadvantaged position with respect to income, working relations, working environment and legal protection. However, their earnings formed a substantial share of the family income. Neither group had control over their income. The self-employed were at the mercy of the consumers. In case of contract workers, wage agreements were between the sub-contracting company and the contractors or middlemen. Women had no control over these agreements. And as pointed out earlier, the longer the chain of middlemen, the smaller the amount left with or paid to women. For higher incomes, women needed to work for longer hours and also had to seek help of other members of the family. If the unit contracting work was very small, women approached the employer directly, but even in such cases the employer decided the quantum of work and payment to be made to the women workers.

Working relations either between self-employed workers and their consumers or contract workers and their employers and middlemen were very informal and based on mutual trust. Because of this informality, wages too were agreed upon verbally. Women had the flexibility to work any number of hours, at any time of the day and night. They may get work either continuously or intermittently or even seasonally. From the worker's point of view, the biggest advantage was that the work was done at home. But, with inadequate ventilation, air and light, the environment within their homes was far from satisfactory. This made them vulnerable to occupational diseases. While the self-employed depended on their own savings for purchase of equipment and raw materials they needed, contract workers were provided equipment by the contractor or trader occasionally but raw materials always.

(b) Domestic Workers

As mentioned earlier, a large number of women in the urban informal sector were trapped in menial services like domestic work, sweeping and hawking. These occupations provided easy entry and most importantly did not demand either formal education or training. Domestic work included washing clothes, pots and pans and cleaning the house of the employer. For most women this work was an extension of housework and could be done without spending time learning the tasks. Second, women with little or no education could not afford to wait for better income opportunities and had limited occupations to choose from. That the number of women entering domestic work has declined over time in urban India and Mumbai was clear from the National Sample Survey Organisation (NSSO) 43rd and 50th Round data (NSSO 1990 and 1997; 1987–8 and 1993–4 for Mumbai). The decline was not surprising given the occupation's low social status. Wages paid to domestics have increased but not enough to compensate for the price rise and certainly not for the fall in status caused by the growth, however inadequate, of higher status employment. Sweeping is commercialised in most cities and women sweepers do find their way to better paid jobs in the formal sector. But sweeping too is a dead-end occupation and stigmatised because it is done mostly by scheduled castes.

(c) Vendors

Hawking offered employment to the less educated and the illiterate. Hawkers could be divided into three types. The first type consisted of women who operated a small shop from their own home from where they often sold items like vegetables, coconuts, biscuits, cheap chocolates, cigarettes, pins, pencils, erasers, soaps and detergents. All members of the household managed the shop.[6] The problem with such petty shops was that there were far too many of them in every slum, which lowered profit margins of all who participated in the activity.

The second type of hawking was done by women at market places located close to their slums. Most sold vegetables but there were some who sold snacks, which have a ready market all over Mumbai. Of the two types of vendors, those operating from home and those selling goods in the market, the latter were much better off particularly if they added value to the product by processing it.

The third category of hawkers was itinerant vendors who vended mostly vegetables, stainless steel utensils and fish. The poorest of the poor women were engaged in the recycling trade and were either rag-pickers or 'batliwalis' who bought old bottles from door to door and sold them to traders engaged in recycling activities.

All women vendors were constrained by initial lack of capital to start the business. During our personal conversations with such workers, it was clear that they bought the goods on cash or credit from wholesalers or bigger vendors at high prices or rates of interest. Their bargaining position was extremely weak in all these situations.

3. AN OVERVIEW OF CURRENT POLICIES FORMULATED FOR WOMEN IN URBAN INDIA

The Department of Women and Child Development currently implements many programmes which are expected to both supplement and complement the general development programmes relating to social sectors like health, education and rural development. The ultimate objective of all these programmes is to ensure that women are empowered, economically and socially. Most of them are implemented through non-governmental organisations (GOI, 1995–6).

The following programmes are relevant for poor women living in urban India. They are: 1) Funding of Hostels for Working Women, 2) Scheme of Training-cum-Employment-cum-Production centres, 3) Socio-economic Programme providing work and wages to the needy/destitute/widows and deserted women, 4) Programme of Condensed Courses of Education and Vocational Training (CCEVT), 5) Nehru Rozgar Yojana (NRY), 6) Mahila Samriddhi Yojana (MSY), and 7) Rashtriya Mahila Kosh (RMK).

We shall review each of these programmes to understand their applicability to women in the urban informal sector especially those living in poor neighbourhoods.

3.1 Funding of Hostels for Working Women

The programme of funding for hostels for working women is definitely a well-meaning one and will go a long way in solving problems of accommodation faced by young, educated women who migrate to urban centres for employment. The programme might not have relevance for illiterate and less educated women, working in the urban informal sector.

3.2 The Scheme of Training-cum-Employment-cum-Production Centres

Funded by the Norwegian Agency for International Development (NORAD) this scheme is designed to impart training to women belonging to weaker sections of society and qualify them for employment on a sustained basis. Training is imparted in selected non-traditional trades such as electronics, watch manufacturing/assembly, printing and binding, garment making, beauty culture, typing, shorthand etc. The scheme is likely to benefit fresh entrants to the urban labour force with some basic education and seems to be more relevant to urban rather than rural areas. Assistance under the scheme is confined to Rs 8,000 per beneficiary, but the actual expenditure per beneficiary was much less. Between 1982–3 and 1994–5, it was Rs 5,459 per beneficiary and the amount sanctioned in 1995–6 was even lower at Rs 4,592 per beneficiary (GOI, 1995–6, p. 51).

In short, the expenditure was spread too thinly over many women and even the actual per capita expenditure was less than the official provision under the scheme. In 1995–6, a total of 13,500 women were to be trained of which barely 510 (3.8 per cent) were in Maharashtra. Needless to say, not many could be from Mumbai which often is excluded from the scope of most programmes because it is a rich city. Curiously enough, over the period of twelve years of the scheme's existence, the number of women trained per year was 5,458, too small a number relative to the educated women who entered the urban labour force during this period. Since the scheme was formulated initially to benefit the weaker sections of society, it would be interesting to see whether the beneficiaries fulfilled this requirement and whether the trained women were able to get sustainable employment. This would clearly indicate the feasibility of the programme, especially for those who are in the informal sector. Despite these limitations, the scheme should be pursued in urban India by approaching other agencies, if necessary, for funding.

3.3 The Socio-Economic Programme

This programme gives financial assistance to NGOs to undertake income generating activities or opportunities for 'Work and Wage' to needy women who are poor, downtrodden, widowed, destitute, disabled etc. The scheme is currently applicable to rural women in economically backward areas. It is not clear what kind of industrial and self-employment units have been set up under the scheme. Somehow one feels that there is an underlying presumption that there are no needy women in urban areas! A recent study of poverty shows that incidence of poverty is marginally higher in urban India than in rural India (GOI, 1993). Some thought should be given to reformulate the scheme to extend it to urban areas too.

3.4 The Scheme of Condensed Courses of Education and Vocational Training Programme for Women (CCEVT)

The CCEVT conducts courses for women aged fifteen years and above. Since 1990–1, grants have been given to voluntary organisations to conduct courses of two or three years duration to enable women to pass the secondary, middle and primary level examinations. Under the vocational training programme, women are trained in different vocations for employment or self employment. It is indeed a laudable scheme and could be extended to poor working women in the urban informal sector.

3.5 The Nehru Rozgar Yojana (NRY)

The scheme is aimed at creating employment opportunities through schemes such as wage employment, micro-enterprises and improvement of shelter for and environment of the urban poor. The budgetary provision for it aims at achieving social goals such as community development, employment generation, skills upgradation and shelter upgradation. In the five years from 1995 it was expected to benefit over five million urban poor in 345 Class II cities. Its achievements are not known. The programme is not addressed to Class I cities and much less to mega-cities like Mumbai.

3.6 Mahila Samruddhi Yojana (MSY)

This is an ingenious scheme started in 1993, to inculcate the habit of thrift among poor rural women who generally do not think of their future and spend all their meagre earnings on current consumption. Uptil March 1996, 16.91 million accounts were opened under the scheme in which Rs 1,724.2 million was deposited giving an average of Rs 102 per account. Though the amount seems meagre at present, with increase in rural incomes it could be expected to increase. This scheme should be extended to women employed in the informal sector in urban India. In the absence of old age benefits, these savings could be precious for them.

3.7 Rashtriya Mahila Kosh (RMK)

This scheme was set up in 1993 to meet credit needs of poor women workers in informal employment who do not own any assets. It aimed at setting up a credit base to provide credit to poor women through NGOs, Women Development Corporations, Co-operative Societies and other agencies who have an infrastructure for disbursement and recovery of credit. The major objectives of the RMK are to provide women access to sources of credit, promot thrift, mobilise savings and channel them for productive activities. The scheme is implemented through NGOs who promote self-help groups, which in turn build a thrift fund that can be revolved among members. The groups act like mini banks for women who have surplus fund but cannot approach a regular bank or ensure security of funds in their own homes. The most important effect of the scheme was that women learned to handle funds and deploy them to increase their income. Women have utilised the money lent to them for various activities, prominently for running petty shops, vending vegetables, fruit, flowers and garments, dairying and catering, doing embroidery, weaving fishing nets and making garlands. The scheme should be pursued vigorously in urban India to provide credit to self-employed women.

Though the scheme is in operation since, it continues to be financially weak. According to the information available from the Department of Women and Child Development, till March 1996, only 103 NGOs were involved in the scheme. Ever since its inception, the total amount allocated per beneficiary amounted to Rs 1,820 of which Rs 1,138 (63 per cent) was actually disbursed to the beneficiary. In 1995–6, the last year for which data was available to us, the amount sanctioned and disbursed per beneficiary had increased to Rs 2,298 and Rs 1,503 respectively. These amounts are too small to start any meaningful sustainable activity that could promise women an escape from poverty. Yet the scheme could prove to be extremely useful to self-employed women in the urban informal sector.

Having briefly examined the programmes currently implemented by the Department of Women and Child Development and other agencies of the central government, we have tried to indicate as follows, policies that could be formulated to help working women especially the poor among them in urban India. They are neither original nor universally applicable. Good policies would be based on a thorough knowledge of the occupations the poor follow and the difficulties they face. We feel that the poor themselves know better than planners how best to solve their own difficulties and hence we would restrict the role of the policy maker to providing them the means to do so.

4. POLICY IMPLICATIONS

The policies which we suggest below are basically of three types:

(a) Policies that are addressed to home-based workers who belong to different activities with differing needs. As noted earlier, there are different kinds of home-based workers and they differ in their needs. So must the policies addressed to them.

(b) Policies that are addressed to women who are currently concentrated in dead-end menial jobs but would like to shift to some other kind of work. These would have to be in keeping with the educational endowments of these women.

(c) Policies that are designed to impart training but would go beyond training to inculcate skills among trainees to enable them to start their own small independent units.

4.1 Policies addressed to Home-based Workers

For this group of women, the following policies could be recommended:

(a) The self-employed, unable either to update their techniques or to expand their activities because of insufficiency of funds, should be provided credit on easy terms. This could be done through the RMK. NGOs, Mahila Mandals and activist groups could play an important role not only in formation of self-help groups of women doing the same kind of work but also in creating access to credit facilities and identifying markets for their finished products. This in fact would be a replication of Annapurna, an organisation that has been operating in Mumbai to help women providing food items or 'khanawalis'. Similar organisations are functioning in Ahmedabad where the Self-employed Women's Association (SEWA) has done excellent work. The policy could be implemented through Mahila Mandals in the slums. Though initially the NGOs and grassroot level workers may help women either in getting credit or in marketing, women should be trained to handle all the operations themselves. The experience of Annapurna and SEWA shows that this is not at all impossible.

(b) The main problem that confronts contract workers who are a part of the putting-out system, is the existence of contractors, middlemen or traders between the employer of the manufacturing unit that puts-out work and the women who work for them. Existence of middlemen often works to the disadvantage of the home-based workers. Since the latter are distributed over space even in the same slum, women rarely get to know who their fellow workers are. NGOs could intervene and find out how many women in the slum work for the same employer or contractor or middleman or trader. It is very important that such women come together and work under the same roof. They could meet and work either in gymnasiums, Mahila Mandals or any other community centre in the slum. Closer contacts between contract workers would eliminate many malpractices that middlemen indulge in. Trade unions or activists so far have not been able to organise workers in manufacturing units in the informal sector.

Organising home-based workers poses a greater challenge. If home-based workers could work from a common place, organisations like trade unions could emerge with the help of NGOs. These organisations could then, by eliminating middlemen directly, establish contact with the principal employer for getting work.

(c) In order to frame appropriate policies, there is a need to form a database that would provide the number of middlemen, number of home-based workers and the linkages between the two. An intensive study of the chain of middlemen which operates in urban labour markets between home-based work for women and employers in manufacturing units which put-out work is long overdue. We do not know how many middlemen there are, who they are and how they operate. Unfortunately, we do not know the magnitude of home-based work in different industries and services in Mumbai either. The government could collect this data when they conduct the Economic Census by canvassing a special questionnaire to firms to find how many firms sub-contract work and to whom the work is given. We need to understand the linkages between the contractors and the home-based workers to frame appropriate policies. As liberalisation proceeds, the tendency to put out work would increase. Unfortunately, we know very little about it. In Indonesia, for instance, a number of studies have been conducted to find out not only how many home workers there are in different industries but also how the putting-out system operates in each industry. With these detailed studies, the government has been able to exercise some control over middlemen. The valuable knowledge which the contractors, middlemen, and traders have should be exploited by the government for improving the productivity and welfare of women home-based workers (ILO, 1992).

4.2 Policies Addressed to Women in Menial Services

The following set of policies could be suggested for this group of women with very little education for enhancing their incomes.

(a) Attempts have been made in many cities to organise domestic workers into unions so that they could get higher wages. Not many women domestics in Mumbai are members of unions. Second, unionisation does not help them move to an occupation that enjoys a higher social status. Given their educational levels, one could only think of alternative occupations that are related to housework.[7]

(b) Many women could be given lessons in advanced cookery and encouraged to set themselves up in vending hygienically prepared food, take-away lunches and snacks from road side kiosks all over Mumbai but concentrated in the Central Business District (CBD). This will require co-operation from municipal authorities, lending agencies and producers of kitchen equipment that could devise suitable hire purchase arrangements for such enterprising women.

(c) We pointed out earlier that many women sold articles of daily consumption particularly vegetables, cigarettes, sweets, etc. from home. We also noted that there were far too many of them than was good for their trade in the same slum. These women could be encouraged and trained to run their business on a co-operative basis with the help of NGOs. Women may be encouraged to buy in bulk and specialise in some lines of trade so that their profit are maximised. The co-operatives may even be helped to run fair price shops in slums to sell foodgrains from the public distribution system. These are currently run by retail traders, who allegedly indulge in unfair trade practices.

(d) It is surprising that though women work as contract workers in the garment industry, hawkers who sell garments in Mumbai are all men. It may be fruitful to explore the possibilities of involving women in this trade. That could be an additional occupation for many in the informal sector in Mumbai. Women who are currently working as contract workers could themselves be involved in this activity. As noted earlier, if firms in the garment industry which sub-contract work are identified at the instance of the government, NGOs could be involved in initially acting as middlemen between the women who would want to sell garments and the firms producing readymade garments. As stated earlier, the Department of Women and Child Development could prevail upon the appropriate authorities regarding issue of licenses to women. One could go further and suggest that certain areas could be reserved for women hawkers who could sell all kinds of goods in the reserved areas. This would especially help many older and less educated women to shift from some of the menial trades to more satisfying and higher paying trades where job opportunities exist but have not been exploited.

4.3 Policies Regarding Training of Women

The following policies for training women could supplement those which are currently in force:

(a) In the light of the observations made earlier, we feel that the training programme assisted by NORAD is indeed excellent despite some of the limitations that we have pointed out. The major limitation, as we could see it, was that the funds available from the programme were too inadequate to meet the need. Very few young girls had access to the programme. Not much can be achieved unless more funds are made available. Therefore, alternate funding agencies could be approached for financing such programmes.

(b) It is time to evaluate the programme particularly to see how the women trained under it have been able to find sustainable employment after completing the training imparted to them. More importantly, it would be crucial to know whether women could utilise their training in the jobs they actually did. This would throw light on the feasibility of the programme for the labour market. In view of these findings, the training programme could, if necessary, be revised to suit the needs of the labour market.

(c) Programmes currently conducted by the government in vocational training of any type would have to be complemented by instruction and counselling in the organisational and managerial aspects of business operation. This is an aspect which needs urgent attention. The current level of skills and knowledge is not adequate for women to start small enterprises on their own. As noted earlier, this is so whether we take the self-employed or contract workers operating from home or other less educated women in menial occupations. Hence, it is not unusual to find women trained under the NORAD scheme working as casual or contract employees. That has been the drawback also of most formal courses elsewhere in developing countries (Fluitman, 1989). These business skills are to be taught not only to women currently undergoing training but also to women who are already in the labour market. For the latter, programme content, timing, duration and location should be devised to ensure accessibility to women. Provisions for retraining and upgrading the skills may be required.

(d) In many countries, non-formal training has been adopted as an alternative to formal training. This is imparted through apprenticeships and training centres. A review of these courses has revealed that their course content, like formal courses, was primarily oriented towards giving women income-generating skills but not essential business skills. These trainees too could at best be employed as contract workers but had no insight into processes of decision making and organisation and management of production to enable them to start small enterprises on their own. Addition of business skills to course content in vocational programmes conducted on a non-formal basis would go a long way in helping women improve their productivity and income but most importantly their total personality so that they learn to maintain good business relations, and are in a better position to face discrimination and hostility.

(e) The third approach to training has been to target the programme to specific groups of workers. In this case, the programmes have been designed in accordance with the felt needs of the target group by undertaking comprehensive studies on the nature of their occupations and finding out their training needs. Experience, however, showed that most of the content of the training courses was incomprehensible and therefore inappropriate for the less educated who form the majority in the informal sector. Most disturbing was the finding that a majority of women were not applying their acquired skills and knowledge to the activities they were engaged in. Evaluation of the actual working of the programmes thus becomes crucial to their reformulation.

(f) Finally, one could design training programmes by adopting a sectoral approach. The approach is adopted by SEWA. The starting point would be to conduct detailed studies of the sector including profiles of women and their business and the problems they face in gaining access to critical resources, discrimination and harassment experienced by them, poor working conditions etc. These detailed reports were used by SEWA to plan the training of women in specific trades. Depending upon the nature of the problems faced, they were either tackled at the policy or institutional levels or as specific interventions to improve access to credit, markets, raw materials or support services. Training was one of the elements in the process of self-improvement and development, which also included credit schemes, maternity benefits, child care, legal and social security, marketing assistance etc. Training therefore covered organisational skills, technical know-how, knowledge of production, marketing, and management skills which enable women to expand and improve income earning opportunities. The process has helped women improve their position in the labour market as workers, producers and managers. This is the most successful approach to training, and needs to be replicated wherever possible.

We have given possible interventions that the government could make either directly or indirectly through voluntary agencies in the informal sector where the majority of poor women work. Urban labour markets are segmented and women form one of the vulnerable groups. They are doubly disadvantaged; first, because they are women and second, because they form a flexible labour category. Nowhere is this more obvious, and very painfully so, than in slums.

ENDNOTES

1. Women rolled *bidies*, made flower garlands to sell from home or in the market located close to their slum and provided meals to single men and migrants who had migrated alone leaving their families in their native place. Some women stitched garments or cloth bags or embroidered garments for small-scale garment units in the vicinity, while others made paper bags or ground spices for traders nearby. Some took to domestic work, which like home-based work, provided an easy entry into the labour market.
2. However, certain aspects of both slums need to be borne in mind while analysing these trends. Closure of textile industries in the late 1980s had curtailed wage employment opportunities for most workers in the Slum 1 region. In contrast, the emergence of the Export Promotion Zone near Slum 2 enhanced wage employment opportunities and growth in that region.
3. A woman worker had worked for about thirteen years at the time of the survey. Years of participation in the labour market did not change their occupational pattern much. An overwhelming majority was still engaged in home-based work, domestic service and factory employment.
4. Surprisingly, when other variables in the earnings function were held constant, training lowered earnings. This odd result was due largely to intense competition from similarly trained women, particularly in tailoring, living in the same neighbourhood.
5. For instance, women involved in preparing food for others would benefit by using simple household gadgets like pressure cookers, mixers, processors and even refrigerators. These gadgets would help them expand their business, but none had money to invest in them.
6. Such enterprises existed in all slums of Mumbai, because they met the daily needs of all sections of the slum population, young and old, women and men. Availability of an item of daily consumption in the vicinity turned consumers to these petty shops, while for the women the shop was a source of supplementary income, which they earned without leaving the home.
7. A maidservant, for instance, works for many households. Normally, she washes pots and pans, and clothes, and sweeps and wipes the floor. She rushes from one house to another and is hard pressed to complete her paid work and still have time to do her own domestic work. Many households own domestic appliances like vacuum cleaners, washing machines and dishwashers but do not let the maids operate them. They could be trained to handle the equipment so that their productivity and incomes increase. In the not too distant future many co-operative housing societies may find it cheaper to set up washing machines in the premises and they would require maids to operate them. In course of time, many may choose to specialise in ironing clothes which today is a man's

occupation. Maids could be given courses in cookery so that they can graduate from very low paid to slightly better paid jobs.

REFERENCES

Deshpande, Sudha and A. Deshpande, 1998. *Impact of the NEP on Women Workers in Slums of Mumbai*, Report on the Research Project funded by The Department of Women and Children, Ministry of Human Resource Development, Government of India.

Fluitman, Fred, 1989. *Training for Work in the Informal Sector*, ILO, Geneva.

Goodale, Gretchen, 1989. 'Training for Women in the Informal Sector', in Fluitman, Fred, 1989. *Training for Work in the Informal Sector*, ILO, Geneva.

Government of India (GOI), 1980. *Shramashakti, Report of the National Commission on Self Employed Women and Women in the Informal Sector*, New Delhi.

______, 1993. *Report of the Expert Group on Estimates of Proportion and number of Poor*, Planning Commission, New Delhi.

______, 1995–6. *Annual Report Part IV 1995–6*, Department of Women and Children, Ministry of Human Resource Development, New Delhi.

Hart, K., 1973. 'Informal Income Opportunities and Urban Employment in Ghana', in Jolly, Richard *et al.*, *Third World Employment Problems and Strategy*, Penguin, Education.

International Labour Office (ILO), 1992. *Homeworkers in Southeast Asia: Struggle for Social Protection in Indonesia*, ILOs Regional Office for Asia and the Pacific, Bangkok, Thailand.

National Sample Survey Organisation (NSSO), 1990. 'Results of the Fourth Quinquennial Survey on Employment and Unemployment (All India)', NSSO 43rd Round (July 1987–June 1988) in *Sarvekshana, Special Number*, New Delhi, September.

______, 1997. *Employment and Unemployment in India, 1993–4*, Results of the Fifth Quinquennial Survey NSS Fiftieth Round (July 1993–June 1994), Department of Statistics, Government of India, New Delhi, March.

______, 1987–8. Results of the Fourth Quinquennial Survey on Employment and Unemployment, NSSO 43rd Round (July 1987–June 1988) for Mumbai, Maharashtra State Sample (Unpublished).

______, 1993–4. Results of the Fourth Quinquennial Survey on Employment and Unemployment, NSSO 50th Round (July 1993–June 1994) for Mumbai, Maharashtra State Sample (Unpublished).

Self, J. and Girling, R.H., 1983. *Reaching Poor Women: A Training Plan for Organisational Development in India*, Washington D.C., ICRW, as quoted in Goodale, G. 1989. op. cit.

Todaro, M.P., 1969. 'A Model of Labour Migration and Urban Unemployment in Less Developed Countries' in *American Economic Review*, March.

chapter 4

Human Poverty and Income Poverty: Linkages and Implications

• *K Seeta Prabhu and Sangita Kamdar*

1. INTRODUCTION

Defining poverty and identifying the poor have been issues engaging the attention of academics and policy-makers in India for over three decades. The pioneering work by Dandekar and Rath (1971) on Indian poverty has been carried forward in a number of directions and the currently available measures provide data on not only the number of poor but also the depth and severity of poverty (Tendulkar and Jain, 1993, Ravallion and Datt, 1996). A common feature of these measures is that they define poverty mainly in terms of inadequacy of income to procure a minimum amount of calories. Thus, deprivation is identified largely with respect to income while deprivation in other basic needs such as education, health and housing are ignored.

The issue of widening the definition of poverty was considered by the Expert Group constituted by the Planning Commission to 'look into the methodology for elimination of poverty at the national and state levels and also to go into the question of redefining the poverty line if necessary' (Planning Commission, 1993, p. 2). The Report of the Expert Group stated that 'while quantifying poverty, it is desirable that we not only consider the calorie needs of an individual but also give due weightage to the basic needs of shelter and health and other needs like education and transport, which would help him/her in living a "normal" and "effective" existence' (p. 31, emphasis as in the original). The Expert Group recommended the consideration of several specific factors while defining the poor. They are a) the dominant characteristics of the poor population in terms of their distribution by region, social group and family characteristics b) nutritional status including anthropometric measurements and activity patterns by age, sex and socio-economic categories c) health status including mortality, morbidity, access to and use of health services and costs d) educational status comprising school enrolments, reach and quality of public education services and costs, and e) living environment including density of settlements, living space per head, type of houses, access to amenities, safe drinking water and sanitation. Despite these recommendations, there has been no concerted effort either at the official level or by independent researchers to extend the concept of poverty to include dimensions other than income.

Meanwhile, the United Nations Development Programme (UNDP), as part of the continuing efforts to shift the norms of judging development from per capita income to other non-income measures, proposed a different concept of poverty which was centred on deprivation in capabilities, particularly those of education, health and nutrition. Commenting on the inadequacy of the income measure of poverty, the *Human Development Report, 1996*, stated, '... 'income poverty' is only part of the picture. Just as human development encompasses aspects of life much broader than income, so poverty should be seen as having many dimensions' (UNDP, 1996, p. 27). In order to distinguish the new concept of poverty from the traditional concept of income poverty, it was termed initially as capability poverty and subsequently as human poverty. Two measures to reflect such deprivation, viz., the Capability Poverty Measure (CPM) and a Human Poverty Index (HPI) were introduced in the annual Human Development Reports in the years 1996 and 1997 respectively, with the former focusing on percentage population lacking in basic capabilities and the latter including, in addition, provision[1] of social sector services (UNDP, 1996,1997).

It may be noted that the concept of human poverty is similar to the indices used to measure well-being that were developed much earlier by Buchanan and Ellis (1955), Adelman and Morris (1967), Morris (1979), and Dasgupta (1993). For example, Morris (1979) included in the Physical Quality of Life Index (PQLI) the indicators, life expectancy at birth, infant survival rate and adult literacy rate whereas Dasgupta (1993) constructed an index comprising the indicators, per capita income, life expectancy at birth, infant mortality rate, literacy rate, index of political rights and index of civil rights. However, the new concept of the UNDP is cast in terms of poverty rather than quality of life, as the intention is to focus on deprivation and to indicate that poverty has several dimensions apart from income deprivation. Unlike in the Human Development Index (HDI) where per capita income is an important dimension contributing to human development along with education and health attainment, in the HPI, human deprivation is characterised by non-income deprivations alone and is thus quite different from the HDI as well as the common perception of what constitutes poverty.

One way of sorting out this lack of correspondence of dimensions used in measures of attainment and deprivation is to include income poverty along with deprivation in education and health in the HPI in order to arrive at an integrated measure of poverty. Such a measure was developed by Haq (1997) in the South Asia Human Development Report. The Human Deprivation Measure suggested therein captured deprivation in the same three dimensions as the Human Development Index, viz., income, educational attainment and health attainment, the advantage being the uniformity of dimensions being considered, whether it be attainment or deprivation. The procedure provided by Haq seems more acceptable than the measures using only non-income deprivations, since poverty has traditionally been associated with income deprivation and a measure that does not include such deprivation cannot, in popular perception, define *poverty*. However, using a measure based on non-income indicators alone has the advantage that it enables one to juxtapose and distinguish between deprivations in income with deprivations in education and health more explicitly. Such an exercise may be particularly important in instances where reduction in income poverty may not necessarily imply a reduction in human deprivation. The strength of the linkages between the two has important implications for policy. This also leads to the issue of the factors that determine the levels of human poverty and the role of private incomes and public action in its alleviation.

The present paper explores some of these issues within the context of Indian states. More specifically, the main objectives of the paper are (a) to construct a measure of human deprivation in terms of a human poverty index, (b) to identify the links between income-poverty and human poverty and (c) explain the main factors that contribute to the incidence of human poverty.

2. HUMAN POVERTY INDEX (HPI) AND ITS MODIFICATIONS

In this paper, the HPI for Indian states was constructed using the indicators suggested by UNDP as well as after modifying it to include only indicators representing final outcomes. The Human Poverty Index (HPI) provided by UNDP included deprivation in three dimensions, viz., deprivation in knowledge, longevity and deprivation in decent living standard.

Deprivation in longevity was represented by the indicator, percentage of people not expected to survive up to age 40 (P_1) and deprivation in knowledge by the percentage of people who were illiterate (P_2). Deprivation in decent living standard was considered from the point of view of deprivation in public as well as private provisioning. Deprivation in public provisioning was represented by the indicators; a) percentage population without access to health services and b) percentage population without access to safe drinking water. Deprivation in private provisioning was represented by the variable, percentage of moderately and severely malnourished children. The composite variable, P_3 was constructed by taking a simple average of the three variables. P_{31}, P_{32}, and $P_{33.}$ The HPI was arrived at as a power mean of the three dimensions as follows:

$$HPI = [1/3\ (P_1^{\ 3} + P_2^{\ 3} + P_3^{\ 3})\ ]^{1/3}$$

The earlier measure, Capability Poverty Measure (CPM), also measured deprivation in the capacity to be well nourished and healthy and the deprivation in education. The variables used were a) the proportion of children under-nourished b) percentage of births unattended by trained health personnel and c) female illiteracy. The CPM was a composite index of these three deprivations wherein the indicators were given equal weights. It is evident that the index considered mainly deprivations suffered by women and children as individuals. As Haq (1997) rightly observed, the measure tends to exaggerate the overall extent of deprivation in South Asia as women and children carry the main burden of such deprivation in this region.

It is obvious that though the CPM and the HPI are measures of deprivation, the dimensions that they take into account are rather limited. It has been pointed out that since the HPI is aimed at capturing the denial of choices to people, ignoring important dimensions of such denial limits the utility of the index. For example, an important dimension that has been omitted is the difference between parliamentary democracies with universal adult franchise and authoritarian regimes. Ranking of all countries on a synthetic index irrespective of the political regimes prevailing therein does not make sense (Krishnaji, 1997).

In both the CPM as well as the HPI, several doubts have been raised about the choice of variables as well as the reliability of data.[2] A common shortcoming of both the measures is that they do not distinguish between (a) outcome, process and input indicators,[3] and (b) individual, household, community and regional level deprivations.[4] An additional shortcoming is that the indicators used are of differing dimensions.[5] Furthermore, whereas the CPM was based on individual level deprivations, the HPI comprised indicators reflecting individual, household as well as regional deprivations. The dimensionality of the variables included in the indices was also quite different[6] with the problem extending also to the processes that get reflected in outcome indicators.[7]

In view of the mixed nature of indicators used in the HPI, we considered it necessary to make some changes in the ones selected for computing a HPI for Indian states. As a prelude to subsequent analysis, we examined the extent of relationship between input and outcome indicators included in the HPI using data from 15 major Indian states for the period around the year 1991. The analysis revealed that the percentage of population without access to health services and safe drinking water explained 74 per cent of the variation in the indicator, probability of dying before the age of 40. Even when the composite indicator of provisioning, which included, in addition to the above variables, percentage children who were undernourished, the variation explained was fairly high at 63 per cent.[8] All the coefficients were significant at 1 per cent level. This reaffirmed our reasoning that it is pointless to include both input as well as outcome indicators in the same index.

Since there are valid objections to the inclusion of both input and output indicators in the index, we relied on only final outcome indicators in order to construct a Modified Human Poverty Index (HPIM). The three indicators used were a) illiteracy to represent deprivation in knowledge, b) probability of not surviving up to age 40 to represent health deprivation and c) children under age 4 who are undernourished (weight for age, -2SD) to represent nutritional deprivation.[9] In order to verify the extent to which these changes affected the values that the states obtained, the index was also computed using indicators suggested by the UNDP. The variables used are set out in Annexure I. The procedure for the calculation of the HPIM was similar to that adopted by the UNDP (1997).

Results

The data used in the computation of the HPI for Indian states is given in Table 1 and values of states on the modified HPI (HPIM) are presented in Table 2. The analysis indicated that the average level of human poverty at the all-India level as per HPIM was 45 per cent as compared to the 41 per cent obtained by using the HPI indicators (Table 2). The fact to note is that both computations yielded somewhat similar magnitude of deprivation in capabilities and point to the high average levels of deprivation at the national level.

The range within which the value of human poverty fluctuated across major Indian states was 28 and 52 per cent for the HPI and 20 and 55 per cent for the HPIM. In both exercises, predictably, Kerala with the lowest levels of human poverty and Bihar with the highest, represented two ends of the spectrum. Significantly, though there was not much difference in the average levels of human poverty in both the indices, the situation was quite different at the disaggregated level. Ten out of 15 states recorded higher levels of poverty on the HPIM as compared to the HPI.

The difference between the two estimates was due to the elimination of the indicators, percentage population without access to health services and percentage population without access to safe drinking water in the third dimension pertaining to provisioning in the HPIM. Due to these changes, the only indicator that represented the third dimension, viz., percentage children undernourished, acquired an equal weight along with the other two indicators used in the HPIM. Hence, states with higher levels of child under-nutrition but relatively better levels of health and drinking water facilities could end up with higher levels of HPIM as compared to the HPI. The difference in ranking on the HPI and the HPIM could also be taken as a reflection of the fact that mere provisioning cannot be equated with better outcomes. Given the familiar scenario where much of the publicly provided health infrastructure remained unutilised,[10] this is not surprising. The HPIM value was higher than the HPI value by 6 to 9 percentage points in the case of Karnataka, Maharashtra, Punjab, Tamil Nadu and West Bengal. Interestingly, the states of Assam, Kerala and Rajasthan reported lower levels of human poverty as per the HPIM. The difference was particularly high (over 7 percentage points)

TABLE 1. DEPRIVATION INDICATORS USED IN THE CONSTRUCTION OF HUMAN POVERTY INDEX FOR INDIAN STATES: 1989–1993

(Per cent)

No.	States	Health (Probability of dying before 40)	Education (Illiteracy Rate)	Children not fully immunised	Deliveries not in institutions	No access to health services	No access to safe water	Childre under age 4 undermourished (weight for age)*	Provisioning
		1989–93	1991	1992–93	1992–93		1992–93	1992–93	
(1)	(2)	(3)	(4)	(5)	(6)#	(7)	(8)	(9)	(10)+
1	Andhra Pradesh	14.88	55.91	17.5	67.2	42.35	36.6	49.1	42.68
2	Assam	21.81	47.11	43.6	88.9	66.25	56.8	50.4	57.82
3	Bihar	19.48	61.52	53.5	87.9	70.70	36.4	62.6	56.57
4	Gujarat	16.75	38.71	18.9	64.4	41.65	24.9	50.1	38.88
5	Haryana	15.37	44.15	17.5	83.3	50.40	27.0	37.9	38.43
6	Karnataka	15.68	43.96	15.2	62.5	38.85	24.4	54.3	39.18
7	Kerala	5.14	10.11	11.4	12.2	11.80	79.0	28.5	39.77
8	Madhya Pradesh	25.34	55.80	34.4	84.1	59.25	44.2	57.4	53.62
9	Maharashtra	12.27	35.13	7.5	56.1	31.80	21.5	54.2	35.83
10	Orissa	22.33	50.91	28.0	85.9	56.95	49.1	53.3	53.12
11	Punjab	13.87	41.19	17.5	75.2	46.35	1.4	45.9	31.22
12	Rajasthan	19.88	61.45	48.5	88.4	68.45	42.7	41.6	50.92

(Table 1 contd...)

13	Tamil Nadu	13.45	37.24	3.3	36.6	19.95	25.4	48.2	31.18
14	Uttar Pradesh	22.24	58.40	43.3	88.8	66.05	25.7	59.0	50.25
15	West Bengal	14.82	42.30	22.4	68.5	45.45	15.1	56.8	39.12
	India	17.99	47.79	30.0	74.5	52.25	31.8	53.4	45.82
	Mean	16.89	45.59	25.50	70.00	47.75	34.01	49.95	43.91
	S.D.	4.91	12.73	15.08	21.25	16.99	18.09	8.52	8.68
	C.V.	29.09	27.92	59.13	30.35	35.58	53.18	17.05	19.76

Notes: 1. *Anthropometric index weight for age, –2SD. also includes children who are below –3 standard deviation from the International Reference Population median.
2. #Column 7 is an arithmetic mean of Columns 5 and 6.
3. +Column 9 is an arithmetic mean of Columns 7, 8 and 9.

Sources: 1. Column 3: Registrar General, 1996, SRS Based Abridged Life Tables 1989–93, SRS Analytical Studies Report No. 1 of 1996, New Delhi.
2. Column 4: Census of India, 1991, Final Population Totals: Brief Analysis of Primary Census Abstract, Series 1, Paper 2 of 1992, Office Registrar General, New Delhi.
3. Column 5, 6, 8, 9: International Institute of Population Studies, National Family Health Survey 1992–93, India, Bombay.

in the case of Kerala. A perusal of the reasons for the same indicated that the exclusion of the variable, population without access to safe drinking water, was responsible for this difference. In the case of two states, Haryana and Orissa, both HPI and HPIM yielded the same level of human poverty.

Due to the above mentioned differences in the levels of human poverty as per the two computations, the ranking of states on HPIM was considerably different from that on the HPI, particularly for the states of Assam (11 in HPI and 7 in HPIM), Haryana (7 in HPI and 2 in HPIM), Maharashtra (3 in HPI and 6 in HPIM), and West Bengal (6 in HPI and 9 in HPIM). However, as observed earlier, there was no difference in the top and bottom ranking states with Kerala belonging to the former category and Bihar to the latter category unambiguously.

The HPI and HPIM were calculated using more recent data for the years ranging between 1993-2001.The data used for the computation of the HPI using UNDP method and the modified HPIM is presented in Annexure 2. The value of the HPI and the HPIM in 1993-2001 was lower than that recorded for the years 1989-93. The HPI for the latter period shows no major changes in the ranking of the states. However, Kerala with the lowest HPI value in 1989-93 lost its position to Tamil Nadu in 1993-2001. The HPIM in 1993-2001 at 36.45 was higher than the HPI value of 31.09.The HPIM indicated no major changes in the rankings of the states. The state with the lowest value of HPIM in 1993-2001 was Kerala and that with the highest value and correspondingly highest rank was Bihar in the time periods 1989-93 and 1993-2001. It is interesting to note that Maharashtra's rank on HPIM slipped from 6 in 1989-93 to 9 in 1993-2001. The HPIM also shows the improvement in the rank of Andhra Pradesh from 11 in 1989-93 (HPI) to 6 in 1993-2001.

3. HUMAN POVERTY AND INCOME POVERTY

In this section,[11] the situation of states with respect to per capita income, human poverty and income poverty is compared with a view to understanding the linkages between these variables. More specifically, the question that is sought to be answered is whether (a) higher levels of per capita SDP are associated with lower levels of human poverty, and (b) whether lower levels of income poverty are associated with lower levels of human poverty. These questions acquire importance in the context of development strategies that presume that there is an automatic link between rise in average levels of income and reduction in income poverty on the one hand and low levels of income poverty and low levels of human poverty on the other.

Since the methodology for the computation of the two dimensions of poverty is different, a comparison of the proportion of population in income poverty and human poverty may not be appropriate. Hence, only the ranks of states on per capita SDP, income poverty and human poverty were compared. In the first instance, ranks of states on current levels of the three indicators were compared. However, in the case of income poverty, two important considerations led to a comparison of ranks of income poverty in 1987-88 with ranks of human poverty in 1989-93. The first consideration was that the incidence of income poverty may be a prior constraint on the prevalence of human poverty and hence it may be meaningful to relate current levels of human poverty to past levels of income poverty. The second consideration was to test the robustness of the relationship between income and human poverty. The estimates of income poverty used were those of the Expert Group of the Planning Commission which are derived from the Quinquennial surveys on consumer expenditure by the National Sample Survey Organisation (NSSO). There has been some controversy regarding the reliability of NSSO estimates in general (Suryanarayana, 2000) and those of 1993-94 in particular (Deaton and Tarozzi, 1999).[12] In view of this controversy, it was deemed prudent to examine the relationship between human and income poverty using the estimates of income poverty for 1987-88. However, the problem with the 1987-88 estimates was that the data pertain to a drought year and hence could exaggerate the extent of income poverty in agricultural states such as Andhra Pradesh. These limitations need to be borne in mind while examining the implications of the analysis that follows. In any case, given the small number of observations, the conclusions are more indicative than definite in nature.

Table 2 presents a comparison of ranks of states on headcount ratio of poverty for 1987-88 and 1993-94 with those of human poverty for 1989-93. It may pointed out that poverty being a negative indicator, the ranking was inversely related to values, with the state reporting the lowest incidence of poverty being ranked first and the state with the highest incidence of poverty being ranked the lowest. A perusal of the ranks of states on income and human poverty (HPIM) indicates a sharp difference for Andhra Pradesh. The state ranked second only to Punjab in income poverty in 1993-94 though in 1987-88, the state's rank was third after Punjab and Haryana. Whatever the reference year for income poverty, the rank of the state on income poverty was more

TABLE 2. RANKING OF STATES ACCORDING TO HPI, HPIM, IPOV AND PCSDP

No	*States*	*HPI Value 1989–93*	*HPI Rank*	*HPIM Value 1989–93*	*HPIM Rank*	*IPOV Value 1987–8*	*IPOV Rank*	*IPOV Value 1993–4*	*IPOV Rank*	*PCSDP Value 1990–3*	*PCSDP Rank*
(1)	*(2)*	*(3)*	*(4)*	*(5)*	*(6)*	*(7)*	*(8)*	*(9)*	*(10)*	*(11)*	
1	Andhra Pradesh	44.02	9	46.23	11	25.86	3	22.19	2	5334.00	7
2	Assam	46.83	11	42.36	7	36.21	7	40.86	12	4645.67	10
3	Bihar	51.98	15	54.50	15	52.13	14	54.96	15	2873.67	15
4	Gujarat	34.34	5	39.75	5	31.54	4	24.21	3	6762.00	4
5	Haryana	36.55	7	36.35	2	16.64	2	25.05	4	8440.00	2
6	Karala	36.76	8	43.62	8	37.53	8	33.16	7	5604.33	6
7	Kernataka	27.74	1	20.09	1	31.79	5	25.43	5	5036.00	9
8	Madhya Pradesh	48.59	13	50.18	13	43.07	11	42.52	13	4257.67	12
9	Maharashtra	31.21	3	40.84	6	40.41	9	36.86	10	8425.67	3
10	Orissa	46.05	10	46.13	10	55.58	15	48.56	14	3699.33	14
11	Punjab	32.50	4	38.35	4	13.2	1	11.77	1	9822.00	1
12	Rajasthan	49.86	14	47.02	12	35.15	6	27.41	6	4596.00	11
13	Tamil Nadu	30.41	2	38.11	3	43.39	12	35.03	8	5917.33	5
14	Uttar Pradesh	48.25	12	51.74	14	41.46	10	40.85	11	3999.67	13
15	West Bengal	35.90	6	44.38	9	44.72	13	35.66	9	5213.67	8
	India	41.29		44.66		38.86		35.97			

Notes: 1. In HPI and HPIM, the state with the lowest value is ranked 1.
2. For PCSDP, the state with the highest value is ranked.

Source: Tasble 1.

favourable as compared to the rank on HPIM where the state ranked 11 with only the states of Rajasthan, Madhya Pradesh, Uttar Pradesh and Bihar obtaining lower ranks. This situation was mainly on account of the high level of illiteracy in the state with more than 55 per cent of the population over 7 years of age being illiterate in 1991 (Table 1). In fact, the illiteracy rate was marginally higher than that prevailing in Madhya Pradesh.[13] A similar situation prevailed in Rajasthan whose ranking on HPIM was much worse than the situation in terms of income poverty. The relative performance of states such as Gujarat and Punjab as well as the low income state of Uttar Pradesh was poorer on HPIM as compared to that on income poverty.

The reverse situation of relatively low levels of human poverty and hence the rank on human poverty being more favourable than that on income poverty in 1987-88 as well as 1993-94 was reported by states such as Kerala, Maharashtra, Orissa and Tamil Nadu. Among these, Maharashtra was the only high-income state (with per capita income levels substantially higher than the national average) that reported high levels of income poverty, the others being middle and low income states. With respect to Kerala, the high levels of social attainments despite relatively low per capita income levels[14] and prevalence of poverty demonstrated the role of non-income factors in determining social attainments. This also is reflected by the low rank correlation of 0.568 between income poverty (1993-94) and human poverty (HPIM of 1989-93). The rank correlation for income poverty in 1987-88 and HPIM (1989-93) was even lower at 0.493 indicating that current levels of income and human poverty are related more closely.

A comparison of the ranks of states on Per Capita State Domestic Product (PCSDP) and HPIM also proved instructive. The high-income states of Punjab, Maharashtra and Gujarat performed poorly on HPIM as compared to their ranks on PCSDP. Other states in a similar predicament included Andhra Pradesh, Karnataka, Madhya Pradesh, Rajasthan, Uttar Pradesh and West Bengal. Only four states, viz., Assam, Kerala, Orissa and Tamil Nadu, recorded better performance on human development than expected on the basis of their per capita SDP.

Overall, at the all-India level the proportion of population affected by education deprivation exceeded the proportion that was under income poverty during the early 1990s. This makes it abundantly clear that deprivation in education was not confined to the poor alone. Also evident was the fact that higher levels of income need not necessarily imply lower income poverty and human poverty. This raises several questions as to the links between per capita income, income poverty and human poverty across regions.

4. FACTORS AFFECTING HUMAN POVERTY

4.1Theoretical Framework

It is possible to identify atleast three sets of factors at the macro level that could influence human poverty levels in a region at any given time. These are (a) structural factors, (b) level of per capita income of the region, and (c) political commitment of the concerned government towards goals of human development.

(a) Structural factors

Structural factors affect human poverty levels by critically limiting the access to and utilisation of social sector services by people. Among structural factors, it is possible to distinguish between (i) inequalities in asset and income distribution, and (ii) inequalities between males and females in society.

Inequalities in asset and income distribution result in the division of households into rich and poor.[15] In instances where public provision of education and health services is inadequate, the ability to demand and utilise private sector services could be critical in determining the level of social attainments of individuals. Since the rich have better access to private sector services, their social attainments are likely to be higher than that of the poorer sections of population. The poor, on the other hand, lack the means to acquire education and health and their low levels of attainment of these crucial capabilities limits their opportunities in the job market as well.

It has also been argued that the role of the education system in capitalist societies is to 'reproduce existing capitalist relations by legitimating the stability of intergenerational occupational status and developing different sets of personality traits among different groups in society necessary for a hierarchical occupational structure' (Hinchcliffe, 1985, p. 1664). Under such conditions, the initial advantage that children from richer households enjoy gets perpetuated. It is likely that in the absence of appropriate government policy that aims at correcting these inequities, the gap between the rich and poor widens over time.

The other set of structural factors that critically influence human development outcomes is gender inequality, which is mainly a reflection of the operation of social and cultural norms in society. While economic factors such as participation in employment could over time change the existing norms, such participation itself is governed by social and cultural factors. Social factors determine the extent of participation of women in education and the importance given to health problems of women. It has been observed that in regions where women's status is high, acquisition of education by females is relatively high which in turn contributes to an overall high rate of literacy. The example of Kerala is often cited in this context (Jefferey, 1993). The reverse situation of low women's status, low social attainments despite higher average levels of per capita income is provided by the states of Punjab and Haryana.

(b) Per capita Income

Given structural constraints, the level of income of the region is critical in influencing its social attainment levels. Higher average income levels are expected to be associated with lower levels of human poverty. This association may be due to the two factors explained below: (i) Given the prevalent pattern of distribution of assets and income, a higher level of income implies a higher capability of households to demand and utilise private sector services for education and health. (ii) A second implication of higher incomes is that it enables the concerned governments to spend relatively higher amount per capita on provision of education and health services. This includes capital expenditure on creation of social infrastructure as well as revenue expenditure incurred on its maintenance.

(c) Political Commitment

The third set of factors that were considered was the political commitment of government towards reduction in human poverty which is reflected in allocations made to these sectors and in ensuring the quality of services provided.

4.2 Empirical Analysis

In the empirical analysis that follows, the effect of structural constraints was sought to be captured through the variable gini coefficient of consumption expenditure (GINI) to reflect inequalities in asset holding and income respectively. Gender inequality was represented through the Female-Male Ratio (FMR) in 1991. Ideally, the FMR ought to be adjusted for migration. However, due to non-availability of such data, unadjusted FMR was used.[16] As the extent of variation in the variable is very low, FMR square was used in the empirical analysis. Per Capita State Domestic Product (PCSDP) was used as a proxy for average income levels of states. The data used was a three year average of real per capita SDP for the years 1990-91 to 1992-93 deflated by state specific implicit SDP deflators to take care of the impact of differing price levels across states. The underlying assumption that State Domestic Product represents state income, holds generally true in the case of most Indian states except Kerala where evidence suggests that income levels could be between 15 to 30 per cent higher than the recorded level of SDP on account of substantial inflow of foreign remittances (Krishnan, 1994).

The average levels of income in a state were considered to affect the ability of the government to incur expenditure on the creation of social infrastructure as well as its maintenance. However, the actual expenditure incurred depends also on the political commitment of the concerned governments. The impact of both these factors was reflected in the level of social infrastructure created in the state and the level of revenue expenditure incurred on such sectors. The variable used to represent government expenditure was the real per capita revenue expenditure on social services (SSER). The deflator used was state specific SDP deflator and the data was an average for 1985-1990. Social infrastructure was represented by an index of education, health and nutrition facilities in 1988-91. The variable was a sum of scores obtained on infrastructure indices constructed using the Principal Components method for the sectors of education, health and nutrition across major Indian states. The variables included in the analysis and their sources are reported in the Annexure 3 to this paper.

The results of our exercise, reported in Table 3, lead us to the following inferences.

The average level of per capita income was not an important factor in explaining variations in human poverty across Indian states. The sign of the variable was negative as expected though the variable was not statistically significant at 10 per cent level. Though per capita income was not an important variable, SSER, with which it had a high and positive correlation, emerged as an important variable explaining a substantial proportion of the variation in human poverty. The variable had the expected negative sign, was statistically significant at 1 per cent level and singly explained over 48 per cent of the variation in human poverty. The importance of the variable was retained even

TABLE 3. REGRESSION RESULTS

No. of observations: 15

No	*Constant*	*PCSDP*	*GINI*	*SINF*	*SSER*	*FMR^2*	*Adj. R^2*	*S.E. of regression*
1	53.6806 (−8.805)	−0.002 (−1.898)					0.1568	7.4771
2	74.5091 (3.507)						0.0826	7.7958
3	71.9508 (3.371)		−100.8534 (−1 377)				0.0601	7.891
4	51.1116 (16.931)			−1.1317 (−3.542)*			0.452	6.0251
5	65.9733 (10.405)				−0.1666 (−3.778)*		0.4867	5.8313
6	85.7771 (4.217)					−0.0001 (−2.127)	0.2011	7.2751
7	103.6622 (7.783)				−0.1589 (−4.598)*	−0.00004 (−3.048)*	0.6866	4.5564
8	86.3684 (6.012)			−1.0332 (−3.752)*	(−3.752)*	−0.00004 (−2.426)**	0.6017	5.1366
9	69.7913 (13.071)	0.0047 (3.362)*		−0.4714 (−1.490)	−0.3572 (−4.085)*		0.7435	4.1222
10	83.9689 (4.088)	0.0036 (1.241)			−0.3465 (−2.236)**	−0.00002 (−0.554)	0.7001	4.4575
11	98.5746 (7.3899)			−0.4694 (−1.392)	−0.1113 (−2.333)**	−0.00004 (−2.946)*	0.7093	4.3884

Notes: 1. Figures in parentheses indicate t-values.
2. **represents 1 per cent and *represents 5 per cent level of significance respectively.

after controlling for per capita SDP. This implies that the level of income by itself is not important for ensuring lower levels of human poverty unless it translates into higher government expenditure on social services. Thus, political commitment, apart from fiscal ability, seems to be important. In view of this result, we used SSER rather than PCSDP in further analysis.

Next in importance was SINF which was also a reflection of the level of income as well as political commitment of the government to social sectors. The variable also accounted singly for 45 per cent of the variation in human poverty. In view of the high correlation between SINF and SSER, it was considered prudent to use only one of the variables in subsequent regressions.

The variables representing structural constraints were GINI and FMR. Of these, GINI did not yield satisfactory results. The variable had the negative sign as expected but had very low explanatory power. However, the variable representing gender inequality, the FMR emerged important and which singly accounted for 20 per cent of the variation in human poverty across states. The importance of the variable was retained even after controlling for SSER or SINF.

Thus, SINF, SSER and FMR in that order were the most important variables that together explained between them 60 to 70 per cent of the variation in human poverty across Indian states.

5. CONCLUSIONS AND IMPLICATIONS

The paper attempted to construct a Human Poverty Index (HPI) for Indian states using the UNDP methodology as well as a Modified Human Poverty Index (HPIM) using only outcome indicators. A juxtaposition of the levels of the two types of poverty indicated that only four states, Assam, Kerala, Orissa and Tamil Nadu had higher ranks on the HPIM as compared to their SDP rankings, indicating better than expected performance of these states on the human development front.

The implications of the empirical analysis are quite clear. Given unequal structural relations, the role of per capita income in reducing human poverty is rather limited. What matters is that higher per capita income needs to be translated into higher levels of social infrastructure and government expenditure on social services which in turn lead to a reduction in the levels of human poverty. Gender inequality emerged very strongly as an explanatory variable when variations in human poverty were examined. Thus, gender inequality as captured by the

FMR is an important dimension to which attention needs to be focused if human poverty levels are to be lowered.

The analysis points to the rich insights which can be obtained once the concept of poverty is expanded to include deprivation in education, health and nutrition. Notwithstanding the fact that the measurement of income poverty is problematic and the measurement of human poverty is still at a preliminary stage and many more refinements, both in terms of the variables included as well as the methodology used for constructing indices are needed, the analysis opens up newer areas for further research. It is evident that much more sustained work is necessary to unravel the interrelationship between economic growth, income poverty and human poverty. Our own limited exercise points to the need to look beyond income poverty as lower levels of income poverty do not necessarily signify lower human deprivation.

The relatively low importance of levels of income and other macro variables alongside the relatively high explanatory power of variables pertaining to gender inequality and political commitment in explaining variations in human poverty indicate the directions in which government policy should proceed in order to alleviate human poverty levels in the coming decades. Relevant in this context is UNDP's grim prediction in 1996 that India will take a century to join the group of high human development countries. It is only concerted public action on a variety of fronts that can extricate India from this dire predicament.

ANNEXURE 1

In our exercise for Indian states, we relied on life tables as reported in Sample Registration System's Analytical Studies Report No. 1 of 1996 for the purpose of deriving the values of percentage population not expected to survive upto age 40 ($P_{1)}$. Data on illiteracy rate was for population aged 7+ (P2), and was obtained from the population census of 1991. In the case of the third indicator, whereas in our exercise we used only percentage children under 4 years of age who were undernourished (weight for age), data for which was available from the NFHS (1994), in the UNDP exercise two other variables, percentage population without access to safe drinking water and percentage non-institutional births were also included. For the indicator, proportion of people without access to safe drinking water, we used the data pertaining to access to drinking water from pipes and pumps available. This excludes other sources such as wells and ponds, which may constitute important sources of drinking water, particularly in states such as Kerala. However, in view of the lack of consensus on what constitutes 'safe drinking water', we preferred to confine ourselves to the data set that was readily available. Data on non-institutional births was available from the NFHS (1994).

In the case of the Revised HPI and HPIM, the sources of data were as follows: Life tables as reported in Sample Registration System's Abridged Life Tables 1992–96 and 1993–97 were used to calculate percentage population not expected to survive upto age 40. Data on illiteracy rate for population 7 and above was obtained from population census 2001. The NFHS-2 (1998–99) provided data on children not fully immunised, non-institutional deliveries, households without safe drinking water and undernourished children (under age 4) (weight for age).

ANNEXURE 2

TABLE A1. DEPRIVATION INDICATORS USED IN THE CONSTRUCTION OF HUMAN POVERTY INDEX FOR INDIAN STATES

No.	States	Health (Probability of dying before 40) 1993–97	Education (Illiteracy Rate) per cent 2001	Children not fully immunised per cent 1998–99	Deliveries not in institutions per cent 1998–99	No access to health services per cent 1998–99	No access to safe water pwe xwnr 1998–99	Childre under age 4 undermourished (weight for age) per cent 1998–99	Provisioning per cent 1998–99
(1)	(2)	(3)	(4)	(5)	(6)#	(7)	(8)	(9)	(10)+
1	Andhra Pradesh	0.15776	38.89	4.5	50.2	27.4	21.5	37.7	28.9
2	Assam	0.23989	35.72	33.2	82.4	57.8	39.9	36.0	44.6
3	Bihar	0.22738	52.47	16.8	85.4	51.1	24.6	54.4	43.4
4	Gujarat	0.16999	30.03	6.6	53.7	30.2	15.5	45.1	30.3
5	Haryana	0.17783	31.41	9.9	77.6	43.8	12.0	34.6	30.1
6	Karnataka	0.15545	32.96	7.7	48.9	28.3	13.0	43.9	28.4
7	Kerala	0.0539	9.08	2.2	7.0	4.6	80.1	26.9	37.2
8	Madhya Pradesh	0.26038	35.89	13.9	79.9	46.9	36.5	55.1	46.2
9	Maharashtra	0.13254	22.73	2	47.4	24.7	18.1	49.6	30.8
10	Orissa	0.23906	36.39	9.4	77.4	43.4	34.7	54.4	44.2
11	Punjab	0.1498	30.05	8.7	62.5	35.6	1.1	28.7	21.8
12	Rajasthan	0.20358	38.97	22.5	78.5	50.5	30.2	50.6	43.8

(Table A1 contd...)

(Table A1 continued)

No.	States	Health (Probability of dying before 40) 1993–97	Education (Illiteracy Rate) per cent 2001	Children not fully immunised per cent 1998–99	Deliveries not in institutions per cent 1998–99	No access to health services per cent 1998–99	No access to safe water pwe xwnr 1998–99	Childre under age 4 undermourished (weight for age) per cent 1998–99	Provisioning per cent 1998–99
(1)	(2)	(3)	(4)	(5)	(6)#	(7)	(8)	(9)	(10)+
13	Tamil Nadu	0.1364	26.53	0.3	20.7	10.5	15.0	36.7	20.7
14	Uttar Pradesh	0.32985	42.64	29.5	84.5	57.0	14.4	51.7	41.0
15	West Bengal	0.15504	30.78	13.6	59.9	36.8	10.7	48.7	32.1
	India	0.19634	34.62	14.4	66.4	40.4	22.1	47.0	36.5
	Mean	0.19	32.97	12.05	61.07	36.56	24.49	43.61	34.88
	S.D.	0.07	9.69	9.83	23.69	15.85	18.82	9.51	8.54
	C.V.	35.52	29.39	81.59	38.80	43.35	76.86	21.81	24.47

**Notes:* 1. Columns 7 and 10 are arithmetic mean of cols. 5 & 6 and 7, 8 & 9 respectively.

2. Safe water data refers to households without drinking water facilities from pipes or hand pump.

3. Anthropometric index weight for age, -2SD includes the children who are below -3SD standard deviation from the International Reference Population median.

Sources: 1. Column 3: Registrar General, 2000, SRS Based Abridged Life Tables 1992–96 and 1993–97, SRS Analytical Studies Report No. 1 of 2000, New Delhi

2. Column 4: Biswas Samir Kumar, 2001, Provisional Population Totals, Paper-1 of 2001, Series 28, Maharashtra, Census of India 2001, Director of Census Operations, Maharashtra

3. Column 5,6,8,9: International Institute of Population Studies, 2000, National Family Health Survey (NFHS-2) 1998–99, India, International Institute for Population Studies (IIPS) and ORC Macro, IIPS, Mumbai

Table A2. Human Poverty Index (UNDP Method) and Human Poverty Index, Modified (HPIM) 1993–2001

No.	States	Health (Probability of dying before 40) 1993–97	Education (Illiteracy Rate) per cent 2001	Children not fully immunised per cent 1998–99	Provisioning per cent 1998–99	HPI Value per cent 1993–2001	HPI Rank pwe xwnr	HPIM Value per cent 1993–2001	HPI Rank per cent
(1)	(2)	(3)	(4)	(5)	(6)#	(7)	(8)	(9)	(10)+
1	Andhra Pradesh	0.15776	38.89	37.7	28.85	30.22	9	33.46	6
2	Assam	0.23989	35.72	36.0	44.57	35.49	10	31.33	5
3	Bihar	0.22738	52.47	54.4	43.37	42.23	15	46.69	15
4	Gujarat	0.16999	30.03	45.1	30.25	26.33	5	34.09	7
5	Haryana	0.17783	31.41	34.6	30.12	26.89	6	28.90	4
6	Karnataka	0.15545	32.96	43.9	28.40	26.95	7	34.24	8
7	Kerala	0.0539	9.08	26.9	37.20	25.92	4	18.89	1
8	Madhya Pradesh	0.26038	35.89	55.1	46.17	36.40	13	41.44	13
9	Maharashtra	0.13254	22.73	49.6	30.80	23.90	3	35.46	9
10	Orissa	0.23906	36.39	54.4	44.17	35.51	11	41.16	12
11	Punjab	0.1498	30.05	28.7	21.80	23.21	2	25.67	2
12	Rajasthan	0.20358	38.97	50.6	43.77	36.26	12	39.77	11
13	Tamil Nadu	0.1364	26.53	36.7	20.73	20.95	1	28.32	3
14	Uttar Pradesh	0.32985	42.64	51.7	41.03	36.56	14	41.58	14
15	West Bengal	0.15504	30.78	48.7	32.05	27.45	8	36.40	10
	India	0.19634	34.62	47.0	36.50	31.09		36.45	

Note: For HPI and HPIM, the state with the lowest value has been ranked 1.

ANNEXURE 3

(A) Education Infrastructure Indicators

1. No. of primary schools and secondary schools per 100 sq.kms.: (1990).
2. No. of primary schools and secondary schools per lakh population: (1990).
3. No. of teachers (Primary + Secondary; both trained and untrained) per 10, 000 students (primary + secondary) (1990).

(B) Health Infrastructure Indicators

1. No. of dispensaries per 100 sq. km. (1989).
2. No. of primary health centers per 100 sq. km. (1989).
3. No. of hospital beds per lakh population (1989).
4. No. of dispensaries per lakh population (1989).
5. No. of primary health centre per lakh population (1989).
6. No. of doctors per lakh population.
7. No. of nursing persons per lakh population.

(C) Nutrition Infrastructure Indicators

1. Fair price shops per lakh population.
2. Per capita foodgrains production (Kg.) (3 year average) (1988–91).
3. Per capita production of milk (Kg.) (1989–90).
4. Per capita production of fish (Kg.) (1989–90).

Sources of Data for Regression Analysis

1. Centre For Monitoring Indian Economy (Vol. II): States; Various Issues.
2. Central Statistical Organisation, Statistical Abstract of India, Various Issues.
3. Gini co-efficient of per capita consumption expenditure, 1987–88: National Sample Survey, 43rd Round 1987–88 Special Tabulation by Dr. P.V. Srinivasan, Indira Gandhi Institute of Development Research, Bombay as available in Dreze and Sen, 1995, 'India: Economic Development and Social Opportunity', New Delhi Oxford University Press.

4. Female-Male ratio, 1991: Nanda, A.R., 1992, 'Final Population Tables: Brief Analysis of Primary Census Abstract', *Census of India 1991*, Series Paper 2 of 1992, Office of the Registrar-General, New Delhi, also available in Dreze and Sen, 1995.
5. Per Capita State Domestic Product, 1990–93: Government of India, 1998, *Economic Survey 1997–98*, Economic Division, Ministry of Finance, New Delhi.
6. Social Infrastructure Index, 1988–91: Prabhu, K. Seeta and S. Chatterjee, 1993, *Social Sector Expenditure and Human Development: A Study of Indian States*, Department of Economic Analysis and Policy, Reserve Bank of India, Bombay.
7. Social Services Revenue Expenditure: compiled from RBI, various reports.

ENDNOTES

1. The Human Poverty Index developed in the 1997 Human Development Report included three indicators viz., survival deprivation represented by people not expected to survive upto the age of 40, deprivation in education and knowledge represented by the adult illiteracy and the deprivation in economic provisioning which was a combined index of the indicators of population without access to safe water, health services and undernourished children below age 5. The three variables were accorded equal weights.
2. As Krishnaji (1997) pointed out, the percentage of population without access to 'safe' drinking water was given as 3 and 19 per cent in Bangladesh and India in the UNDP (1997) report. In view of the wide prevalence of water-borne diseases in these countries, it is difficult to believe that an overwhelming proportion of the population had access to safe drinking water.
3. Of the three indicators used in the CPM in 1996, adult illiteracy and percentage undernourished children are outcome indicators whereas the proportion of non-institutional births is a variable that influences maternal mortality and infant mortality rates. In the HPI of 1997, of the three indicators, two, viz., probability of not surviving up to age 40 and illiteracy rate represent final outcomes and reflect survival and educational deprivations. In the third dimension representing provisioning, the indicators, percentage population without access to health services and safe drinking water are input indicators whereas undernourished children is an outcome indicator.
4. For details regarding the regional and community level factors affecting women's development in the Indian context, see Hirway and Mahadevia, 1996.
5. Education and health deprivations are represented by individual level indicators whereas the third indicator dealing with provision of basic services comprises the individual level indicator, percentage of undernourished children below age 5, the household level deprivation indicator, population without access to drinking water and a regional/community level indicator, population without access to health services. The average of these three deprivations is considered to reflect deprivation in basic services. The mixed nature of the indicator however, makes it difficult to draw inferences regarding requisite remedial policy
6. The problem is particularly acute in the CPM. While adult illiteracy pertains to the whole population, the indicator, undernourished children, takes into account only the population of children even as percentage of births not attended to by medical personnel pertain only to total births. In the HPI, the inclusion of undernourished children as a variable in the third indicator that is intended to capture the lack of access to public services leads to a similar problem.
7. Thus, Krishnaji (1997) commenting on the HPI states, 'adult illiteracy as observed now is the result of neglect in the past, covering several decades. ... Prospects of survival to the age 40 are computed, however,

at current age-specific mortality rates, varying widely across the countries and over time, such measurements of survival rates, without reference to the actual course of decline in mortality and how it was brought about in the different countries can be misleading' (Krishnaji, 1997, p. 2204).

8. This is not surprising as percentage undernourished children is an outcome indicator.
9. It may be noted that even the HPIM is not free from the dimensionality problem referred to earlier. However, it is relatively neat conceptually as it represents only outcome indicators at the individual level.
10. The under-utilisation of public health infrastructure is particularly glaring in the case of Primary Health Centres (PHCs). The National Council of Applied Economic Research (NCAER, 1992) reported that, on an average, at the all-India level, PHCs accounted for only 8.2 and 5 per cent of all cases treated in rural and urban areas respectively.
11. We benefited a great deal from the comments of Jean Dreze on this section.
12. It has been argued that the use of Laspeyres indices in the expert group methodology typically exaggerated the impact of inflation and failed to notice the substantial reduction in rural poverty. The difference that a change in methodology can cause to the estimates was demonstrated by Deaton and Tarozzi who arrived at alternative estimates of rural and urban poverty by using the same NSSO data but adopted Tornqvist indices rather than Laspeyre's indices for computation. For details that this makes to the estimated reduction in poverty, see Deaton and Tarozzi, (1999).
13. The situation is not very different even if the literacy rate in 2001 is considered. The literacy rate for that year in Andhra Pradesh was 61.11 per cent as compared to 64.09 per cent in Madhya Pradesh, indicating the slow progress of literacy in the state (Registrar General of India, 2001).
14. It has been pointed out that the per capita income levels of Kerala have been underestimated. If account is taken of the remittances from abroad, the state's average per capita income is estimated to be higher by atleast 15 to 30 per cent (Krishnan, 1994).
15. We ignore in the present analysis the presence of middle class households.
16. This is not expected to make much difference to the analysis as earlier studies have shown that, on an average, the extent of migration is limited in extent, a reason that has prompted several researchers to use unadjusted sex ratios in the analysis (Agarwal, 1997).

REFERENCES

Adelman, I., and Cynthia T. Morris, 1967, *Society, Politics and Economic Development: A Quantitative Approach*, Maryland, The John Hopkins Press, USA.

Agarwal, W., 1997. 'Small Schools: Issues in Policy and Planning', Occasional Paper 23, New Delhi National Institute of Educational Planning and Administration, NIEPA, New Delhi.

Buchanan, N., and H.S. Ellis, 1955, *Approaches to Economic Development*, New York, Twentieth Century Fund.

Central Statistical Organisation (CSO), 1998, *Statistical Abstract of India*, New Delhi, Government of India.

Dandekar, V. M. and N. Rath, 1971, *Poverty in India*, Indian School of Political Economy, Pune.

Dasgupta, P., 1993, *An Inquiry into Well-Being and Destitution*, Oxford, Clarendon Press.

Deaton, A. & A. Tarozzi, 1999, *Prices and Poverty in India*, Princeton University, Research Programme in Development Studies, *http//www.deaton@princeton.edu/*.

Haq, Mahbub ul, 1997, *Human Development in South Asia*, Oxford, Oxford University Press.

Hirway, Indira and Darshini Mahadevia, 1996, 'Critique of Gender Development Index', *Economic and Political Weekly*, XXXI (43): WS 87–96, 26 October.

Hinchlifffe, K., 1985, 'Employment and Education', in Torsten Husen and T.N. Postlethwaite, *The International Encyclopaedia of Education: Research and Studies*, Oxford, Pergamon Press.

International Institute for Population Sciences (IIPS), 2000. 'National Family Health Survey (NFHS) 1998–99', October, Mumbai, India.

Jeffrey, Robin, 1992, *Politics, Women and Well-Being: How Kerala Became a Model*, Basingstoke and London, Macmillan.

Krishnaji, N., 1997, 'Human Poverty Index: A Critique', *Economic and Political Weekly*, 32 (35): 2206–5.

Krishnan, T.N., 1994, 'Foreign Remittance, Consumption and Income', A.K.G. Centre for Research and Studies, as cited in Ramachandran, V.K. 'On Kerala's Development Achievements', in Jean Dreze and Amartya Sen, 1998, *Indian Development: Selected Regional Perspectives*, Delhi, Oxford University Press, pp.: 205–356.

Morris, M.D., 1979, *Measuring the Condition of the World's Poor: The Physical Quality of Life Index*, New Delhi, Promilla and Co. Publishers.

National Council for Applied Economic Research, (NCAER), 1992, *Household Survey of Medical Care*, New Delhi, NCAER.

Planning Commission, 1993, *Report of the Expert Group on Estimation of Proportion and Number of Poor*, New Delhi, Planning Commission.

Ramachandran, V.K., 1998, 'On Kerala's Development Achievements', in Jean Dreze and Amartya Sen, *Indian Development: Selected Regional Perspectives*, Delhi, Oxford University Press, pp.: 205–356.

Ravallion, Martin and Gaurav Datt, 1996, 'India's Checkered History in Fight against Poverty: Are There Lessons for the Future?' *Economic and Political Weekly*, XXXI (35,36 & 37): 2479–85, Special Number, September.

Registrar General of India, 2001. *Provisional Population Totals* Census of India, Series 1, Paper of 2001. *http://www.censusindia.net/results/webed.html.*

Suryanarayana, M.H., 2000, 'How Real is the Secular Decline in Rural Poverty?' *Economic and Political Weekly*, June, 17, 35(25):2129–40.

Tendulkar, S.D. and L.R. Jain, 1993, *Poverty in India 1970–71 to 1988–89* ARTEP Working Papers, New Delhi, International Labour Organisation.

United Nations Development Programme (UNDP), 1996, 1997, *Human Development Report*, Oxford University Press, New York.

part two

Nutrition

chapter 5

Foodgrain Production, Prices and Rural Poverty in India

• *B.L. Mungekar*

1. INTRODUCTION

It is indeed distressing to observe that the fiftieth anniversary of India's Independence should coincide with nearly one-third of its population remaining below the poverty line. In a way, it is also an indictment on India's strategy of planned economic development over four and a half decades. During this period, the emphasis of economic policy changed from time to time. Political considerations not only intermingled with but also influenced economic programmes. For instance, the slogan of 'Garibi Hatao' raised by Indira Gandhi, the then Prime Minister of India, during the fifth general election to the Lok Sabha was more political than economic in content. But it was in the early 1980s, that it clearly dawned on both the political leadership as well as economic planners that the mainstream growth process inherent in economic planning was by itself inadequate to tackle the problem of poverty. Therefore, specially designed 'Poverty Alleviation Programmes' (PAPs) were needed to meet the challenge of poverty.

The abundant literature on poverty in India had two main features. First, the literature almost entirely dealt with rural poverty. Second, it remained preoccupied with the problems of measurement of poverty

The author is grateful to Tirtharaj Samant and Ravindra Tambe for prompt and sincere computer assistance in the preparation of this paper.

mainly with calorie norms and deflators (Ahluwalia, 1978; Bardhan, 1970 and 1973; Dandekar and Rath, 1971; Minhas, 1970; Ojha, 1970; Rajaraman, 1975; and Vaidyanathan, 1974). In view of the necessity of framing an appropriate poverty alleviation policy that also had financial implications, the importance of correct quantification of poverty can hardly be underestimated. But in the process, to one's dismay, the other equally, if not more important question 'Why Poverty?' remained sidelined. Thus, as against the late 1960s and the entire 1970s when measurement of poverty dominated the debate on poverty in India, the 1980s and the 1990s came to witness an attempt to identify the factors causing poverty (Ahluwalia, 1986; Kakwani and Subbarao, 1990; Mellor, 1986; Ravallion and Datt, 1996; Abhijit Sen, 1996; and Amartya Sen, 1986). This shift in focus was indeed gratifying.

There are a number of factors that can, *a priori*, explain the existence of poverty, particularly rural poverty, understood in the sense of 'lack of assets' or income or food (i.e. calorie intake) or any other relevant unit chosen for the measurement of poverty. Such factors, among others, may include low rate of overall economic growth and unequal distribution of its gains; inequality in the ownership of land and other related productive assets; low levels of agricultural productivity and production; low or non-availability of irrigation; low levels of farm and non-farm employment; inflation, particularly high levels of absolute and relative food prices; low levels of real agricultural wages, and so on. These are by and large economic variables. There are socio-cultural factors such as caste and gender discrimination, which have a large bearing on economic variables directly determining poverty. In fact, not only do they influence the determinants of poverty at a point of time, but also form a vicious circle of poverty and thus, serve as a mechanism for the inter-generational transmission of poverty.

This paper seeks to examine the relationship between foodgrain production, prices and rural poverty in India during the period 1971–2 to 1991–2. Some studies have preceded this attempt, and almost all of them have provided new insights into the determinants of rural poverty in India. The aim here, therefore, is to ascertain some of the findings of these earlier studies and simultaneously try to make a few new observations, which have some policy implications.

The next section outlines the main trends in foodgrains production in India while Section 3 sets out the analytical frame. This is followed by an analysis of the results of econometric exercises conducted (Section 4) and the impact of economic reforms on rural poverty (Section 5). The last section discusses the conclusions emerging from the study.

At the outset, it would be appropriate to provide the socio-economic profile of rural poverty in India. The information given in Table 1 clearly shows that poverty is much more extensive among agricultural as well as other labourers, scheduled castes and scheduled tribes, and female-headed households in rural areas (while the same is true in the urban areas except 'other' labourers.) It needs to be further emphasised that the proportion of poor among the scheduled castes and the scheduled tribes, as also among agricultural labourers, is much higher than their respective share in the total population both in rural and urban areas.

TABLE 1. PROFILE OF RURAL POVERTY IN INDIA (HEAD-COUNT RATIO) 1987–88

Groups	*Rural*		
	Population share	*Per cent Poor*	*Per cent of Total Poor*
Self-emp in Agri.	44.3	38.3	37.9
Self-emp in non-Agri.	12.5	39.0	10.8
All self-emp.	56.7	38.5	48.7
Agri. Labour	27.1	62.7	41.8
Other Labour	8.1	48.7	9.2
Others	7.9	26.4	4.5
Scheduled Castes	18.4	56.1	22.9
Scheduled Tribes	10.5	62.7	14.7
All households	100.0	44.9	100.0

Source: B. Ozler, G. Datt and M. Ravallion (1996).

The next section examines the trends in foodgrain production in India in the post-Independence period.

2. TRENDS IN FOODGRAIN PRODUCTION

Notwithstanding the reservations that have been expressed about the desirability of the green revolution in India, it seems to be an indisputable fact that it broke the 'low productivity syndrome' that had characterised Indian agriculture till the mid-1960s (Blyn, 1966). Table 2 explains this.

As is evident from the Table, during the period from 1949–50 to 1964–5 i.e., the pre-green revolution period, total foodgrain production in the country increased at the annual rate of growth of 2.82 per cent. The main feature of this increase was that it was secured through an expansion of area under cultivation which grew at the rate of

TABLE 2. ALL INDIA COMPOUND GROWTH RATES OF AREA, PRODUCTION AND YIELD OF FOODGRAINS, 1949–50 TO 1994–95

Crop	*1949–50 to 1963–64*			*1967–68 to 1993–94*		
	A	P	Y	A	P	Y
Rice	1.21	3.50	2.25	0.56	2.87	2.30
Wheat	2.69	3.98	1.27	1.62	4.81	3.14
Jowar	0.99	2.51	1.49	-1.05	0.98	2.06
Bajra	1.08	2.34	1.24	-0.85	0.61	1.47
Maize	2.67	3.88	1.18	-0.03	1.60	1.63
Coarse Cereals	0.90	2.25	1.23	-1.19	0.66	1.76
Total Cereals	1.25	3.21	1.77	0.06	2.91	2.40
Total Pulses	1.72	1.41	-0.18	0.21	0.88	0.69
Foodgrains	1.35	2.82	1.36	0.09	2.63	2.16

Note: A-Area, P-Production, and Y-Yield.
Source: Government of India (1996).

1.35 per cent annum, increase in productivity (yield per hectare) being 1.36 per cent per annum. The green revolution changed this scenario. Thus, during the post-green revolution period from 1967–8 to 1994–5, an 2.63 per cent increase in foodgrains production was brought about through nearly twice the increase in foodgrains productivity, as the increase in the area under cultivation remained virtually stagnant. The magnitude of increase of 3.14 per cent in wheat productivity in the latter period was stupendous as compared to 1.27 per cent growth in the earlier period. It is gratifying to observe that, of late, even coarse cereals like *jowar*, *bajra* and maize have witnessed an increase in productivity. Production of pulses, the main source of protein for the poor, has been a cause for concern in the country. But on that front too, one notices an 0.90 per cent increase in the latter period compared to an annual fall of 0.18 in their production in the earlier period. Thus, of late, the green revolution has spread to new food crops as also to hitherto bypassed regions, which may be a consoling feature of India's pattern of growth in foodgrains production (Bhalla and Singh, 1997; Sawant and Achyuthan, 1995; Thamarajakshi, 1997).

Among other things, the green revolution-induced increase in foodgrains, particularly cereal production, relieved the country of the need to import foodgrains. Thus, as against the excessive reliance of the country's public distribution system (PDS) on foodgrains import during the late 1950s and the whole of the 1960s, the PDS, in the post-green revolution period, has come to be sustained almost entirely by the increase in domestic foodgrains production. Regretfully, this exemption from foodgrains import was erroneously considered by academicians and policy-makers as constituting self-sufficiency in foodgrains production.

3. ANALYTICAL FRAMEWORK AND DATABASE

It is against this background that we turn to examine the relationship between foodgrains production, prices and rural poverty in India. We have attempted to do this through an econometric specification. The explanatory variables and their *a priori* relationship with rural poverty are as follows:

(a) Rural Poverty (RPOV)

The dependent variable was the head-count ratio for RPOV for the period from 1971–2 to 1991–2. Since estimates of head-count ratio were not available for each of the years covered in the period, these were obtained through interpolation wherever necessary.

(b) Per Capita Availability of Foodgrains (PCNAFD)

Per Capita Availability of Foodgrains (Kg per person per year) was used as a proxy for foodgrains production, because along with changes in foodgrains production, it also accounts for the increase in population and changes in net import. Since our study covered the post-green revolution period, PCNAFD very closely approximates the domestic production scenario. Thus, PCNAFD is expected to have a negative impact on RPOV through a negative effect on foodgrain prices and a positive effect on real agricultural wages.

(c) Irrigation (IRGN)

Irrigation has been one of the major ingredients that brought the green revolution to Indian agriculture. It made possible the use of productivity-raising improved varieties of seeds, chemical fertilizers, and pesticides. It also increased cropping intensity. In the process, it helped generate more employment, particularly in the irrigated tracts of the country.

Thus, increase in the extent of irrigation would represent increase in foodgrains productivity and production, and fall in foodgrain prices, as also increase in the volume of agricultural employment. We therefore postulate IRGN to have a negative impact on RPOV.

(d) Real Agricultural Wages (RAWGS)

Real Agricultural Wages are assumed to depress RPOV. This is because, as evident from Table 1, the extent of poverty among agricultural labourers is very high and therefore, in the Indian context, they are rightly described as the poorest among the poor. Second, the main source of calories for the poor is foodgrains, with some change in their consumption pattern being evident only in recent times. Third, increase in RAWGS suggests an improvement in the purchasing power of agricultural labourers and the rural poor in general. It is for this reason that relative prices of foodgrains were not considered as an explanatory variable in the model. Thus, in the limited context of rural poverty, changes in RAWGS can be used in place of relative food prices with only one difference; relative food prices are expected to be positively related to rural poverty while real agricultural wages tend to be inversely related.

(e) Procurement of Foodgrain as Percentage of Net Availability (PROFD)

One would expect the PDS to be one of the variables having a negative impact on RPOV. There are however a number of studies pointing out that the scope of the PDS in rural areas is limited and that its overall functioning has been far from satisfactory (Mahendra Dev, 1996 and Mahendra Dev and Suryanarayana, 1991). Again, the non-poor seem to draw substantial benefits from the PDS, which is against the intentions of the scheme (Sawant, 1995). We have therefore used PROFD as one of the explanatory variables, which presumably has a negative impact on RPOV. The rationale for this argument is as follows:

The increase in PROFD indicates both the intention and the capacity of the government to intervene in the foodgrains market with the objective of ensuring a steady supply of foodgrains and maintaining the stability of their prices. In other words, an increase in PROFD is expected to check the capacity of private trade to charge unduly high prices for foodgrains and ultimately to have a negative impact on RPOV.

Thus, the multivariate model that seeks to explain the behaviour of rural poverty in India is as follows:

RPOV= f (PCNAFD, IRGN, RAWGS, PROFD)

The results of the empirical estimation of the model are presented in Table 3.

TABLE 3. ALL INDIA RURAL POVERTY EQUATION (DEPENDENT VARIABLE. HEAD-COUNT RATIO)

Variable	*Coefficient*	*t statistics*
CONSTANT	109.70	31.72
PCNAFD	-0.06	-3.04
IRGN	-0.54	-12.06
RWGD	-0.89	-2.75
PROCPN	-0.22	-2.18

Notes: No. of observations = 20.
R Square = 0.99.
D.W. Statistics = 2.03.
F Statistics = 386.96.

The results in Table 3 show that the specification of our model is satisfactory. As postulated, regression coefficients of all explanatory variables bear the expected i.e., negative signs and satisfactory t values. D.W.statistics point to the absence of autocorrelation. Lastly, the model explains 99 per cent of the variation in India's rural poverty.

4. ANALYSIS OF RESULTS

We now attempt to offer an explanation regarding the determinants of rural poverty in India over two decades from 1971–2 to 1991–2. The following observations are in order:

(a) It is quite obvious that real agricultural wages emerged as the most potent factor explaining the decline in rural poverty. But before we deliberate on the issue, let us briefly examine the available literature that provides the background for explaining this relationship.

Amartya Sen (1981) in his seminal contribution brought to the centre-stage the role of prices as a crucial determinant of entitlement of the poor to food. Dharm Narain used food prices as the most important variable explaining rural poverty. In his model, he used the consumer price index for agricultural labourers and the index of wholesale foodgrains prices as variables (Amartya Sen, 1986) to explain rural poverty. He found that rural poverty was inversely related to agricultural labourers' output per head of rural population and positively to the level of foodgrains prices. Thus, Dharm Narain's model was a pioneering attempt in establishing a causal relationship between rural poverty on the one hand, and foodgrains output and prices on the other.

Dharm Narain's poverty equation was however criticised on the grounds that it included absolute or nominal prices of foodgrains, which made his specification incorrect (Ahluwalia, 1986). This point is worth considering (Amartya Sen 1986). 'But Dharm Narain's genius lay in developing a simple but insightful equation to drive home his point.' (Desai, 1986). He was trying to capture 'some important aspects of a complex reality (i.e. rural poverty) in a simple and elegant way' (Amartya Sen, 1986). Thus, the novelty of Dharm Narain's analysis was his emphasis on price change in explaining the variations in rural poverty (Amartya Sen, 1986).

Instead of real foodgrain prices, we used real agricultural wages in our rural poverty equation for the reasons explained earlier. Considerable research has gone into examining the variations in All-India and state-wide real agricultural wages in India. These studies covered different time periods, used different sources of data and adopted different methodologies. Obviously, they came to different and sometimes conflicting conclusions. And yet, there was a broad conclusion, viz. till 1980–1, with annual fluctuations, real agricultural wages in India, by and large, remained stagnant (Mungekar, 1992). As against this, notwithstanding fluctuations, since the early 1980s they have shown a consistent increase (Acharya, 1989 and Jose, 1988). Thus, during the decade 1981–91, real agricultural wages at the All-India level increased at an annual trend rate of growth of 4.91 per cent, as against a meagre 0.33 per cent during the preceding decade.

Had nominal foodgrain prices in the country not increased as they did, mainly in response to the demand of surplus farmers for continuously higher support or procurement prices which pushed market foodgrain prices upwards (Raj Krishna and Roychaudhuri, 1980; Mitra, 1978; and Mungekar, 1992); had the various state governments been somewhat serious in rigorously implementing the Minimum Wages Act and periodically revised agricultural wages as the Act stipulated; and had the agricultural labourers themselves been more organised, real agricultural wages would have been still higher and would have caused a more pronounced negative impact on rural poverty.

(b) Irrigation emerged as the next important factor having a negative impact on rural poverty. This seems logical. As mentioned earlier, irrigation was one of the major factors that helped bring about the green revolution in Indian agriculture. Thus, as against 305.9 million hectares irrigated area under food crops in 1970–1, it increased to 416 million hectares in 1986–7 i.e., at the rate of 1.9 per cent annum. During the same period, the extent of irrigation under rice increased from 149.2 to 178 million hectares, the increase being 1.1 per cent per annum. In the case of wheat, there was a quantum jump in the use of irrigation from 98.3 to 178.8 million hectares making 77.3 per cent of the area under its cultivation irrigated with an annual increase of 3.8 per cent. Again, during the same period, irrigated area under non-foodgrains increased from 79.6 to 140.4 million hectares, registering an increase of 3.6 per cent per annum.

This overall increase in the use of irrigation increased the cropping intensity of Indian agriculture. The same was true of the cropping pattern whose index increased from 96.3 to 105.4 during the period under consideration. Such a rise in cropping intensity leads to an increased demand for labour by increasing the number of agricultural operations (Mellor, 1986). Irrigation ought to have a price-depressing or at least price-stabilising effect through the increase in productivity and production of foodgrains. All these linkages of irrigation seemed to have a negative effect on rural poverty.

(c) In our equation, procurement of foodgrains (mainly that of rice and wheat) had a negative effect on poverty. This may be explained as follows:

In the post-green revolution period, the volume of procurement of foodgrains increased considerably. Not only did it almost entirely sustain the country's PDS, but since the mid-1980s, it even exceeded the quantity of grains distributed through the PDS. For instance, procurement increased from 0.5 million tonnes in 1961 to 8.9 million tonnes in 1971, and further to 19.6 million tonnes in 1991. (It reached 28 and 26 million tonnes respectively in 1993 and 1994). In 1971 it was 9.43 per cent of the national net availability, which increased to 12.35 per cent in 1991. Again, in some of the years during this period, the quantity distributed through the PDS was less than the quantity procured and as a result, the government came to possess sizeable stocks of foodgrains. Thus, as continuously rising support or procurement prices had a positive effect on market prices of foodgrains (Mitra,1978; and Mungekar, 1992), so also did the ever-increasing quantity of procurement seem to have checked the capacity of private trade to raise prices further, due to the fear of potential unloading of stocks of foodgrains through the PDS.

(d) Foodgrain production, represented by per capita net availability, had a negative impact on rural poverty, but among all the four variables, its effect was minimal. Two main explanations are in order.

First, the highly unequal distribution of land, the major source of foodgrains (agricultural) production and other productive assets in the rural areas does not make growth in foodgrains (agricultural) production directly relevant to the poor. Not only are agricultural labourers and rural artisans purchasers of foodgrains, but almost all marginal farmers and the majority of small and even medium farmers in the dry and semi-arid regions are net purchasers of foodgrains. Second, and what follows from the first, the vast body of the rural poor therefore depends upon (a) the volume of farm as well as non-farm employment, and (b) the level of real wage (and any other) income.

Thus, the inegalitarian agrarian structure accompanied by all kinds of social and cultural inequalities, seems to reduce the efficacy of growth in foodgrains production in making a meaningful impact on rural poverty.

5. CONTEXT OF ECONOMIC REFORMS

From the point of view of the present theme, a brief mention has to be made of two policy changes relating to reforms in agriculture that have a crucial bearing on food security and poverty in India. These are attempts to equalise domestic agricultural prices to world prices, and provide a thrust to agricultural exports including foodgrains. Let us quickly elaborate these points.

(a) Equalising Domestic Agricultural Prices to World Prices

An argument is sought to be made, particularly after the country has initiated wide-ranging economic reforms based on globalisation, liberalisation, and privatisation since mid-1991, that equalising domestic agricultural prices with world prices through trade will integrate Indian agriculture into the world economy, This measure is expected to raise the level of domestic prices from their present levels; provide incentives to producers; step-up investment in the agricultural sector, and ultimately raise overall growth in that sector.

Due to the peculiar characteristics of agricultural production, agricultural output, unlike industry, is unaffected by demand and prices in the short-run (Patnaik, 1996). On the other hand, so far as foodgrains are concerned, any rise in their prices is certain to harm the poor. The implications of such a measure for poverty are clear for all to see.

(b) Export of Agricultural Products

Being enthusiastic about their role as one of the engines of economic growth, the post-liberalisation period has come to witness a more rigorous thrust on exports, including agricultural exports. So far as exports of foodgrains are concerned, one can hardly question the export of superior quality of rice such as *basmati*. But the same cannot be said about the export of other foodgrains such as ordinary quality rice and wheat. Their export, however, seems to be defended on grounds of the so-called self-sufficiency argument; and also on the grounds that in the days of deficiency, the country may import the necessary amount of foodgrains (Tyagi, 1990). As far as self-sufficiency is concerned, with respect to foodgrains, we have argued above that it is not genuine, but the sheer result of lack of purchasing power with the poor. If that is not the case, the explanation for the large stocks of unsold foodgrains is rather awkward, viz. India's poor have improved their dietary level to such an extent that they do not require any more foodgrains. In reality, this is far from true. Second, export of ordinary quality rice and wheat will reduce their domestic availability proportionately and consequently raise their prices, again harming the interests of the poor.

In this context, it is also pertinent to observe that after liberalisation of trade, both agricultural growth and cropping patterns have undergone considerable changes. For instance, during the five years after liberalisation, i.e., 1991–2 to 1995–6, the average annual growth rate in the production of rice, wheat, coarse cereals, pulses, and all foodgrains was 1.94, 1.52, 0.27, 0.90, and 1.27 per cent, respectively. On the other hand, oilseeds production increased by 4.93 per cent per annum (Utsa Patnaik, 1996 and 1997). Again, during 1990–1 to 1995–6, area under cereals, wheat, and coarse pulses declined annually by 3.5 per cent, 13.2 per cent, and 3.24 per cent respectively. On the other hand, area under oilseeds grew at the annual rate of 9.1 per cent. This growing commercialisation of India's agriculture, among other things, may affect the level of foodgrain production, particularly in view of the relatively slow pace of seed technology advances (Sawant, 1997), harm the country's food security and ultimately adversely affect the poor.

6. CONCLUSION

It is now time to recapitulate the main findings of this paper. They are mainly three.

(a) In a country like India where land, the most important source of livelihood in rural areas, and other productive assets are highly unequally distributed, the efficacy of an increase in foodgrains production in making a meaningful dent on rural poverty is seriously impaired. This is further thwarted by a sustained increase in prices of foodgrains, prompted among other factors, by the pressure exerted by surplus farmers to get continuously higher support or procurement prices. The entire arrangement of the PDS, particularly in rural areas, is far from satisfactory. In other words, the rural poor suffer from the lack of adequate access to both production of foodgrains and their distribution; the first due to unequal rural property relations, and the second due to defective arrangements for distribution.

(b) A sustained increase in real agricultural wages and expansion of irrigation facilities seem to be more significant factors for reducing rural poverty in India.

(c) Any attempt on the part of the country to equalise the domestic prices of foodgrains with world prices and to export foodgrains of ordinary quality in response to the process of globalisation may seriously jeopardise the already fragile state of food security in the country.

REFERENCES

Acharya, S., 1989. 'Agricultural Wages in India: A Disaggregated Analysis,' *Indian Journal of Agricultural Economics*, XLIV (2): 121–39.

Ahluwalia, M.S., 1978. 'Rural Poverty in India: 1956–7 to 1973–4', Occasional Papers, World Bank Staff Working Paper, Washington D.C.

______, 1986. 'Rural Poverty, Agricultural Production, and Prices. A Re-examination', in Mellor and Desai (eds.), *Agricultural Change and Rural Poverty*, Oxford University Press, New Delhi.

Bardhan, Pranab, 1970. 'On the Minimum Level of Living and The Rural Poor', *Indian Economic Review*, VI (1): 78–87.

______, 1973. 'On The Incidence of Poverty in Rural India in the Sixties,' *Economic and Political Weekly*, 8(4–6): 245–54.

Bhalla, G.S. and G. Singh, 1997. 'Recent Developments in Indian Agriculture: A State Level Analysis,' *Economic and Political Weekly*, 32(13): A2–A18.

Blyn, George, 1966. *Agricultural Trends in India 1891–1947: Output, Availability and Productivity*, University of Pennsylvania Press, Philadelphia.

Centre for Monitoring Indian Economy, 1994. *World Economy and India's Place In It*, Mumbai, October.

Dandekar, V.M. and N. Rath, 1971. *Poverty in India*, Indian School of Political Economy, Pune.

Dantwala, M.L., 1967. 'Incentives and Disincentives in Indian Agriculture,' *Indian Journal of Agricultural Economics*, 22(2): 1–25.

______, 1983. 'Prices: Not Quite a Magic Wand,' *Economic and Political Weekly*, 18(26): A46–A47.

Desai, Gunwant M., 1986. 'Trends in Rural Poverty: An Interpretation of Dharm Narayan', in Mellor and Desai (eds.), *Agricultural Change and Rural Poverty*, Oxford University Press, New Delhi.

Dholakia, Bakul H., 1997. 'Impact of Liberalisation on The Growth of Indian Agricultural,' in B.M. Desai (ed.), *Agricultural Development Paradigm for the Ninth Plan Under New Economic environment*, Oxford & IBH Publishing Co. Pvt. Ltd., New Delhi.

Government of India, 1996. *Estimates of Area, Production and Yield of Principal Crops in India, 1993–4 to 1994–5*, Ministry of Agriculture, Directorate of Economics and Statistics, New Delhi.

Jose, A.V., 1988. 'Agricultural Wages in India,' *Economic and Political Weekly*, 23(26): A46–A58.

Kakwani, N. and K. Subbarao, 1990. 'Rural Poverty and Its Alleviation in India,' *Economic and Political Weekly*, 25(13): A2–A16.

Minhas, B.S. 1970. 'Rural Poverty, Land Distribution and Development Strategy: Facts and Policy', *Indian Economic Review*, V (16): 97–128.

Mahendra Dev S., 1988. 'Poverty of Agricultural Labour Households in India: A State Level Analysis,' *Indian Journal of Agricultural Economics*, 31(1): 14–25.

______, 1996. 'Food Security: PDS vs EGS, A Tale of Two States,' *Economic and Political Weekly*, 31(27): 1752–64.

______, and M.H. Suryanarayana, 1991. 'Is PDS Urban-Biased and Pro-Rich? An Evaluation,' *Economic and Political Weekly*, 26(41): 2357–66.

Mellor, John W., 1986. 'Departments of Rural Poverty: The Dynamics of Production, Technology and Price', in Mellor and Desai (eds.), *Agricultural Change and Rural Poverty*, Oxford University Press, New Delhi.

Mitra, Ashok, 1977. 'Terms of Trade and Class Relations,' Frank Cass, London.

Mungekar, B.L., 1992. *'The Political Economy of Terms of Trade,'* Himalaya Publishing House, Mumbai.

Ojha, P.D., 1970. 'A Configuration of Indian Poverty: Inequality and Levels of Living,' *Reserve Bank of India Bulletin*, 24(1):16–27.

Olson, R.O. 1960. 'Impact and Implications of Foreign Surplus Disposal on Under Developed Economies', *Journal of Farm Economics*, 42(5): 1042–5.

B. Ozler, G. Datt and M. Ravallion. 1996. 'Database on Poverty and Growth in India', The World Bank, cited in Abhijit Sen,' Economic Reforms, Employment And Poverty', *Economic and Political Weekly*, 31(35–7): 2479–85.

Patnaik, Prabhat, 1996. 'Should Domestic Prices Be Equated to World Prices?' *Economic and Political Weekly*, 31(35–7): 2425–8, Special Number.

Patnaik, Utsa, 1996. 'Export-Oriented Agriculture and Food Security in India', *Economic and Political Weekly*, 31(35–7): 2429–50, Special Number.

———, 1997. 'Political Economy of State Intervention in Food Economy,' *Economic and Political Weekly*, Special Number.

Raj Krishna and G.S. Raychaudhuri, 1980. *'Some Aspects of Rice and Wheat Price Policy in India'*, World Bank Staff Working Paper No. 381, Washington D.C.

Rajaraman, Indira, 1975. 'Poverty, Inequality and Economic Growth in Punjab. 1960–1 To 1970–1', the *Journal of Development Studies*, 1(4):278–90.

Ravallion, M. and G. Datta, 1996. 'India's Checkered History in Fight Against Poverty: Are There Lessons For The Future?' *Economic and Political Weekly*, 31(35–37): 2479–85, Special Number.

Sen, Abhijit, 1996. 'Economic Reforms, Employment and Poverty: Trends and Options', *Economic and Political Weekly*, 31(35–37): 2459–78, Special Number.

Sen, Amartya, 1981. *'Poverty and Famines: An Essay on Environment and Deprivation'*, Clarendon Press, Oxford.

———, 1986. 'Dharm Narain on Poverty: Concepts and Broader Issues', in Mellor and Desai (eds.), *Agricultural Change and Rural Poverty*, Oxford University Press, New Delhi.

Sawant, S.D., 1995. 'Public Distribution System in India: Why to Revamp It?' in K.R. Gupta (ed.), *Issues in Indian Economy*, Atlantic Publishers and Distributors, New Delhi.

———, 1997. 'Foodgrains Output Growth in India. Emerging Trends and Perspectives for Technology Development Policies', in B.M. Desai (ed.), *Agricultural Development Paradigm for Ninth Plan under New Economic Environment*, Oxford & IBH Publishing Co., New Delhi.

——— and C.V. Achyuthan, 1995. 'Agricultural Growth Across Crops and Regions: Emerging Trends and Patterns,' *Economic and Political Weekly*, 30(12): A2–A13.

Srinivasan, T.N., 1986. 'Agricultural Production Prices, Entitlements and Poverty', in Mellor and Desai (eds.), *Agricultural Change and Rural Poverty*, Oxford University Press, New Delhi.

Thamarajakshi, R., 1997. 'Economic Reforms and State Intervention In Foodgrain Market', *Economic and Political Weekly*, Vol. 32, No. 30, p. 1894–900.

Tyagi, D.S., 1990. 'Managing India's Food Economy: Problems and Alternatives', Sage Publications, New Delhi.

Vaidyanathan, A., 1974. 'Some Aspects of Inequalities in Living Standards in Rural India', in T.N. Srinivasan and P.K. Bardhan (eds.), *Poverty and Income Distribution in India*, Statistical Publishing Society, Calcutta.

chapter 6

Targeting Food Subsidies

• *Shikha Jha and P.V. Srinivasan*

1. INTRODUCTION

Riddled with problems such as low income support, ineffective targeting of subsidies to the poor and substantial leakage from the Public Distribution System (PDS), the Indian government initiated a new scheme in June 1997 called Targeted PDS (TPDS), to directly target the subsidy to the poor. How well is this scheme likely to work? What are the problems associated with targeting? Does a re-evaluation of the existing PDS show any positive signs of a pick-up? Can it be revived and improved to do away with the need for a finely targeted programme? These are some of the questions addressed by this paper. We evaluate the PDS in terms of its successes and failures, focusing especially on recent years (after the mid-1990s) to obtain insights and provide an agenda for change. The paper comments on the recently revamped and targeted food subsidy programmes and their efficacy. It also discusses the feasibility and appropriateness of moving away from universal provision to direct targeting, keeping in view the past record of administrative efficiency of states while drawing lessons from the experiences of other countries.

2. THE BACKGROUND

Foodgrains constitute one of the most important items distributed under the PDS. Under this system, which runs parallel to a free market, any individual with a registered residential address is eligible to get a 'ration card'. Each ration card holder is entitled to a buy a fixed quota of grains supplied through 'fair price' shops (FPSs) at subsidised 'ration' or 'issue' prices. The system at present has a countrywide network of about .45 million FPSs in rural and urban areas (GOI, 1999).[1] The central government makes PDS allocations to state governments at Central Issue Prices (CIP). The state governments then fix the 'retail end' prices after adding transportation cost and dealers' commission and subtracting state subsidy, if any. As a result, the state level issue price can be higher or lower than the CIP. The PDS prices in some states such as Arunachal Pradesh, Karnataka (for the 'tri-colour' cards), Mizoram and Tamil Nadu (for rice) are lower than the CIP. On the other hand, Maharashtra and Gujarat top the list in terms of charging the highest ration prices to their consumers.

The supplies for the PDS are purchased from producers who supply a part ('levy') of their marketable surplus at pre-announced 'procurement' prices (often lower than the prevailing market prices) to public procurement agencies. Procurement prices are based on support prices announced by the Department of Agriculture and Co-operation and are meant to provide, during good crop years, remunerative prices to farmers as an incentive to increase production. The Food Corporation of India (FCI) and state agencies carry out procurement operations in consultation with state governments. In addition to procurement, the central government imports grain when necessary to fulfil its requirements. The FCI also maintains a buffer stock of grains and handles other aspects of the system such as distribution, imports and exports on behalf of the central government. These stocks are meant to satisfy the minimum requirement for food security, act as operational stocks for monthly releases for PDS supply and meet the requirement for release in the open market for price stabilisation. The expenses of the FCI, net of its sales realisation, are reimbursed to it by the central government in the form of what is usually referred to as 'food subsidy'.

3. EVALUATING THE PERFORMANCE OF PDS

The performance of PDS in India can be judged on three broad counts, viz., its effectiveness in providing food security to the poor given the universal nature of the programme, the level of effective protection in general to consumers and producers, and the costs of operation. As we shall see, most of the available studies on PDS are based on NSS (National Sample Survey) data for 1986–7. The findings, therefore, cannot be generalised to very recent years. In particular, we find some improvement in the functioning of the existing PDS from the mid-1990s.

Recent literature shows that the leakage in the system is substantial and the subsidies are not effectively targeted to the poor. Approximately 35–40 per cent of rice and wheat meant for distribution through the FPSs does not reach consumers while the poor receive less than their fair share of the amount distributed (Table 1). There are some exceptions such as Kerala and Andhra Pradesh where the poor have better access to the PDS. On an average, it costs the central government Rs 4.27 to transfer one rupee to the poor (Radhakrishna *et al.*, 1997).

TABLE 1. LEAKAGE FROM AND SHARE OF POOR IN PDS QUANTITIES

(per cent)

State/ UT	*Leakage as a proportion of PDS Distribution*		*Overall Targeting Effectiveness*
	Rice	*Wheat*	
Andhra Pradesh	25.70	40.30	20.20
Assam	68.50	97.60	5.90
Bihar	73.80	83.30	9.60
Gujarat	43.70	52.50	14.00
Haryana	44.40	100.00	1.10
Himachal Pradesh	—	—	22.00
Jammu & Kashmir	—	53.40	21.80
Karnataka	31.00	44.00	13.20
Kerala	26.90	—	19.20
Madhya Pradesh	45.90	—	11.60
Maharashtra	40.60	36.40	12.60
Orissa	88.00	77.60	0.80
Punjab	—	80.60	1.60
Rajasthan	—	32.20	17.50
Tamil Nadu	49.50	7.50	12.30
Uttar Pradesh	18.10	—	7.90
West Bengal	36.60	36.60	13.10
All India	36.90	37.80	NA

Notes: 1. These numbers are based on a consumer expenditure survey carried out by the National Sample Survey Organisation (NSSO) for the year 1986–7.
2. Leakage is defined as quantity distributed minus quantity actually purchased.
3. Targeting effectiveness is the ratio of amount reaching the bottom 20 per cent of households to total amount supplied to PDS.

Sources: Ahluwalia (1993) and Parikh (1994).

The system appears to have failed to transfer grains from surplus to deficit states (such as Bihar, Orissa and Madhya Pradesh) which have a high incidence of hunger and poverty. This has resulted in a stagnant or declining trend in cereal and calorie intake (Radhakrishna and Rao, 1994). There has not been any marked improvement in the per capita availability of cereals since the 1980s. Using more recent data for 1995 based on selected village studies in four states, Radhakrishna (1996) finds that inter-regional biases in distribution of PDS supplies persist and that the efficacy of PDS distribution in backward states is poor. Even after fifty years of independence, per capita consumption of the poorest sections of population remains far below recommended nutritional levels (Sarma, 1988; World Bank, 1986 and World Bank, 1997). This is despite India having achieved self-sufficiency in foodgrains production, reduced dependence on imports and a system of distributing grains at subsidised prices. All these findings show that the PDS is not effective as an anti-poverty instrument. Further, the off-take of foodgrains across states is found to be unrelated to existing poverty levels and, even within states, the incidence of subsidies is not very progressive (World Bank, 1997). Survey data also reveals a weak correlation between access levels to the poor and incidence of poverty across regions (Srinivasan, 1997).

However, it is worth noting that despite these weaknesses, there are many positive aspects to the system. In most states, the PDS has a much higher pro-poor bias than many other public services such as provision of safe drinking water, health services of various types and electrification of residences (Table 2). While there is wide variation in accessibility of FPSs to consumers across states, there has been an improvement in access over time in all the states (Table 3), as judged by an index of accessibility constructed by Howes and Jha (1992).[2]

TABLE 2. PRO-POOR BIAS IN ACCESS TO RURAL PUBLIC SERVICES

State/ UT	*PDS Rice*	*PDS Wheat*	*Drinking Water*	*Family Planning Services*	*Electrified Dwellings*	*Pediatric Care*
Andhra Pradesh	0.17	−0.05	0.16	0.07	−0.29	−0.06
Assam	0.19	0.33	−0.12	−0.08	−0.36	−0.35
Bihar	0.06	0.02	−0.01	−0.04	−0.26	−0.03
Gujarat	0.14	0.39	−0.12	0.00	−0.26	−0.35

(Table 2. contd...)

Haryana	0.35	—	0.04	−0.14	−0.17	−0.24
Jammu & Kashmir	0.27	0.21	−0.24	−0.37	−0.18	−0.28
Karnataka	0.05	0.03	0.05	−0.07	−0.17	−0.28
Kerala	0.05	−0.06	−0.09	0.03	−0.23	−0.10
Madhya Pradesh	0.12	0.07	0.00	−0.08	−0.19	−0.15
Maharashtra	0.00	0.04	0.01	−0.03	−0.24	0.01
Orissa	−0.28	−0.71	0.00	0.07	−0.34	−0.04
Punjab	—	3.54	0.19	0.13	−0.23	−0.60
Rajasthan	0.25	0.35	−0.03	−0.17	−0.25	−0.32
Tamil Nadu	0.14	−0.15	−0.05	0.10	−0.21	−0.06
Uttar Pradesh	−0.13	−0.41	0.14	0.22	−0.53	−0.25
West Bengal	0.14	−0.11	0.05	−0.05	−0.64	−0.17

Notes: 1. These numbers are based on a consumer expenditure survey carried out by the National Sample Survey Organisation (NSSO) for the year 1986–7.

2. Pro-poor Bias is defined as $[(P_a/P)/(T_a/T)-1]$ where P_a and P are respectively the number of poor who have access to the service and the total number of poor. Similarly, T_a and T are the total number of people who have access and the total number of people respectively.

Source: Srinivasan (1997).

TABLE 3. ACCESSIBILITY OF RATION SHOPS

State/ U.T.	*a = 0.25*		*a = 0.5*		*a = 0.75*	
	1978	*1995*	*1978*	*1995*	*1978*	*1995*
Andhra Pradesh	2.92	6.39	1.23	2.30	0.52	0.83
Assam	5.81	5.24	2.29	2.60	0.90	1.29
Bihar	5.08	8.97	1.74	2.43	0.60	0.66
Goa	3.67	6.79	1.35	2.30	0.50	0.78
Gujarat	1.88	3.22	0.78	1.23	0.33	0.47
Haryana	3.52	7.11	1.29	2.40	0.48	0.81
HP	2.34	3.39	1.22	1.61	0.64	0.77
Karnataka	2.66	4.73	1.13	1.75	0.48	0.65
Kerala	8.72	11.14	2.65	3.21	0.81	0.92
Madhya Pradesh	1.59	2.60	0.76	1.13	0.36	0.49
Maharashtra	3.35	5.55	1.33	1.99	0.53	0.72
Manipur	0.99	4.78	0.53	2.44	0.29	1.24
Meghalaya	3.37	5.36	1.73	1.66	0.89	0.51
Mizoram	0.99	3.22	0.70	1.95	0.49	1.18
Orissa	2.15	6.99	0.98	2.68	0.45	1.03

(Table 3. contd...)

(Table 3. continued)

State/ U.T.	a = 0.25		a = 0.5		a = 0.75	
	1978	1995	1978	1995	1978	1995
Punjab	8.27	10.46	2.89	3.43	1.01	1.12
Rajasthan	1.21	2.53	0.60	1.12	0.30	0.50
Tamil Nadu	2.57	7.06	0.87	2.16	0.30	0.66
Tripura	2.35	4.78	0.97	1.78	0.40	0.66
Uttar Pradesh	2.91	6.45	1.00	2.14	0.35	0.71
West Bengal	5.88	8.21	1.79	2.34	0.54	0.67
Delhi	26.81	62.71	5.14	9.40	0.99	1.41
A&N Islands	1.49	2.91	1.00	1.61	0.68	0.89
Chandigarh	23.52	57.80	4.68	9.11	0.93	1.43
Daman & Diu	3.67	10.82	1.35	3.18	0.50	0.93
Pondicherry	9.00	24.22	2.27	5.12	0.57	1.08
All India	2.83	5.86	1.13	2.09	0.45	0.74

Notes: 1. Accessibility of a ration shop in a State i is defined as $X_i = P_i\,(1/C_i)a(1/D_i)(1\text{-}a)$, as per Howes and Jha (1992). P refers to the proportion of population covered by the system, C to crowding in the ration shops and D to 'average' distance of a residence from a ration shop. Accessibility improves with better coverage, lower crowding and shorter distance of ration shop. a is the weight assigned to crowding and (1-a) to distance.
2. Given the exorbitantly high 'P' in Bihar and Meghalaya, accessibility in these states has been calculated by taking the coverage to be 1.16, the national average.

Sources: 1. The number of households and or ration cards are taken from GOI (1997a)
2. Total number of ration shops is taken from GOI (1997b) and their distribution across states from GOI (1991).
3. State-wise area is obtained from data on population and density from GOI (1997b).

Another useful role of the PDS has been in containing prices and preventing the development of localised food shortages. This has been documented for the drought years 1979–80 and 1987–8 by, among others, Ahluwalia (1991) and Tyagi (1990). The PDS also plays a role in the stabilisation of food prices since the quantity distributed is enhanced during bad crop years. However, as Thamarajakshi (1997) suggests, expansion of irrigation facilities and technology can be a cheaper and more sustainable way of achieving price stability as compared to the instrument of PDS.

In order to run the PDS, the government has been following a policy of procuring foodgrains from wheat farmers and rice millers. Since the procurement prices mostly acted as support prices, this policy has been largely successful in providing price incentives to suppliers of both rice and wheat (Radhakrishna and Indrakant, 1988).[3]

Maintenance of large grain stocks has been a drain on the government's resources (GOI, 1991) mainly due to the high operating costs of the FCI. According to a report of the Bureau of Industrial Costs and Prices (GOI, 1991), the storage costs of FCI can be slashed by as much as 30 per cent simply by economising on its staff strength which accounts for more than 70 per cent of the total. Moreover, the FCI can more than double its rate of capacity utilisation to operate at optimal levels. Jha and Srinivasan (1997) calculate that these two measures together can cut down its storage costs by more than half. In addition, the FCI can also reduce its costs of procurement, distribution etc., by improving its efficiency of operation and reducing its margins. A large part of the government's expenditure on account of food subsidy thus goes to cover up rising costs of the FCI rather than benefiting the consumer. Per unit costs of FCI's operations have been substantially higher compared to that of private traders (Gulati *et al.*, 1996). Unfortunately, despite such evidence, the government so far seems to be wary of private trade. This is reflected in recurrent moves such as selective credit control to effect a credit squeeze and the imposition of limited stock holdings on traders (Table 4).

TABLE 4. OPERATIONAL COSTS OF FCI AS PERCENTAGE OF PROCUREMENT PRICE

Year	*Procurement Incidentals*	*Distribution Cost*	*Carrying Cost*	*Total Cost*	*Procurement Price (Rs/q)*
		(as percentage of procurement price)			
		RICE			
1989–90	9.39	22.90	16.76	49.05	276
1990–1	12.62	24.38	14.10	51.10	306
1991–2	11.79	21.08	20.27	53.13	343
1992–3	7.01	21.78	21.71	50.51	403
1993–4	14.79	23.61	20.19	58.59	437
1994–5	7.42	21.77	21.60	50.80	537
1995–6	4.32	19.31	17.20	40.84	597
1996–7	4.98	15.26	20.08	40.32	662
1997–8	4.81	21.28	24.36	50.46	686
1998–9	4.25	22.04	22.03	48.31	776

(Table 4. contd...)

(Table 4. continued)

Year	Procurement Incidentals	Distribution Cost	Carrying Cost	Total Cost	Procurement Price (Rs/q)
	(as percentage of procurement price)				
			WHEAT		
1989–90	21.91	34.54	25.28	81.73	183
1990–1	11.91	34.70	20.12	66.73	215
1991–2	19.58	32.13	30.89	82.60	225
1992–3	15.14	31.92	31.82	78.88	275
1993–4	30.71	31.27	26.73	88.71	330
1994–5	27.61	33.41	33.14	94.16	350
1995–6	27.11	31.78	28.53	87.42	360
1996–7	23.47	28.84	34.96	87.27	380
1997–8	21.02	26.59	36.63	84.24	455
1998–9	28.05	30.37	33.55	91.97	510
			AVERAGE		
1989–90	14.38	27.54	20.16	62.08	230
1990–1	12.33	28.64	16.58	57.55	261
1991–2	14.87	25.45	24.48	64.80	284
1992–3	10.31	25.90	25.81	62.01	339
1993–4	21.64	26.90	23.00	71.55	384
1994–5	15.39	26.36	26.16	67.91	444
1995–6	12.89	24.00	21.46	58.36	479
1996–7	11.72	20.20	25.51	57.43	521
1997–8	11.28	23.41	29.25	63.94	570
1998–9	13.68	25.33	26.60	65.62	643

Notes: 1. The figures for 1998–9 are estimates.

2. Since data on procurement price of rice is not available after 1995–6, we assume procurement incidentals to be at the average level (Rs 33/ quintal) during 1989–90 to 1995–6 (except for 1993–4, when it was Rs 65/ quintal). The procurement price is then obtained as the residual from the sum total of purchase cost and procurement incidentals.

Source: Updated from Jha and Srinivasan (1997).

Nevertheless, putting together the numbers from Table 4, it is easy to check that the average unit cost of FCI (for rice and wheat together) as a percentage of procurement price has fallen in the latter half of the 1990s. While it constituted 64.22 per cent of procurement price during the first five years from 1989–90 to 1993–4, it reduced to 62.73 per cent during the next five years from 1994–5 to 1998–9.[4] This may be due to measures implemented on the basis of suggestions from various studies such as those mentioned earlier. This has resulted in lowering of the cost-benefit ratios for the PDS that have, hitherto, been very high (Table 5). Thus, based on macro data, there seems to be considerable scope for cutting down the costs of the FCI.

4. NEW SCHEMES AND ASSOCIATED PROBLEMS

The real expenditure on food subsidy by the government doubled between 1980–1 and 1994–5 (Radhakrishna *et al.*, 1997). In order to curb the increasing food subsidy bill and simultaneously provide greater food security to the poor, it has initiated a few new schemes to strengthen the existing universal or untargeted PDS (UPDS). The basic premise behind these schemes is that costs of providing subsidy to the poor are increasing due to universal provision and therefore subsidy has to be targeted to the needy. Hence, the focus on special interest groups. In the UPDS, the extent to which a household can benefit depends on its purchasing power. In particular, ultra-poor households below the poverty line (BPL) cannot purchase the entire quota they are eligible for and hence do not benefit from subsidies to the maximum extent possible. This situation could be corrected in principle by 'targeted PDS' since BPL households are charged very low prices under this scheme.

4.1 The Revamped Public Distribution System (RPDS)

The Revamped Public Distribution System (RPDS) was established in January 1992 and subsequently merged with the Integrated Tribal Development Program (ITDP) in June 1992. This scheme is meant to serve households located in tribal, hill and arid areas having poor infrastructure and covering 1,775 blocks and 170 million people. Under RPDS, rice and wheat are allocated to states and union territories with a quota of 20 kg per family per month at prices lower by 50 paise per kg than the CIP for UPDS. In addition to foodgrains, RPDS also

TABLE 5. BENEFIT-COST CALCULATIONS FOR INTERVENTION IN GRAIN MARKETS

Year	*1990–91*	*1991–92*	*1992–93*	*1993–94*	*1994–95*	*1995–96*	*1996–97*	*1997–98 (P)*
			RICE (Rs/quintal)					
a. Market price	480	586	672	718	794	893	989	1095
b. CIP	377	377	437	537	537	537	537	537
c. Procurement price	306	343	403	437	537	597	662	686
d. Administrative cost	113	113	116	168	157	141	134	179
e. Storage cost	43	70	88	88	116	103	133	167
I. Consumer benefit (a–b)	103	209	235	181	257	356	452	558
II. Producer loss (a–c)	174	243	269	281	257	296	327	409
III. Government cost (c+d+e–b)	85	148	170	156	273	304	392	494
Consumer benefit (govt. cost + producer loss)	0.40	0.53	0.54	0.41	0.48	0.59	0.63	0.62
			WHEAT (Rs/quintal)					
a. Market price	293	348	387	431	465	460	566	696
b. CIP	280	280	330	402	402	402	402	402
c. Procurement price	215	225	275	330	350	360	380	455
d. Administrative cost	100	116	129	205	214	212	199	217
e. Storage cost	43	70	88	88	116	103	133	167
I. Consumer benefit (a–b)	13	68	57	29	63	58	164	294
II. Producer loss (a–c)	78	123	112	101	115	100	186	241
III. Government cost (c+d+e–b)	78	131	162	221	278	273	310	436
Consumer benefit (govt. cost + producer loss)	0.08	0.27	0.21	0.09	0.16	0.16	0.33	0.43

Notes: 1. Consumer benefit is the difference between market price and issue price.
2. Producer loss is the difference between market price and procurement price. Since rice is procured from rice millers, producer loss in this case should be read as 'millers' loss.
3. Government cost is the sum of procurement, storage and administrative costs minus sales realisation.

Source: Updated from Jha and Srinivasan (1997).

supplies items like tea, soap, pulses and iodised salt. The Economic Survey 1995–6 provides further details on this (GOI, 1996).

4.2 The Targeted Public Distribution System (TPDS)

The Targeted Public Distribution System (TPDS) based on the recommendations of the Chief Ministers' Conference in July 1996, is another scheme that was launched in June 1997. This scheme is meant to serve families below the poverty line. Under this scheme the states are required to identify these families and provide them 10 kg of foodgrains per family per month, at 50 per cent of the UPDS price. Supply of grain to the states for this purpose is guaranteed by the central government. In addition, workers under the Employment Assurance Scheme (EAS) or the Jawahar Rojgar Yojna (JRY) would also receive food coupons to be exchanged at FPSs for grains at the rate of 1 kg per man-day. The states will be free to provide higher quotas or price subsidies by adding from their own resources. The population above the poverty line (APL) would continue to receive foodgrains as per the normal UPDS. However, the proposal is to slowly phase out this part of the programme. It is this particular proposal that could lead to both inclusion and exclusion errors.

The allocation of foodgrains to states for TPDS purpose is based on poverty estimates obtained using the Expert Group (Lakdawala Committee) methodology. While the responsibility for implementing the TPDS rests with the states, the centre has given them broad guidelines regarding the identification of the poor at the micro level. The following specific suggestions have been made (GOI, 1997a). The quinquennial surveys made by the Ministry of Rural Areas and Employment for implementation of IRDP etc. for households living below the poverty line can be a basis for the identification of eligible families. Gram Panchayats and Gram Sabhas should be involved in this process. Identification of vulnerable sections can be based on occupational and asset holding characteristics. For example, these would include landless agricultural labourers, marginal farmers and rural artisans and in urban areas, slum dwellers and daily wage earners such as porters, coolies and pavement vendors.

Based on a study of Latin American countries, Grosh (1995) concludes that incidence of subsidies on the poor is better with targeted programmes and there is no evidence to show that programmes with better incidence necessarily have higher administrative costs. In the Indian case, while schemes using explicit targeting mechanisms are commendable, the question of how much they can achieve is difficult to answer for the following reasons.

(a) There are limits to redistribution. For example, calculations based on regional poverty indices estimated by Dreze and Srinivasan (1996) show that benefits due to geographic targeting cannot be dramatic at low levels of regional disaggregation. If subsidy is distributed in proportion to the number of poor in each region as opposed to the entire population in that region, the fraction of total subsidy reaching the poor increases only by 4 percentage points. This point has also been demonstrated by Datt and Ravallion (1993) who show that removal of disparities in mean consumption expenditure across Indian states through redistribution reduces the overall head-count index by 1.8 percentage points only.

(b) Even if a fair amount of redistribution is possible, direct targeting of the needy classes, as required under the new schemes, could become a futile exercise if informational constraints limit the ability to efficiently and accurately discern the income levels of individuals. Many have expressed doubts regarding successful identification of the poor. See Bevan and Fullerton-Joireman (1997), Swaminathan (1997) and Thamarajakshi (1997).[5]

(c) Costs of identifying the poor can be substantial and recurring. Since poverty is a transient phenomenon for many, means testing will have to be carried out at regular intervals, perhaps annually. If identification costs outweigh the benefits in terms of reduced government expenditure achieved through reduced distribution of grains under TPDS, the purpose of the scheme gets vitiated. Besley and Kanbur (1993) cite examples of such problems that occurred in Sri Lanka and Brazil. In Sri Lanka, when the universal programme of rice subsidy was replaced by food stamps, the eligible group of people was identified only once. This meant that households whose incomes increased beyond the eligibility level continued to benefit from the programme. On the other hand, those who became eligible after the implementation of the programme could not receive the benefits. In Brazil, a finely targeted food distribution programme was reverted to a universal programme—though within selected poverty areas—since it was found that the leakage of benefits to the non-target group was less expensive than the cumbersome targeted programme.

(d) In trying to identify people based on poverty levels, the most important problem is of identifying the poverty line. For, instance, there is a wide variation in estimates of incidence of poverty by the Expert Group and the official estimates according to the Planning

Commission. The difference could be due to the use of different price indices for valuing the calorie norms in the two estimates. This problem adds another dimension of complexity to the problem of identification. For example, in the case of Andhra Pradesh, Parthasarthy and Nirmala (1997) point out that basing the TPDS on the former estimates would be grossly unfair to the state. There is wide variation in the costs of living in different urban regions and the use of a single poverty line for all the urban regions in a state can lead to gross under-estimation of poverty for some of the big cities such as Mumbai.

(e) While TPDS tries to fine-target subsidies, it ignores some of the existing problems. For instance, people without proper residential addresses including the homeless, street children, those under institutional care, the destitute etc. continue to be left uncovered. Due to targeting errors, families that fail to get identified as 'below poverty line' but are otherwise poor and left out of TPDS would become worse off than before if the untargeted PDS is phased out. Since the price of TPDS grain is much lower than the market price, there is an increase in the effective subsidy reaching the ultra poor (whose purchasing power is very low). However, TPDS, by limiting grain distribution based on head-count poverty measure, is likely to miss out, due to identification errors, some of the poor among current beneficiaries. Thus, the net effect due to TPDS on per capita subsidy to the poor is ambiguous.

(f) Apart from the question of feasibility and appropriateness of fine targeting, there is the question of the commitment and ability of state governments to carry out the programmes. Since most states charge different (usually higher) retail end prices than the CIP, the objectives of the central government are not met to the full extent and the purpose of providing grains at highly subsidised prices may be defeated. For instance, the prices charged for rice and wheat under RPDS are higher than the relevant CIP in almost all the states, the exceptions being Andhra Pradesh, Maharashtra and Tamil Nadu in the case of rice (Figure 1), and Karnataka and Maharashtra in the case of wheat (Figure 2). But strangely, even Maharashtra, which seems to cross-subsidise RPDS consumers against the regular PDS consumers, does not fare well in the reforms programme. Swaminathan (1996) finds that while household entitlements and the quantities supplied through the PDS have fallen during the post-reform period, the issue prices of goods sold at the FPSs, including foodgrains, have gone up. Together, these changes have led to a substantial reduction in subsidy to consumers.

FIGURE 1. RICE (COMMON VARIETY) PRICES IN DIFFERENT STATES/UTs. (RS/KG) (AS ON 1 FEBRUARY 1994)

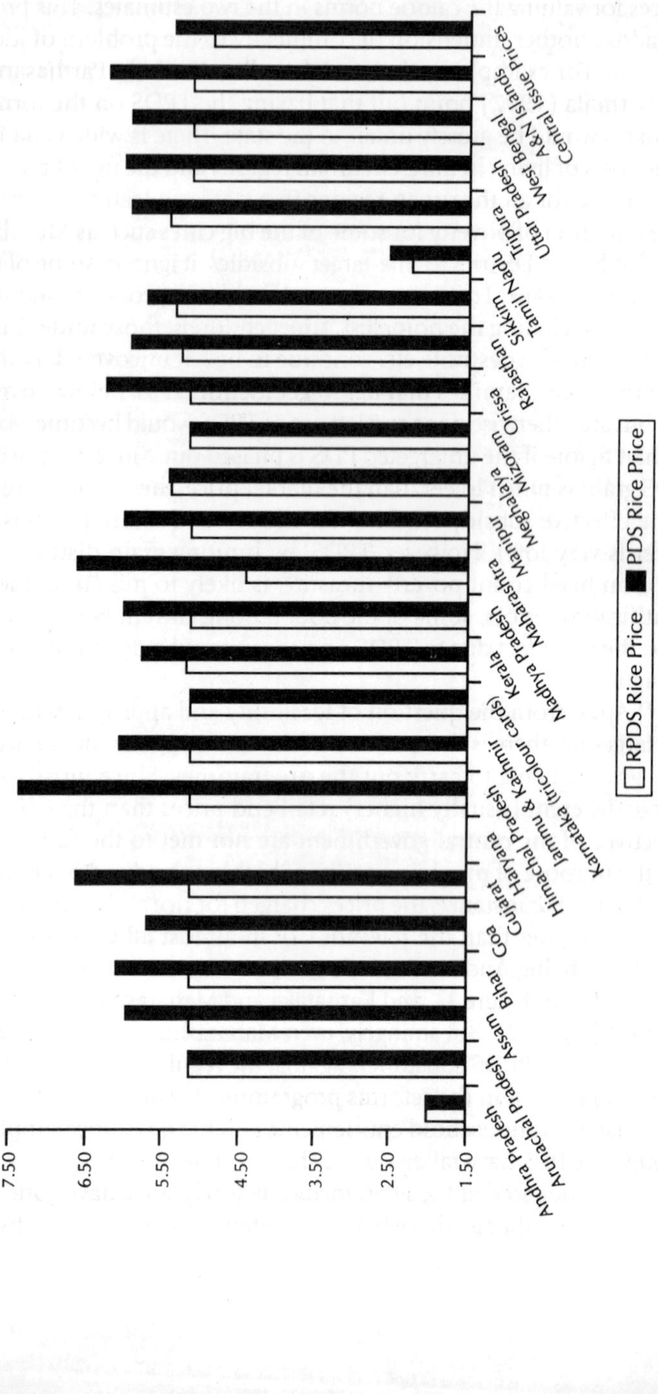

Source: Government of India (1996), Table 5.2, p. 89.

FIGURE 2. WHEAT PRICES IN DIFFERENT STATES/UTS (RS/KG) (AS ON 1 FEBRUARY 1994)

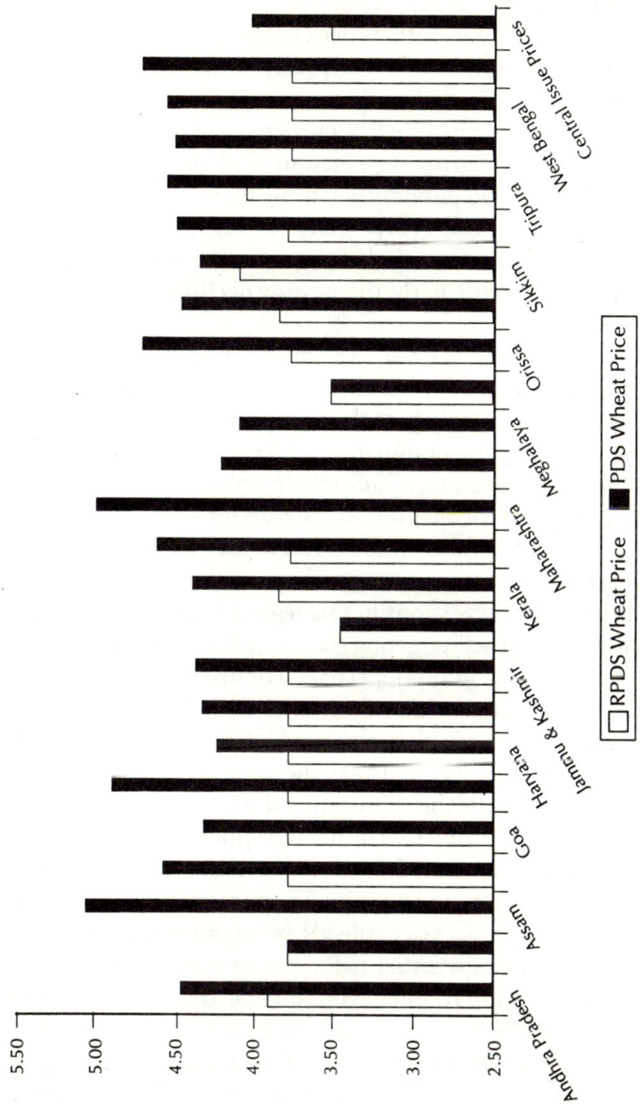

Source: Government of India (1996), Table 5.12, p. 89.

5. EXPERIENCES OF OTHER COUNTRIES

There is a large and expanding literature comparing the experiences of different countries in terms of public spending in general, and food subsidies in particular, with a focus on how to make the spending reach target groups more efficiently (Cornia and Stewart, 1995; Sahn and Alderman, 1995; Tuck and Lindert, 1996 and Van de Walle and Nead, 1995). Analysing the experiences of eight developing countries (including India), Cornia and Stewart find that switching from a universal to a targeted public programme led to a large increase in the number of poor excluded (Type-I error of targeting). But the number of non-deserving classes included (Type-II error of targeting) reduced only marginally. Particularly, the subsidy declined in real terms with targeting.

In a study of food subsidies in Tunisia, Tuck and Lindert (1996) find that along with the high costs of operation of the programme, there is a substantial leakage to the non-poor. Given the possibility of food riots, a complete elimination of food subsidies is likely to be infeasible. Direct targeting of subsidies involves high costs and would require changes in the institutional set-up for which there is usually a high level of political reluctance. Alternative means have to be devised if safety nets for the poor are to be maintained. Tuck and Lindert make interesting suggestions in this regard. They recommend some innovative ways of self-targeting such as different types of packaging for the poor and the non-poor classes. For instance, they suggest that cooking oil sold at subsidised prices could be packaged in 'cheap, unattractive bottles with plain labels, which simply identify their contents as *cooking oil*' (p. 71). Whereas, the same oil if packaged in attractive bottles with clear labels indicating the type of oil sold and other details is likely to be preferred by the non-poor classes even at higher prices. This seems to be an idea that could work very well in India too.

Sahn and Alderman (1995) make an interesting observation in their study of Sri Lanka's rice subsidy programme namely, that food ration can lead to substantial reduction in work effort. Thus while total *utility* of a ration recipient goes up due to additional leisure, its *consumption* bundle may not increase corresponding to 'the objective function of the designer or evaluator of the subsidy scheme' (p. 403). Sahn and Alderman therefore suggest that a lower rise in expenditure than the amount transferred by the government should not be referred to as leakage since it increases the consumer's utility in a strict welfare sense. In particular, they suggest that in addition to studying the two errors of targeting, it is equally important to study the incentive effects of public transfers and to be able to appreciate the disutility of labour especially for those engaged in heavy manual work. This is an important point to be considered in the Indian context in recommending the replacement or linking of the PDS with some employment-based programmes (Parikh, 1994).

6. RECOMMENDATIONS FOR FUTURE REFORMS

Better utilisation of limited subsidies requires minimisation of leakage or maximisation of benefits reaching the intended beneficiaries. Towards this end, direct targeting involves obtaining relevant information on individual characteristics (levels of income, expenditure, asset holdings etc.) and restricting the benefits only to those with eligible characteristics (i.e., low levels of living). However, it can be costly to acquire such information and these costs should not exceed the savings made in terms of lower leakage to the non-poor. Under the TPDS, which is supposed to serve people below the poverty line, the state governments will have the responsibility of identifying the poor and implementing the scheme. The success of TPDS would then depend on the state governments' ability in identifying and reaching the poor.

Past experiences are not very encouraging in this regard. For example, in Andhra Pradesh where the dual ration card scheme exists, around 80 per cent of households have ration cards meant for poor households. In fact, in most states the total number of ration cards is greater than the total number of households; in Bihar the number of ration cards is twice that number, and in Meghalaya almost seven times that of the households! (See GOI, 1997a). By fixing the quantity of foodgrains allocated to the states based on poverty levels, the central government is able to put a cap on food subsidy. However, given the practical difficulties involved in perfect targeting and in estimating the incidence of poverty, some allowance should be made for targeting errors even under TPDS. The central supplies to the states need to be fixed at levels higher than what would follow from the Expert Group's poverty estimates. The effectiveness in extending the subsidy to the poor (i.e., reducing the exclusion error) also depends on the individual states' capabilities in identifying the beneficiaries. If the states' capabilities are limited in this respect, then it is advisable to depend on self-selection and other indirect targeting mechanisms.

6.1 How to Reach the Poor Effectively

Since identifying the poor is in general a difficult and expensive task, it is necessary to look at possible alternatives to direct targeting. Mechanisms that encourage self-selection, such as supply of low-quality grains in the PDS, can keep the non-poor out of the system. It is also generally observed that consumers from lower income groups buy goods in small quantities. Thus, selling goods like cooking oil in loose quantities—without bottling or tinning—is likely to be self-targeted to the poor. Although packaging of foodgrains is not yet very popular in India, suggestions such as simple instead of attractive packaging in order to exclude the non-poor (Tuck and Lindert, 1996) are worth trying out.

Since most of the poor do not have resources to buy quantities in bulk, the quotas should be made available in smaller quantities at more frequent intervals such as a week, a fortnight etc.[6] Further, imposition of an upper limit on how much can be purchased at one go can act as a disincentive to well-off classes. Hence, they may not buy goods from the FPSs even if their requirement is for goods like sugar which is cheaper than but of a very similar quality to what is available in the free market.

Identification based on group characteristics (such as location of residence) is relatively easier and less expensive than that based on individual ones (such as income levels). Schemes such as RPDS are therefore likely to be more effective than TPDS in reaching the poor. While geographic targeting could be done at the micro level (e.g., at the district level), this alone may not suffice since the poor in relatively richer regions would be excluded. In general, whether it is based on individual or group characteristics, it is desirable to base identification on several possible characteristics rather than rely on income indicators alone, in order to minimise the exclusion error. Successful examples of other group-based targeting schemes of the government include the Integrated Child Development Scheme (ICDS), a nutrition and general development scheme targeting pre-school children in the age group 0–6 years and the Mid-Day Meal scheme which targets school-going children.

Since a majority of participants in the Employment Guarantee Scheme (EGS) in the state of Maharashtra in India come from households initially below the poverty line, Dev (1996) recommends targeting of UPDS to workers under the EGS by linking the two schemes.

For non-EGS workers, other targeting mechanisms could be used in conjunction with UPDS. The EGS provides many indirect benefits such as improving agricultural wages, asset creation, insurance, stabilisation of income etc. See also Kanbur *et al.* (1995), who evaluate the success of targeting in poverty alleviation programmes through labour supply, and Gaiha (1997) who gives specific suggestions to improve the diminishing accuracy of targeting and poverty impact of the EGS.

6.2 How can the System be Made Cost Effective

Apart from reducing leakages through better targeting, the system can be made cost effective by making the operations of the FCI more efficient. This could be achieved in several ways. First, the buffer stocks maintained by the FCI can be utilised solely for stabilising prices by de-linking its twin objectives of price stability and income distribution. This will greatly reduce the government's burden of carrying excessive stocks and hence its costs. Second, procurement operations could be carried out locally to reduce transportation costs to the extent that marketable surplus is available for purchase in the states. Third, the requirement for PDS supplies could be met directly from the free market, since private trade margins are lower than that of FCI. The higher purchase cost would be offset by lower transportation and storage costs.

National Sample Survey (NSS) data for 1986–7 shows that universal or untargeted PDS (UPDS) covering foodgrains, edible oils and sugar provides a meagre subsidy of just 1.4 per cent of mean expenditure to the average Indian consumer (Jha, 1992). If the entire amount of this subsidy were targeted (directly or indirectly) to, say, the bottom 30 per cent of the population, it would constitute about 5–7 per cent of the mean expenditure of an average person in this group. If the FCI could economise on its costs as suggested earlier, then without any additional expenses, the price subsidy could be increased substantially to raise the overall subsidy to a respectable proportion of expenditure. Since on an average the FCI's costs are higher than consumer benefits, a given percentage reduction in the former can be translated into a much higher percentage increase in the latter. It is easy to construct an example to see how the benefit-cost ratio can be improved simply by improving cost effectiveness and without affecting the issue or procurement prices. (In fact, issue prices have not been raised in the last few years and the off-take has picked up substantially). Table 6 provides such an example where reducing the FCI (purchase

TABLE 6. EXAMPLE TO SHOW HOW IMPROVED COST EFFICIENCY CAN RAISE BENEFIT-COST RATIO

Rs/ quintal	*Existing Scenario*	*Intermediate Step*		*Final Step*	
		Cost Reduction	*Changed Scenario*	*Reduction in Issue Price*	*Final Scenario*
A. Market Price	100		100		100
B. Issue Price	80		80	–30	50
C. FCI Cost (including purchase price)	120	–30	90 (-25%)		90
I. Consumer Benefit (A-B)	20		20	30	50 (+250%)
II. Net Government Cost (C-B)	40	–30	10	30 (–75%)	40
Benefit-Cost Ratio	0.50		2.00		1.25

price inclusive) cost by 25 per cent can be used to increase consumer benefit by 250 per cent, thereby raising the benefit-cost ratio two and a half times.

Currently, the government is forced to bear the burden of large stocks due to the high price support provided to farmers. Dependence, at least partly, on trade and on buying options could ease this burden. The government, in fact, has removed some of the controls on trade. However, the credibility of such policies needs to be improved. The reluctance on the part of the government to free external trade arises from its apprehension that (a) foreign markets can be unreliable sources of supply and demand and (b) the higher price variability in these markets may make domestic prices unstable (Dantwala, 1993; Nayyar and Sen, 1994 and Pursell and Gulati, 1993). Contrary to this, Jha and Srinivasan (1997) find from simulation exercises that liberalisation of external trade can lead to more stable domestic prices if a sufficient wedge is provided between domestic and international prices. They also find that free trade reduces PDS costs.

CONCLUSION

Based on the earlier discussion on the pros and cons of various reform measures, the following observations can be made. While TPDS can potentially make the incidence of food subsidies more progressive, its implementation is fraught with several problems. It depends very much on the state governments' willingness and ability to identify the poor perfectly since the central government has fixed an upper bound on the number of poor based on poverty estimates of the Expert Group. For each state, two poverty lines are defined—one for urban and one for rural areas. In the preceding estimates, within each of these two categories, the corresponding poverty line is assumed to be the same across all regions of a state. This assumption can lead to unfair distribution of benefits to regions whose poverty lines are higher than the one assumed. Further, the amount of possible redistribution through geographic targeting is limited. The informational constraints and costs of identification could outweigh benefits. Attempts at direct targeting, along with a reduction in government expenditure, can potentially increase the exclusion error, i.e. the error of excluding the needy. It is therefore important that the untargeted portion of the PDS (or UPDS) is not neglected while the poor's access is improved through geographic and other forms of direct targeting. Otherwise, the poor excluded from TPDS would be left at the mercy of market forces. As such, since the introduction of TPDS in June 1997, the off-take of rice and wheat has reduced by 35–40 per cent compared with the off-take during the corresponding months of 1996–7 (CMIE, 1998).

Experiences of some other countries have shown that a shift from universal to targeted provision of subsidies increases the exclusion error. Future reform measures should therefore concentrate on improving the self-targeting feature of the universal system.

While the TPDS emphasises the poverty alleviation objective of food subsidy, other benefits should not be ignored. For example, PDS keeps food prices in check during bad crop years and combats inflationary pressures. Therefore, a case for maintaining universal provision of food subsidies can be made considering the fact that PDS has a macroeconomic impact of reducing inflationary pressures by lowering food prices relative to other commodities. This benefit could possibly compensate for the leakage of subsidies to the non-poor. The extent of subsidies reaching the poor can be increased by increasing the overall coverage under universal provision of subsidies. The consequent rise in the food subsidy bill can be reduced by improving efficiency in the operations of the system, encouraging private trade and storage and deregulating domestic and international trade in foodgrains.

There have been some suggestions regarding replacement or linking of the UPDS with better-targeted systems such as the EGS. However, it has to be noted that these schemes address different issues. While the latter scheme attacks poverty by providing purchasing power through employment creation, the former provides food subsidy since wages adjust to price changes with a time lag. Linking UPDS to EGS would however help in effectively targeting subsidies to the poor. Despite its weaknesses, the UPDS has a better pro-poor bias than many other public services in rural areas. This, together with the large network of FPSs that exists, and improvement in the efficiency of operation of the FCI should be used to improve the quantum of subsidy and the reach of the universal PDS.

Until there is a review and evaluation of the effectiveness of TPDS after its implementation, UPDS should not be phased out and the amount of grains distributed through FPS should not be reduced. TPDS aimed specifically at the poor and UPDS with implicit targeting mechanisms can co-exist at least until the TPDS is streamlined and the costs of administering this scheme are only marginal. In the meanwhile, government costs can be reduced through other means. These include improving the operational efficiency of the FCI, limiting the amount of buffer stocks by restricting the role of the FCI purely to price stabilisation, minimising inclusion errors through self-targeting mechanisms based on location and other household characteristics and improving the administrative efficiency of the state governments. The benefits to consumers, relative to costs to the government and producers, can be increased simply by reorganising and reorienting the FCI so as to improve its cost efficiency.

ENDNOTES

1. However, the evidence of an urban bias in the system raises the question of how well these shops function in rural areas. In this context see, among others, Dreze and Sen (1990), Howes and Jha (1992), Krishnaji (1990) and Radhakrishna and Rao (1994). For further debate on urban bias, see Dantwala (1993) and Howes and Jha (1994).
2. This index is based on three variables—the coverage of population by the PDS, the number of ration shops per square km area and the number of people served by each ration shop.
3. But these benefits are confined only to a few surplus states that contribute most of the total grain procured. In all other states, producers sell to private traders at prices below procurement price [Ray (1994)].
4. This is despite assuming procurement incidentals for rice in the last three years from 1996–7 to 1998–9 to be at the average level (Rs 33/ quintal) for the previous seven years. In the two immediately preceding

years, 1993–4 to 1995–6, these incidentals had actually declined from Rs 65 to Rs 26/ quintal (See the notes to Table 4).

5. According to Sen (1995, p. 18), while looking for indicators for targeting there is a 'case for going beyond income considerations into the type of life led' since the latter will influence the recipients' choices and decisions. The measure of consumption poverty, e.g., will depend upon consumption strategies that in turn will be affected by livelihood system and culture, seasonality or annuality of cropping system, etc.
6. Currently, there is an adverse selection going on because of ration quotas being made available mostly on a monthly basis. Due to this the relatively less poor have better access as compared to poor people who earn on a daily basis.

REFERENCES

Ahluwalia, D., 1991. 'Drought Proofing in the Indian Foodgrain Economy', *Indian Journal of Agricultural Economics*, 46(2): 111–20, April-June.

______, 1993. 'Public Distribution of Food in India: Coverage, Targeting and Leakages', *Food Policy*, February, 18(2): 33–54.

Besley, T. and R. Kanbur, 1993. 'The Principles of Targeting', in Lipton and Van der Gaag (eds.), *Including The Poor*, World Bank, Washington D.C., p. 67–90.

Bevan, P. and S. Fullerton-Joireman, 1997. 'The Perils of Measuring Poverty: Identifying The "Poor" in Rural Ethiopia', *Oxford Development Studies*, 25(3): 315–35.

Centre for Monitoring Indian Economy (CMIE), 1998. 'Monthly Review of the Indian Economy', Economic Intelligence Service, Mumbai, May.

Cornia, G.A. and F. Stewart, 1995. 'Two Errors of Targeting', Chapter 13, in Van de Walle and Nead (eds.), *Public Spending and the Poor: Theory and Evidence*, Johns Hopkins University Press (for World Bank), Baltimore, p. 350–86.

Dantwala, M.L., 1993. 'Agricultural Policy: Prices and Public Distribution System: A Review', *Indian Journal of Agricultural Economics*, 48(2): 173–86, April-June.

Datt, G. and M. Ravallion, 1993. 'Regional Disparities, Targeting and Poverty in India', in Lipton and van der Gaag (eds.), *Including the Poor*, World Bank, Washington D.C., pp. 91–114.

Dev, Mahendra S., 1996. 'Food Security: PDS versus EGS, A Tale of Two States', *Economic and Political Weekly* 31(27): 1752–64.

Dreze, Jean and A. Sen, 1990. 'Hunger and Public Action', Clarendon Press, Oxford.

______, and P.V. Srinivasan, 1996. 'Poverty in India: Regional Estimates 1987–8', *Development Economics Research Programme* Discussion Paper DEP No. 70, STICERD, London School of Economics.

Gaiha, R., 1997. 'Do Rural Public Works Influence Agricultural Wages? The Case of the Employment Guarantee Scheme in India', *Oxford Development Studies* 25(3): 301–14.

Government of India, 1999. 'Economic Survey 1998–9', Ministry of Finance, Economic Division, New Delhi.

______, 1997a. 'Focus on the Poor: Guidelines for the Implementation of the Targeted Public Distribution System', Ministry of Civil Supplies, Consumer Affairs and Public Distribution, New Delhi.

______, 1997b. 'Economic Survey: 1996–7', Ministry of Finance, Economic Division, New Delhi.

______, 1996. 'Economic Survey 1995–6', Ministry of Finance, Economic Division, New Delhi.

______, 1991. 'Report On "The Operations Of The Food Corporation Of India"', Bureau of Industrial Costs and Prices (BICP), Ministry of Industry, New Delhi.

Grosh, Margaret E., 1995. 'Toward Quantifying the Trade-off: Administrative Costs and Incidence in Targeted Programs in Latin America', Chapter 16 in Van de Walle and Nead (eds.), *Public Spending and The Poor: Theory and Evidence*, Johns Hopkins University Press (for World Bank), Baltimore, 450–88.

Gulati, A., P.K. Sharma and Satu Kähkönen, 1996. 'The Food Corporation of India: Successes and Failures in Indian Foodgrain Marketing', IRIS-India Working Paper No.18, IRIS Center, University of Maryland, College Park.

Howes, S. and Shikha Jha, 1992. 'Urban Bias in the Indian Public Distribution System', *Economic and Political Weekly*, 27(19): 1022–30, 9 May.

______, and Shikha Jha, 1994. 'Public Distribution of Food in India: A Comment', *Food Policy*, 19(1): 65–8, February.

Jha, Shikha, 1992. 'Consumer Subsidies in India: Is Targeting Effective?' *Development and Change*, 23(4): 101–28, October.

______, and P.V. Srinivasan, 1997. 'Grain Price Stabilisation Policies in India', mimeo, Indira Gandhi Institute of Development Research, Mumbai.

Kanbur, R., Keen, M. and M. Tuomala, 1995. 'Labour Supply and Targeting in Poverty Alleviation Programmes', Chapter 5 in Van de Walle and Nead (eds.), *Public Spending and The Poor: Theory and Evidence*, Johns Hopkins University Press (for World Bank), Baltimore, 91–113.

Krishnaji, N., 1990. 'Agricultural Price Policy: A Survey with Reference to Indian Foodgrain Economy', Review of Agriculture, *Economic and Political Weekly*, 25 (26): A54–A63, 30 June.

Lipton, M. and J. van der Gaag (eds.), 1993. 'Including the Poor', World Bank, Washington, D.C.

Nayyar, D. and Abhijit Sen, 1994. 'International Trade and Agricultural Sector in India', *Economic and Political Weekly*, 29(20): 1187–203, 14 May.

Parikh, Kirit, 1994. 'Who Gets How Much from PDS: How Effectively does it Reach the Poor?' *Sarvekshana*, 17(3): 1–34.

Parthasarthy, G. and K.A. Nirmala, 1997. 'Lakdawala Estimate of Poverty and Targeted PDS: Injustice to Andhra Pradesh', Commentary, *Economic and Political Weekly*, 32(16): 815–816, 19 April.

Pursell, G. and A. Gulati, 1993. 'Liberalising Indian Agriculture: An Agenda for Reform', Policy Research Working Papers No. WPS 1172, Policy Research Department, World Bank, Washington, D.C.

Radhakrishna, R., 1996. 'Food Trends, Public Distribution System and Food Security Concerns', *Indian Journal of Agricultural Economics*, 51(1&2): 168–83, January-June.

______, and K. Hanumantha Rao, 1994. 'Food Security, Public Distribution and Price Policy', Discussion Paper No. 4, Studies on Human Development in India, Project of the United Nations Development Programme.

______, and S. Indrakant, 1988. 'Effects of Rice Market Intervention Policies in India: The Case of Andhra Pradesh' in: *Evaluating Rice Market Intervention Policies: Some Asian Examples*, Asian Development Bank.

______, and K. Subbarao with S. Indrakant and C. Ravi, 1997. 'India's Public Distribution System: A National and International Perspective', World Bank Discussion Paper No. 380, World Bank, Washington, D.C.

Ray, S.K., 1994. 'Food Management Revisited', *Journal of Indian School of Political Economy*, 6(2): 313–36.

Sahn, D.E. and H. Alderman, 1995. 'Incentive Effects on Labour Supply of Sri Lanka's Rice Subsidy', in Chapter 14: Van de Walle and Nead (eds.), *Public Spending and The Poor: Theory and Evidence*, Johns Hopkins University Press (for World Bank), Baltimore, 387–409.

Sarma, J.S., 1988. 'Administered Prices of Foodgrains in India', in Mellor and Ahmed (eds.), *Agricultural Price Policy for Developing Countries*, Johns Hopkins University Press, Baltimore, MD, 155–68.

Sen, A., 1995. 'The Political Economy of Targeting', Chapter 2 in Van de Walle and Nead (eds.), *Public Spending and the Poor: Theory and Evidence*, Johns Hopkins University Press (for World Bank), Baltimore, 11–24.

Srinivasan, P.V., 1997. 'Regional Poverty and Access to Public Services in Rural India', IRIS-India Working Paper No. 30, IRIS Centre, University of Maryland, College Park.

Swaminathan, M., 1996. 'Structural Adjustment, Food Security, and System of Public Distribution of Food', *Economic and Political Weekly*, 31(26): 1665–72, 29 June.

______, 1997. 'Dangers of Narrow Targeting', *Frontline*, 31 October, 12–16.

Thamarajakshi, R., 1997. 'Economic Reforms and State Intervention in Foodgrain Market', *Economic and Political Weekly*, 32(30): 1894–900, 26 July–1 August.

Tuck, L. and K. Lindert, 1996. 'From Universal Food Subsidies to a Self-Targeted Program: A Case Study in Tunisian Reform', World Bank Discussion Paper No. 351, World Bank, Washington, D.C.

Tyagi, D.S., 1990. 'Managing India's Food Economy: Problems and Alternatives', Sage Publications, New Delhi.

Van de Walle, D. and K. Nead (eds.), 1995. 'Public Spending and The Poor: Theory and Evidence, Johns Hopkins University Press (for World Bank), Baltimore.

World Bank, 1986. 'Poverty and Hunger: Issues and Options for Food Security in Developing Countries', A World Bank Policy Study, Washington, D.C.

______, 1997. 'India: Achievements and Challenges in Reducing Poverty', A World Bank Country Study, June, Washington D.C.

chapter 7

Nutrition Security in India: Issues and Policies

• *M.H. Suryanarayana*

1. INTRODUCTION

The current reform programme lays emphasis on achieving economic growth, *inter alia*, by promoting efficiency in resource allocation at minimum social cost. One important issue which has received little attention relates to promoting growth via an increase in labour efficiency secured by improved nutrition.[1] This is an important policy option, which can take care of objectives with respect to both growth and social cost. Without adequate nutrition, a person will not be able to realise the potential of his or her labour power, as undernourishment would impair the ability to market and sell this asset, hence, the ability to obtain enough food. Since nutritional status cannot be improved without food, the situation would lead to a vicious circle. From this viewpoint, nutritional status is a capital asset. This is a micro-profile with profound macro implications via labour efficiency and productivity. Studies have confirmed the importance of raising calorie intake as an investment in human capital and its role in promoting productivity and growth (Fogel, 1991 and Schultz, 1993). Rural human capital accounts much more than non-human capital in explaining differential growth rates in per capita income among developing countries (Chai, 1995).

In spite of efforts to achieve 'growth with social justice' over fifty

The author would like to thank K. Seeta Prabhu for comments and suggestions on an earlier draft of the paper.

years of independence, India has achieved only limited progress.[2] About 60 million children under four years of age, which amounts to 53 per cent of the corresponding child population, were undernourished (UNDP, 1997a). This should be quite alarming given the findings that nutrition and economic growth are mutually reinforcing (Bhargava, 1996; Glewwe, Jacoby and King, 1996). About 2.20 million infants die every year from preventable causes (UNDP, 1997a).

There are considerable inter-state disparities with regard to nutritional outcome parameters, which cannot be explained solely in terms of income. How do we account for such disparities and what should be the appropriate policy response for them? An understanding of the nature of the nutrition problem, the population groups suffering from or vulnerable to malnutrition and the reasons for them is important for formulating nutrition intervention programmes. However, due to lack of necessary statistical information, these issues are not examined in the present paper. Instead, an attempt is made to quantify and understand the problem at the micro level using available direct survey estimates by rural and urban sectors for all-India and for major states. Such direct estimates, contrary to the macro food balance sheet estimates (Dawson and Tiffin, 1998), show a decline in cereal consumption and calorie intake in India as a whole and in almost all the constituent states (Suryanarayana, 1996).[3] This has happened in spite of some growth in income and reduction in poverty.

The conventional approach examines poverty-nutrition linkage in terms of biological and behavioural variables. In India too, the observed reductions are explained in terms of changes in consumer preferences and resulting increases in cost of calories (Radhakrishna, 1991; Radhakrishna and Ravi, 1992; Perspective Planning Division (PPD), 1993). The present study seeks to examine the poverty-food and nutrition linkage with an all-India perspective and explain the findings in terms of inter-state disparities and intra-state distributions. What distinguishes the analysis in this paper from the conventional approach is that the question of food and nutrition security is examined in a wider context considering changes in institutions and development parameters and also the data generating process.[4] The paper is structured as follows: Section 2 examines the question of food and nutrition security at the all-India level. Section 3 provides a state-wise profile and its implications. Section 4 deals with incidence, depth and severity of calorie deficiency across states and other distributional features. The final section concludes the paper.

2. FOOD AND NUTRITION SECURITY: AN ALL-INDIA PROFILE

Food security has been defined in different ways depending upon whether the question is examined at the global, national or individual level: (i) less world hunger; (ii) stability in foodgrain prices; (iii) ample foodgrain availability in a region or country; (iv) national self-sufficiency in food, and (v) availability of foreign exchange to finance foodgrain imports into a country (Adelman and Berck, 1991). Reutlinger and Knapp (1980) defined food security as a state wherein the probability of a given population's foodgrains consumption falling below a minimal nutritional standard is low. An understanding and appreciation of and policy solutions considered for promoting food security differs depending upon the way the concept is defined and measured. The same applies to the studies on India.[5]

It is now generally agreed that a society is food secure when it has both economic and physical access to food for an active and healthy life (World Bank, 1986). Nutrition security refers to realisation of the potential for food security.[6] In this paper, food and nutrition security is verified by examining actual food and calorie intake with reference to stipulated norms (PPD, 1979; p. 7)—2,400 calories and 2,100 calories per capita per day for the rural and urban sectors respectively—for the following reasons.[7] Food security, as measured by (i) imports as a proportion of domestic food production; (ii) per capita availability of foodgrains; (iii) proportion of per capita income required to buy a unit of food; and (iv) relative increases in per capita income at current prices and prices of items in the food basket, has improved considerably in India (Tyagi, 1990). Alternative measures like changes in the relative prices of food indicate that low-income groups, which spend a larger proportion of their income on foodgrains than the upper income groups, have benefited more than the latter from the Green Revolution in India (Rao, 1994). Estimates of poverty show a decline in the proportion of population having a consumption level below a pre-specified normative minimum in the 1980s in both rural and urban all-India (PPD, 1993; Minhas, Jain and Tendulkar, 1991; Tendulkar, Sundaram and Jain, 1993). The normative minimum is defined in terms of calorie intake and the Indian poor obtain about 85 per cent of their calorie intake from cereals (Bhattacharya *et al.*,

1991; p. 53). Thus, the finding that poverty has declined should confirm the results based on macro parameters. Simultaneously, per capita net foodgrain production increased from 132.43 kg in 1950–1 to 179.13 kg in 1993–4 and per capita net cereal production from 110.41 kg to 166.24 kg during the same period (GOI, 1997a).[8] Government policy measures to ensure better and regular availability of foodgrains through appropriate changes in public stocks and imports of foodgrains seem to have succeeded to some extent. The average availability of cereals as well as foodgrains has been higher than their average net production. The NSS results show an increase in the proportion of households reporting availability of adequate food throughout the year between 1983 and 1993–4. It increased from 81.1 per cent to 94 per cent in rural all-India and from 93.3 per cent to 98.1 per cent in urban all-India (NSSO, 1998; p. 61). All these factors together should imply an improvement in cereal consumption and nutrition intake. However, micro empirical verification does not confirm these findings.

The measures and analyses referred to earlier do not reveal anything about the underlying dynamics of changes in institutional and production structures and their adverse implications on food and nutrition security at the micro level. Over time, during the era of poverty reduction till the mid-80s,[9] landlessness and casualisation of labour increased due to growing demographic pressures on available limited land. As a result, the endowment set of the poor diminished from land and labour to only labour. Simultaneously, agriculture got increasingly commercialised involving changes in cropping patterns. Between 1960–1 and 1989–90 per capita daily availability of rice increased from 201.10 gms to 212.60 gms (by 5.72 per cent), that of wheat from 79.10 gms to 132.90 gms (by 68.02 per cent) while that of other cereals decreased from 119.50 gms to 87.10 gms (by 27.12 per cent) (GOI, 1992; p. 136). The decline in coarse cereal availability, along with changes in production conditions and rural labour markets, necessitated changes in the cereal consumption pattern in favour of superior and costlier cereals. This meant an increase in average cereal cost and hence, reduction in the entitlement set.[10] This seems to have accounted for the decline in total cereal consumption of some of the rural poor decile groups.

The observed changes in the cereal consumption basket could be also due to changes in relative prices in favour of superior cereals under the new production and availability conditions. This must be true of the population groups participating in the food market. The prices of *jowar, bajra, ragi* and other coarse cereals have increased faster relative to those of superior cereals since 1964–5. The market dependent consumers must have responded to the changing relative prices by rearranging their purchases in favour of superior cereals whose relative prices had fallen. As a result, total cereal quantity consumed must have declined because coarse cereals were still cheaper than superior cereals in terms of absolute prices.

Thus, there has been a reduction in economic access mainly in the rural areas in spite of an increase in physical access due to growth in domestic cereal production. The poor's preference for variety in consumption over their nutrient content is another reason for the decline in cereal consumption. Such preference patterns may be the result of growing commercialisation and integration of the rural economy into the market economy (Vaidyanathan, 1994; p. 3,151). For instance, for the poorest decile group, total consumption at constant prices increased by 27.68 per cent between 1977–8 and 1988–9. The commodities which largely accounted for this increase were cereals and cereal substitutes; fruits, vegetables and nuts; durable and miscellaneous goods and services; edible oils; beverages and refreshments; milk and milk products; *paan*, tobacco and intoxicants; fuel and light; pulses, and sugar that ranged between 1.04 per cent to 6.82 per cent (Suryanarayana, 1995; p. 230). Cereal consumer expenditure declined for all the decile groups in the rural sector except the poorest three. When the rural population is considered as a whole, total consumer expenditure increased by 5.99 per cent. The commodities that accounted for such an increase were fruits and vegetables, beverages and refreshments, edible oils, and milk and milk products. The increase ranged between 1.25 per cent and 3.31 per cent (Suryanarayana, 1995; p. 235). The experience of the urban population was similar to that of the rural. Total consumer expenditure at constant prices increased by 14.12 per cent for the poorest decile group during the second period. This was largely accounted for by durable and miscellaneous goods and services; milk and milk products; edible oils; and fruits, vegetables and nuts that ranged between 1.45 per cent and 4.16 per cent (Suryanarayana, 1995; p. 242). These four commodity groups accounted for the bulk of the increases in total real consumption for other decile groups and also for the whole urban population.

As a result, the nutrient intake of the poor as well as the general population in rural and urban India declined (Suryanarayana, 1997a). Cereal consumption of the rural poorest decile group has increased but is marked by large fluctuations. Its level of cereal consumption even today falls short of the subsistence requirement level of 11.58 kg per month recommended by the Indian Council of Medical Research (ICMR) and far below the cereal bundle (15.46 kg per month) corresponding to the class interval enclosing the poverty line for 1973–4 (Suryanarayana, 1997b; p. 214). Monthly per capita cereal consumption of the rural population as a whole and those of the third and fourth poorest rural decile groups have declined since the early 1960s. This has happened in spite of the increases in total expenditure, and levels of cereal consumption which are below the poverty line cereal bundle. As regards the urban sector, monthly per capita consumption of cereals has fluctuated around a stationary level for the poorer decile groups and for the population as a whole. This is surprising, since barring a couple of years, in the early sixties cereal consumption levels for all the decile groups concerned and the urban population as a whole have been below the ICMR norm. The general picture, therefore, is one of decline in cereal consumption in the rural sector and no improvement in the urban sector in spite of an apparent increase in per capita real expenditure (Suryanarayana, 1997a).

The diversification of the consumption basket has been at the cost of calorie intake. Calorie intake has not improved at all between 1972–3 and 1993–4 (NSSO, 1989a and 1997b). The average per capita intake of calorie per diem declined from 2,511 in 1961–2 to 2,266 in 1972–3, increased to 2,328 in 1973–4 but declined to 2,221 in 1983 and further to 2,153 in rural India. The corresponding estimates for urban India are 2,063, 2,107, 2,003, 2,089 and 2,071 respectively (Centre for Development Studies, 1977; NSSO, 1989a and 1997b). The intake of calorie per rural consumer unit per diem was 2,781 calories in 1983 and 2,683 in 1993–4. Between these two years, rural protein consumption declined from 78 gms to 75.0 gms per consumer unit per diem while fat intake increased from 34 gms to 39.1 gms respectively. In urban India, the corresponding estimates are 2,574 (2,542) calories of energy, 70 gms (70.2 gms) of protein and 46 (51.6) gms of fat in 1983 (1993–4). The calorie intake in urban India fell short of the minimum requirement of 2,700 calories per diem per consumer unit. The levels of protein and fat consumption were higher than the minimum required level in both rural and urban areas (NSSO, 1989a; p. 29). The calorie intakes of all the poorer decile groups were below the ICMR recommended daily intake of 2,150 calories and the PPD (1979; p.7) norms of 2,400 for rural India and 2,100 for urban India. In sum, hunger had declined but not malnutrition.[11]

Such reductions in nutritional intake in an era of reduction in poverty and growth in foodgrain production has to be explained. It could be that with development and urbanisation, people consume more food purchased from outside the home. The NSS treats prepared food items as 'beverages'. The NSS estimates show an increase in the proportion of total expenditure (at 1970–1 prices) on 'beverages and refreshments' and 'fruits, vegetables and nuts' for the entire rural population from 2.66 to 4.21 and from 4.82 to 7.24 per cent respectively between 1970–1 and 1988–9. Similar increases could be observed for the rural poorer decile groups also. As regards the urban sector, the increases are perceptible only with respect to 'fruits, vegetables and nuts' (Suryanarayana, 1995). Perhaps with improvements in public health facilities, people tend to use the limited calorie intake more efficiently. All these issues emphasise the need for a careful verification of their cumulative impact in terms of anthropometric measures and other indicators like mortality, morbidity and productivity at work.[12] Available anthropometric evidence from the NNMB repeat surveys for 1975–9 and 1988–90 show some improvement in the nutritional status. The nutritional status of school children as measured by weight-for-age improved significantly. The proportion of normal children had increased (NNMB, 1991). Such improvements could be due to better health care, education and awareness and nutrition support through various welfare programmes.

Still, the problem continues to be serious. Estimates for 1992–3 show that the proportions of underweight (moderate and severe) children in rural and urban India are 55.90 and 45.20 per cent respectively (UNDP, 1997a; p. 49). The all-India picture is only an average picture of the experiences of heterogeneous states which differ widely with respect to growth and development experiences. Hence, the results on stagnant cereal consumption and declining calorie intake has to be examined in terms of a state-wise profile. Therefore, in the following section, an attempt is made to understand the inter-regional dimensions of the problem, its determinants and consequences.

3. STATE-WISE PROFILE

Macro estimates for India show an increase in per capita food production and cereal availability.[13] Yet, for a variety of economic and structural reasons, cereal consumption and calorie intake have declined. At the state level, changes in production and cereal availability have not been uniform in sign and size. As a result, inter-state disparities in production have increased. About 50 per cent of the increase in foodgrains production in the post-green revolution period came from less than 15 per cent of the area under foodgrains (GOI, 1985). The co-efficient of variation in per capita foodgrain production across states increased form 57.21 per cent in 1970–1 to 78.88 per cent in 1987–8 (Suryanarayana, 1996).[14] At a time when casualisation and market dependence of the poor is increasing, what is relevant is disparity in marketed surplus which is much higher than that in production since surpluses are confined to only a few states. For instance, in 1988–9, Punjab alone accounted for 52 per cent of the total foodgrain procurement; the rest coming from Haryana, Uttar Pradesh and Andhra Pradesh (Krishnan, 1992). Yet, thanks to active government intervention and increasing market integration across states, inter-state disparities in physical access to foodgrains in both the rural and urban sectors have declined. For instance, the coefficient of variation in rural per capita cereal consumption across states decreased from 14.98 per cent in 1972–3 to 10.39 per cent in 1987–8; the corresponding decline with respect to the urban sector being from 13.95 per cent to 10.30 per cent (Suryanarayana, 1996). Still, as at the all-India level, there has been a decline in per capita cereal consumption in almost all the states except Kerala (Suryanarayana, 1996).

While the all-India picture aggregates the experiences of states specialised in rice, wheat, *jowar* etc., the regional differences in crop composition, in turn, correspond to the predominant cereal in the consumption pattern of different states. A state-wise analysis for the period 1960–1 to 1990–1 shows that the decline in total cereal consumption in the states of Andhra Pradesh, Gujarat, Karnataka, Maharashtra, Rajasthan and Uttar Pradesh occurred largely on account of a decline in coarse cereal consumption (Suryanarayana, 1996). These are the states where coarse cereal is a major food crop for production and consumption.

Thus, there has been a decline in inter-state disparities in calorie intake with respect to both the rural and urban sectors (Table 1). As regards the rural sector, the range [i.e. (Xmax-Xmin)], which was (3,147–1,631) in 1961–2 decreased to (2,677–1,861) in 1983 and further down to (2,491–1,884) in 1993–4; the corresponding picture for the urban sector being a decline from (2,469–1,554) to (2,255–2,000) during the first period but an increase to (2,261–1,922) during the second period. However, inter-state disparities in calorie intake in both rural and urban sectors have declined since 1972–3. The reduction in the disparities in rural India occurred as a result of an increase in the minimum value and a decrease in the maximum value. The increase in the minimum value could be the result of increases

TABLE 1. AVERAGE CALORIE INTAKE PER CAPITA PER DIEM ACROSS STATES

State	*Rural Sector*			*Urban Sector*		
	1973–74	*1983*	*1993–94*	*1973–74*	*1983*	*1993–94*
Andhra Pradesh	2209	2204	2052	2121	2009	1992
Assam	2105	2056	1983	2031	2043	2108
Bihar	2186	2189	2115	2300	2131	2188
Gujarat	2180	2113	1994	2230	2000	2027
Haryana	2971	2554	2491	2244	2242	2140
Karnataka	2211	2260	2073	1995	2124	2026
Kerala	1534	1884	1965	1760	2049	1966
Madhya Pradesh	2422	2323	2164	2108	2137	2062
Maharashtra	2044	2144	1939	2163	2028	1989
Orissa	2125	2103	2199	2164	2219	2261
Punjab	2818	2677	2418	2355	2100	2089
Rajasthan	2719	2433	2470	2243	2255	2184
Tamil Nadu	2012	1861	1884	2092	2140	1922
Uttar Pradesh	2450	2399	2307	2046	2043	2114
West Bengal	2070	2027	2211	2196	2048	2131
All-India	2328	2221	2153	2003	2089	2071
Coefficient of variation (per cent)	12.04	8.48	7.62	5.40	3.41	4.07

Source: CDS (1975), NSSO (1989a, 1997b), and Sengupta and Joshi (1978).

in physical and economic access to cereals in deficit states like Kerala. The decrease in the maximum value of calorie intake could have resulted from increased cost of cereals in the predominantly coarse cereal consuming states like Rajasthan and diversification of the consumption baskets in the prosperous states like Punjab. But the relative rankings of states in terms of calorie intake varied between years and hence, it is not possible to draw a one-to-one correspondence between the changes in calorie intake and that in the structural and institutional parameters explained in the preceding section. Still it would be worthwhile to explain the inter-state variations in average calorie intake and examine their policy implications.

To begin with, the average calorie intakes of both rural (2,153 calories) and urban populations (2,071 calories) in 1993–4 fell short of their normative minimum (2,400 and 2,100 calories respectively) considered by the Planning Commission Task Force (PPD, 1979). The state-wise dispersion about this average reveals another picture. As regards the rural population, only Haryana, Punjab and Rajasthan had an average calorie intake more than the normative minimum. On the other hand, on the urban front, about seven states consisting of Assam, Bihar, Haryana, Orissa, Rajasthan, Uttar Pradesh and West Bengal had an average calorie intake more than the urban norm of 2,100 calories.

How do we explain such disparities? One obvious choice would be measures of physical access like foodgrain production and of economic access like income/total expenditure and costs of cereals. Select empirical results (for some years till 1983) from Suryanarayana (1996) and the results for 1993–4 are presented in Table 2.

3.1 Rural Sector

The results for the year 1961–2 indicate that foodgrain production and unit cost of cereals, as measured by their unit values, explain about 64 per cent of the variation in calorie intake across states. The coefficients of these two variables were significant and had the expected positive and negative signs respectively. As for 1972–3 and 1973–4, cereal cost emerges as the major and only significant explanatory variable accounting for a substantial part of the inter-state variation in calorie intake. For 1983, in addition to unit cost of cereals, inequality in land distribution and foodgrain production per head of rural population, which together measure foodgrain scarcity in rural areas, emerge as significant variables. Together, they accounted for about 86 per cent of the inter-state variation in calorie intake. The results for 1993–4, though weaker statistically, indicated that cereal availability and cereal costs were important in explaining inter-state variations in calorie intake.[15]

3.2 Urban Sector

For the year 1961–2, state per capita food production, unit cost of cereals and monthly per capita consumer expenditure together explained about 70 per cent of the variation. Cereal cost and availability explained variation in urban calorie intake in 1972–3 to a significant extent. As regards 1973–4, only cereal cost emerged as the significant explanatory variable. The results for 1983 and 1993–4 were statistically perverse.[16]

TABLE 2. ESTIMATED PARAMETERS OF THE MODEL ON INTER-STATE VARIATIONS IN PER CAPITA CALORIE INTAKE: 1993–94

Regressand	*Functional form*	*Intercept*	*Agricultural/Non-Agricultural income per head of rural/urban population (AIPHRP/ NAIPHUP) at current all-India prices*	*Lorenz ratio in operational land distribution*	*Unit values of cereals*	*Foodgrain production per head of rural population (FPPHRP)*	*Average monthly per capita total consumer expenditure (AMPCTCE) at current all-India prices*	*R-square*	*R-square adjusted*
				Rural Sector					
Average per capita calorie intake	Linear	2808.09*** (4.52)	–	(-)8.10 ((-)0.69)	(-)82.46 ((-)1.71)	0.26 (1.52)	0.58 (0.51)	0.54	0.35
"	"	2589.41*** (4.27)	(-)0.09 ((-)1.25)	2.34 (0.22)	(-)94.32** ((-)2.12)	0.60** (1.93)	–	0.59	0.43
"	"	2518.62*** (10.03)	–	(-)1593.30** ((-)2.82)	(-)86.05** ((-)1.97)	0.22 (1.69)	–	0.52	0.44
				Urban Sector					
Average per capita calorie intake	Linear	2332.13*** (11.07)	0.01 (0.69)	(-)55.42 ((-)1.46)	(-)0.06 ((-)0.43)	–	–	0.19	(-)0.06

(Table 2 contd...)

(Table 2 continued)

Regressand	*Functional form*	*Intercept*	*Agricultural/Non-Agricultural income per head of rural/urban population (AIPHRP/ NAIPHUP) at current all-India prices*	*Lorenz ratio in operational land distribution*	*Unit values of cereals*	*Foodgrain production per head of rural population (FPPHRP)*	*Average monthly per capita total consumer expenditure (AMPCTCE) at current all-India prices*	*R-square*	*R-square adjusted*
"	"	2959.27*** (12.10)	-	(-)22.26 ((-)0.93)	0.12 (1.23)	-	(-)1.79 ((-)0.54)	0.58	0.46
"	"	2332.38*** (11.32)	-	(-)41.33 (1.32)	(-)0.01 ((-)0.06)	-	-	0.16	0.02

Notes: (i) Estimates of rural and urban calorie intake are from NSSO (1997b; p. 15).

(ii) Estimates of rural and urban average per capita cereal consumption are from NSSO (1996; p. 33).

(iii) Estimates of rural unit values of cereals are obtained by dividing total consumer expenditure on cereals by cereal quantities consumed from NSSO (1996; pp. A-67–A-99 & A-133–A-165) and urban unit cereals consumption are from NSSO (1996; pp. 100–A-132 & A-166–A-198).

(iv) Estimates of state-wise total agricultural and non-agricultural income are from EPW Research Foundation (1998; pp. 87–111).

(v) Estimates of state-wise total foodgrains production are from GOI (1997b; pp. S-19–S-21).

(vi) Estimates of rural and urban AMPCTCE at state-specific current prices are from NSSO (1996; pp. 25–28).

(vii) Estimates of AIPHRP and MPCTCE at current all-India prices are obtained using price indices from Minhas and Jain (1990; pp. 346–347).

(viii) Estimates of NAIHUP and urban AMPCTCE at current all-India prices are obtained using price indices from Minhas, Jain and Saluja (1990; p. 229).

(ix) Estimates of Lorenz ratio of operational holdings in various states for the year 1981–82 are from NSSO (1997b; p. 26).

(x) Figures in parentheses are t-ratios and (**) indicates significance for a two-tail test at 5 per cent level, and (***) at 1 per cent level.

In sum, economic access as determined by income/expenditure and cereal cost, and physical access to foodgrains as measured by foodgrain production appeared as the major policy variables for reducing inter-state disparities in calorie intake. Hence, an instrument like the PDS, which can ensure adequate foodgrain availability at reasonable and stable prices, can be an effective policy option in addressing issues regarding calorie deficiency and malnutrition.[17] These results only provide us a profile across states. However, to answer concrete questions in terms of magnitudes and trade-offs, we need to have a better understanding of the question of incidence, depth and severity of calorie deficiency, which is attempted in the next section.

4. CALORIE DEFICIENCY: INCIDENCE, DEPTH AND SEVERITY

Estimates of incidence of calorie deficiency, its depth and severity can be meaningfully examined if juxtaposed with estimates for similar dimensions of poverty. Such estimates can be made on the basis of the NSS data available currently for the years 1983 and 1993–4. But the NSS data is available in the form of size distribution of consumer expenditure, calorie intake, etc. Such data do not permit an easy and accurate estimation of the three different aspects of poverty/calorie deficiency under consideration here. In such a context, poverty measures can be estimated either through interpolation by fitting a distribution function to the grouped data or based on parameterised Lorenz curves. Poverty measures can be derived from parameterised Lorenz curves using the following two functions:

Lorenz curve: $L = L(p; \pi)$
Poverty measure: $P = P(\pi/z, \pi)$

where L is the share of the bottom p per cent of the population in aggregate consumption, π is a vector of (estimable) parameters of the Lorenz curve, P is a poverty measure expressed as a function of the average consumption π to the poverty line z, and the parameters of the Lorenz curve.[18]

In this paper, the focus is only on the Foster-Greer-Thorbecke (FGT) (Foster, Greer, Thorbecke, 1984) class of poverty measures given by:

$$P_\alpha = \int_0^z [\frac{x-x}{z}]^a f(x)\, dx \quad \alpha \geq 0 \qquad (1)$$

where x is the household consumption expenditure, f(x) is its density, z denotes the poverty line, and a is a non-negative parameter. We consider the FGT measures for values of (= 0,1 and 2, that is, measures of incidence, depth and severity of poverty respectively).

The Lorenz curve specifications considered for the estimation of these poverty measures are (i) the General Quadratic Lorenz curve (Villasenor and Arnold, 1984, 1989); and (ii) the Beta Lorenz curve (Kakwani, 1980). Between the two specifications of the Lorenz curve, a choice is made on the basis of goodness-of-fit criterion.

The estimates of poverty for both the rural and urban sectors of fifteen selected states for the year 1983 are made with reference to the poverty lines suggested by the Expert Group (PPD, 1993). Poverty is a function of both mean and inequality parameters of the distribution. In the same way, incidence of calorie deficiency also depends on the mean and inequality parameters of the calorie intake distribution. From Tables 4, 5, 8 and 9, it can be seen that in both the rural and urban sectors across states, inequalities in calorie intake distribution are less than half of those in consumer expenditure distribution. This is only to be expected in terms of Engel's law about consumer behaviour. Other results are as follows:

4.1 Rural Sector

The incidence of rural poverty in 1983 in the country as a whole was 43.49 per cent while the depth and severity of poverty were 11.90 and 4.49 per cent respectively (Table 3).[19] Of the fifteen states considered here, six, viz., Bihar, Madhya Pradesh, Orissa, Tamil Nadu, Uttar Pradesh and West Bengal had incidence, depth and severity of rural poverty much above the national rural averages. In Madhya Pradesh, Maharashtra and Orissa, the elasticities of the three rural poverty measures with respect to the rural mean consumption were substantial and exceeded the corresponding national estimate, thus implying scope for a strategy of growth for poverty reduction in these states.[20] On the other hand, the incidence of rural calorie deficiency exceeded half of the rural population in all the states except Punjab and Haryana. While the incidence (67.53 per cent), depth (21.96 per cent) and severity (9.71 per cent) of rural poverty were the highest in Orissa, the corresponding aspects of calorie deficiency were 72.8, 17.56 and 6.02 per cent respectively; that is, the depth and severity dimensions of calorie shortfall were less than those of income shortfall. Tamil Nadu, with an incidence of rural poverty of 53.6 per cent, had a much higher incidence of calorie deficiency at 87.18 per cent involving an aggregate rural calorie shortfall of 27.21 per cent. In rural Bihar, the

TABLE 3. MEASURES OF DIFFERENT ASPECTS OF POVERTY AND CALORIE DEFICIENCY ACROSS STATES: RURAL SECTOR (1983)

State	P_0 *(per cent)*	P_1 *(per cent)*	P_2 *(per cent)*	*Incidence of calorie deficiency* (C_0)	*Calorie Gap index* (C_1)	*Severity of calorie deficiency* (C_2)
Andhra Pradesh	27.05	5.88	1.76	72.18	13.27	3.61
Assam	42.09	8.09	2.25	81.89	16.35	4.37
Bihar	65.19	19.92	8.17	68.92	15.13	4.74
Gujarat	27.07	5.00	1.39	75.50	15.77	4.48
Haryana	19.21	3.63	1.07	49.04	8.02	1.91
Karnataka	35.93	9.63	3.56	64.30	14.30	4.76
Kerala	39.21	9.91	3.50	83.73	25.51	9.80
Madhya Pradesh	48.96	13.61	5.12	64.04	11.43	2.97
Maharashtra	45.28	11.35	3.85	77.99	14.25	3.49
Orissa	67.53	21.96	9.71	72.80	17.56	6.02
Punjab	14.31	2.42	0.65	40.35	7.27	2.13
Rajasthan	34.20	9.15	3.42	58.18	8.75	2.00
Tamil Nadu	53.60	17.02	7.23	87.18	27.21	10.69
Uttar Pradesh	45.51	12.31	4.55	57.51	10.36	2.75
West Bengal	62.24	20.59	9.23	77.36	20.84	8.05
All-India	43.39	11.90	4.49	68.75	14.09	4.15

Note: Author's estimates based on NSSO (1986 & 1989c).

incidence of calorie deficiency exceeded that of poverty by 5.72 per cent; but the depth and severity dimensions of calorie deficiency fell short of their poverty counterparts by 24.05 and 41.98 per cent respectively. The incidence of calorie deficiency, its depth and severity were almost three times the corresponding dimensions of poverty in the rural areas of Gujarat and Punjab. A similar picture was obtained for other states like Andhra Pradesh, Haryana, Karnataka and Kerala implying that nutrition security is not simply a question of economic access to foodgrains.

The aggregate shortfall of calorie intake, as measured by the calorie deficiency depth measure for rural all-India, was only 14.09 per cent. Rural aggregate calorie shortfall exceeded 10 per cent in the states of Andhra Pradesh, Assam, Bihar, Gujarat, Karnataka, Kerala, Madhya Pradesh, Maharashtra, Orissa, Tamil Nadu, Uttar Pradesh and West

Bengal (Table 3). Barring Kerala, all these states had a rural average per capita cereal consumption level more than the ICMR norm of 11.58 kg per month (Table 4). By 1993–4 Gujarat, Kerala, Maharashtra and Punjab reported a rural average per capita cereal consumption level that was less than the ICMR norm (Table 5). That the incidence of calorie deficiency and calorie gap in the rural areas of these states were substantial could be due to inadequate cereal consumption (as a result of either inadequate economic and physical access to cereals or changing consumer preferences).

Between 1983 and 1993–4, as per the Expert Group methodology, rural poverty declined in almost all the states except Assam and Haryana (PPD, 1993, p. 39; GOI, 1997b, p. 26). Rural average intake of calorie per capita per diem declined in all the states and India as a whole; Kerala, Orissa, Rajasthan, Tamil Nadu and West Bengal being the exceptions (Table 1). One important reason, apart from the increasing cost of cereals, is that of diversification of consumption patterns as evidenced by a decline in the expenditure proportion on food and a decline in the relative importance of cereals as a source of calories (Tables 4 and 5).[21] Along with the decline in rural average calorie intake, the inequality in its distribution had declined virtually in almost all the states except Haryana and Maharashtra (Tables 4 and 5). However, incidence of rural calorie deficiency increased in all states except Kerala, Orissa and West Bengal (where it declined between two to six per cent) and Rajasthan (where the reduction was substantial 12.9 per cent) (Tables 3 and 6). However, proportionate shortfall of calories and severity of calorie deficiency declined in the rural sectors at the all-India level, and across seven states (Bihar, Kerala, Orissa, Rajasthan, Tamil Nadu, Uttar Pradesh and West Bengal).

In sum, incidence of calorie deficiency increased in rural India as a whole with a decline in its proportionate gap and severity. There was also a decline in rural average protein intake in all states except Haryana, Kerala, Orissa, Rajasthan and West Bengal; still the average quantity consumed exceeded the normative level in these states. Rural average fat intake, on the other hand, increased in all the states (Tables 4 and 5).

4.2 Urban Sector

The incidence of urban poverty in 1983 in the country as a whole was 38.08 per cent while the depth and severity of poverty were 10.46 and 4 per cent respectively (Table 7). Of the fifteen states considered here,

TABLE 4. MEASURES OF FOOD AND NUTRITION SECURITY ACROSS STATES: RURAL SECTOR (1983)

State	*Monthly Per Capita Consumer Expenditure at current all-India prices*	*Lorenz ratio (per cent) of Consumption Distribution*	*Avg. Calorie Intake Per Capita Per Diem (cal.)*	*Lorenz ratio (per cent) of Calorie Intake Distribution*	*Monthly Avg. Per Capita Cereal Consumption (kg)*	*Percentage of Total Intake of Calories from Cereals*	*Percentage Expenditure on Food*	*Avg. Protein Intake Per Capita Per Diem (gm)*	*Avg. Fat Intake Per Capita Per Diem (gm)*
Andhra Pradesh	131.04	29.68	2204.00	12.75	15.37	79.74	60.19	56	24
Assam	105.59	19.85	2056 00	10.76	14.25	79.73	73.33	52	18
Bihar	84.03	25.93	2189.00	15.22	15.88	81.97	73.65	65	20
Gujarat	122.50	26.05	2113.00	12.78	12.61	64.60	66.66	59	44
Haryana	144.76	27.63	2554.00	15.61	14.63	63.82	63.54	78	47
Karnataka	121.52	30.37	2260.00	16.68	15.11	75.65	63.27	60	26
Kerala	126.27	33.88	1884.00	17.97	10.06	60.96	61.43	47	32
Madhya Pradesh	106.04	29.60	2323.00	14.25	16.03	77.30	65.92	68	25
Maharashtra	104.25	28.84	2144.00	11.21	13.83	73.41	61.17	62	30
Orissa	88.75	27.00	2103.00	15.86	15.62	85.07	73.69	51	13
Punjab	160.22	28.85	2677.00	16.56	13.61	57.46	58.26	79	52
Rajasthan	131.58	34.59	2433.00	13.75	17.37	73.27	60.73	75	42
Tamil Nadu	101.85	32.91	1861.00	19.20	13.07	75.69	64.63	47	22
Uttar Pradesh	112.37	29.41	2399.00	14.86	15.69	73.18	63.48	73	29
West Bengal	190.11	28.84	2027.00	18.07	14.29	80.47	73.92	52	17
All-India	112.68	30.10	2221.00	14.69	14.57	75.16	65.46	62	27

Source: Author's estimates based on Jain and Minhas (1991); Minhas and Jain (1990), NSSO (1986 & 1989b, c).

TABLE 5. MEASURES OF FOOD AND NUTRITION SECURITY ACROSS STATES: RURAL SECTOR (1993–94)

State	*Monthly Per Capita Consumer Expenditure at current all-India prices*	*Lorenz ratio (per cent) of Consumption Distribution*	*Avg. Calorie Intake Per Capita Per Diem (cal.)*	*Lorenz ratio (per cent) of Calorie Intake Distribution*	*Monthly Avg. Per Capita Cereal Consumption (kg)*	*Percentage of Total Intake of Calories from Cereals*	*Percentage Expenditure on Food*	*Avg. Protein Intake Per Capita Per Diem (gm)*	*Avg. Fat Intake Per Capita Per Diem (gm)*
Andhra Pradesh	310.43	28.97	2052.00	11.25	13.27	74.43	59.60	50.80	27.20
Assam	230.66	17.86	1983.00	8.74	13.17	76.46	72.30	49.50	21.00
Bihar	195.26	22.48	2115.00	11.86	14.31	77.51	71.00	60.20	23.00
Gujarat	293.91	24.04	1994.00	11.78	10.70	59.61	67.10	55.60	47.40
Haryana	346.85	31.33	2491.00	15.65	12.92	58.98	60.10	78.40	53.60
Karnataka	278.86	26.97	2073.00	11.93	13.15	72.43	62.00	55.10	28.60
Kerala	337.14	30.20	1965.00	13.95	10.11	59.36	60.50	50.80	32.70
Madhya Pradesh	259.00	28.04	2164.00	11.84	14.20	75.05	61.20	63.00	28.30
Maharashtra	252.40	30.65	1939.00	11.92	11.39	66.80	59.50	54.80	33.50
Orissa	210.35	24.55	2199.00	10.75	15.93	83.31	68.10	52.70	14.80
Punjab	390.09	28.34	2418.00	12.17	10.78	50.68	57.90	74.70	59.80
Rajasthan	345.17	26.56	2470.00	11.08	14.85	67.11	62.30	79.40	52.80
Tamil Nadu	292.45	31.25	1884.00	13.19	11.72	71.32	62.80	46.80	24.70
Uttar Pradesh	301.91	28.16	2307.00	11.65	13.91	68.68	61.50	70.40	35.50
West Bengal	224.64	25.47	2211.00	10.61	14.96	77.59	66.80	54.80	21.40
All-India	281.40	28.54	2153.00	11.33	13.40	71.03	63.20	60.20	31.40

Note: Author's estimates based on Minhas and Jain (1990), NSSO (1996 & 1997b).

TABLE 6. MEASURES OF CALORIE DEFICIENCY ACROSS STATES: RURAL SECTOR (1993–94)

State	*Incidence of calorie deficiency* (C_0)	*Calorie Gap index* (C_1)	*Severity of calorie deficiency* (C_2)
Andhra Pradesh	82.52	16.77	4.62
Assam	91.68	17.81	4.61
Bihar	75.01	14.86	4.26
Gujarat	83.90	18.90	5.51
Haryana	51.46	9.33	2.44
Karnataka	76.74	16.22	4.67
Kerala	81.98	20.44	6.90
Madhya Pradesh	72.84	13.73	3.64
Maharashtra	89.12	21.28	6.34
Orissa	68.42	11.86	3.19
Punjab	52.77	8.16	1.90
Rajasthan	45.19	6.72	1.50
Tamil Nadu	88.11	23.09	7.75
Uttar Pradesh	62.93	10.23	2.32
West Bengal	72.14	11.74	2.77
All-India	74.50	13.75	3.57

Note. Author's estimates based on Minhas and Jain (1990), NSSO (1996 & 1997b).

the states of Bihar, Karnataka, Kerala, Madhya Pradesh, Orissa, Tamil Nadu and Uttar Pradesh had incidence, depth and severity of urban poverty much above the all-India urban average. The incidence of calorie deficiency exceeded half of the urban population in all the states except Haryana, Orissa and Rajasthan. While the incidence of urban poverty was the highest in Madhya Pradesh (51.42 per cent), Kerala ranked first in terms of its depth (15.08 per cent) and severity (6.35 per cent). Once again, Tamil Nadu, whose urban poor proportion was only 44.56 per cent, topped the calorie deficiency list with an incidence of 75.34 per cent, calorie gap of 18.97 per cent and severity of calorie deficiency of 6.49 per cent. The aggregate shortfall of calorie intake, as measured by the calorie deficiency depth measure for urban all-India, was only 10.5 per cent. The incidence of urban calorie deficiency exceeded that of urban poverty by less than 2 per cent in

TABLE 7. MEASURES OF DIFFERENT ASPECTS OF POVERTY AND CALORIE DEFICIENCY ACROSS STATES: URBAN SECTOR (1983)

State	P_0 *(per cent)*	P_1 *(per cent)*	P_2 *(per cent)*	*Incidence calorie deficiency* (C_0)	*Calorie index* (C_1) *Severity of calorie deficiency* (C_2)	*Severity of calorie deficiency* (C_2)
Andhra Pradesh	36.74	9.78	3.72	65.28	10.74	2.75
Assam	23.44	5.15	1.62	56.76	9.13	2.45
Bihar	49.64	14.39	5.52	50.18	8.26	2.09
Gujarat	37.75	8.27	2.54	62.96	10.71	2.74
Haryana	19.62	3.98	1.24	41.52	7.28	2.66
Karnataka	40.26	12.28	5.09	52.45	10.27	2.94
Kerala	48.26	15.08	6.35	63.90	16.25	5.54
Madhya Pradesh	51.42	14.24	5.22	52.54	6.58	1.18
Maharashtra	37.55	11.32	4.64	67.82	11.06	2.52
Orissa	48.79	14.14	5.53	40.24	6.37	1.83
Punjab	22.60	4.85	1.51	54.51	11.13	3.36
Rajasthan	38.31	10.12	3.78	41.40	5.59	1.47
Tamil Nadu	44.56	13.51	5.64	75.34	18.97	6.49
Uttar Pradesh	49.32	14.26	5.43	61.71	9.81	2.25
West Bengal	30.71	7.75	2.77	57.91	9.95	2.76
All-India	38.08	10.46	4.00	60.83	10.50	2.67

Note: Author's estimates based on NSSO (1986 & 1989c).

the states of Bihar and Madhya Pradesh; but the depth and severity dimensions of calorie deficiency are about 40 to 50 per cent less than the corresponding dimensions of urban poverty in these two states. The urban aggregate calorie shortfall exceeded 10 per cent in the states of Andhra Pradesh, Gujarat, Karnataka, Kerala, Maharashtra, Punjab and Tamil Nadu. Barring Gujarat, Kerala, Maharashtra, Punjab and Tamil Nadu, all the states had an average per capita cereal consumption level more than the ICMR norm of 11.58 kg per month (Table 8).

By 1993–4, urban poverty declined in all the states in India (PPD, 1993, p. 39; GOI, 1997b, p. 26). Yet, urban average intake of calorie per capita *per diem* increased only in the states of Assam, Bihar, Gujarat, Orissa, Uttar Pradesh and West Bengal; it decreased in the remaining

TABLE 8. MEASURES OF FOOD AND NUTRITION SECURITY ACROSS STATES: URBAN SECTOR (1983)

State	*Monthly Per Capita Consumer Expenditure at current all-India prices*	*Lorenz ratio (per cent) of Consumption Distribution*	*Avg. Calorie Intake Per Capita Per Diem (cal.)*	*Lorenz ratio (per cent) of Calorie Intake Distribution*	*Monthly Avg. Per Capita Cereal Consumption (kg)*	*Percentage of Total Intake of Calories from Cereals*	*Percentage Expenditure on Food*	*Avg. Protein Intake Per Capita Per Diem (gm)*	*Avg. Fat Intake Per Capita Per Diem (gm)*
Andhra Pradesh	182.17	31.82	2009.00	12.41	11.96	68.03	55.27	50	32
Assam	154.39	26.54	2043.00	11.47	12.81	71.56	64.07	52	25
Bihar	135.77	30.82	2131.00	12.61	13.66	72.14	66.20	61	26
Gujarat	155.26	27.76	2000.00	11.99	9.69	53.60	62.08	55	53
Haryana	183.79	31.79	2242.00	14.53	11.72	58.41	55.89	67	49
Karnataka	173.85	34.52	2124.00	15.19	11.77	62.88	60.88	55	36
Kerala	164.11	39.34	2049.00	21.45	10.20	56.41	59.86	51	38
Madhya Pradesh	160.27	30.32	2137.00	10.50	12.42	65.71	60.36	62	36
Maharashtra	166.71	34.80	2028.00	13.36	10.00	55.84	57.67	56	45
Orissa	147.07	30.65	2219.00	12.66	14.21	73.39	66.25	56	24
Punjab	192.73	33.92	2100.00	15.88	10.05	53.72	55.95	63	49
Rajasthan	160.66	30.93	2255.00	12.71	13.03	64.26	56.75	69	47
Tamil Nadu	161.63	36.37	2140.00	29.29	10.41	54.93	59.62	45	29
Uttar Pradesh	155.64	32.32	2043.00	12.08	11.78	64.87	59.32	62	34
West Bengal	184.11	34.49	2048.00	12.84	11.85	65.49	60.82	55	31
All-India	115.02	34.08	2089.00	14.85	11.42	61.43	59.01	57	37

Note: Author's estimates based on Jain and Minhas (1991), Minhas, Jain and Saluja (1990) and NSSO (1986 & 1989b, c).

states and India as a whole (Table 1, 8 and 9). Cereals as a source of calories declined in importance in the urban sector also (Tables 8 and 9).[22] The inequality in urban calorie intake distribution declined in all the states. Incidence of urban calorie deficiency increased only in the states of Haryana, Karnataka, Kerala, Madhya Pradesh and Maharashtra (Tables 7 and 10). Proportionate shortfall of calories and severity of calorie deficiency declined in the majority of the states except Madhya Pradesh. In sum, incidence, depth and severity of calorie deficiency decreased in urban India as a whole between 1983 and 1993–4. The pattern of variation with respect to protein and fat intake differed across states; yet their levels exceeded the normative limits in all states.

The results based on the NSS are confirmed by the NNMB repeat survey for the year 1988–90. The NNMB results show that in addition to Kerala, Gujarat and Madhya Pradesh also enjoyed some improvement with respect to average nutritional intake (NNMB, 1991 and 1996). However, as regards distribution of nutrition security, it was only in Kerala that the incidence of both protein and calorie deficiency had declined, though marginally. A similar marginal improvement in nutritional security could be found in Gujarat. Madhya Pradesh was the only state where there was a marked decline in incidence of calorie deficiency (NNMB, 1991 and 1996). These findings for Madhya Pradesh may not be reliable because of the small sample size. As for a recent picture, the NNMB survey for 1993–4 reported that 47.70 per cent of rural households across eight states had an inadequate calorie intake.[23]

Chronic energy deficiency (CED), as measured by body mass index (BMI),[24] among adults exceeded 50 per cent in six states; the exceptions being Kerala and Tamil Nadu (NNMB, 1996; p. 40).[25] CED was maximum among agricultural labourers (53.1 per cent) followed by marginal (49.5 per cent), small (47.8 per cent) and large farmers (45.9 per cent). Across social groups, CED was 60.9 per cent among the Scheduled Tribes, 53.2 per cent among the Scheduled Castes and 46.8 per cent among others (NNMB, 1996). Among the eight states, severe and moderate forms of malnutrition (body weight less than 75 per cent of standard) among the most vulnerable social groups (pre-school children of 1–3 years) was the least in Kerala (26 per cent) and highest in Gujarat (65 per cent) (NNMB, 1996; p. 26). Contrary to the general impression, the NNMB survey reported a lesser extent of growth retardation among girls than boys; the 'weight status for age' is normal for a larger percentage of girls as compared to that for boys (NNMB, 1996; p. 31). In sum, Kerala stands out in

TABLE 9. MEASURES OF FOOD AND NUTRITION SECURITY ACROSS STATES: URBAN SECTOR (1993–94)

State	*Monthly Per Capita Consumer Expenditure at current all-India prices*	*Lorenz ratio (per cent) of Consumption Distribution*	*Avg. Calorie Intake Per Capita Per Diem (cal.)*	*Lorenz ratio (per cent) of Calorie Intake Distribution*	*Monthly Avg. Per Capita Cereal Consumption (kg)*	*Percentage of Total Intake of Calories from Cereals*	*Percentage Expenditure on Food*	*Avg. Protein Intake Per Capita Per Diem (gm)*	*Avg. Fat Intake Per Capita Per Diem (gm)*
Andhra Pradesh	444.13	32.36	1992.00	10.57	11.30	65.30	53.80	49.60	34.90
Assam	415.19	29.00	2108.00	9.44	12.05	65.62	59.70	53.50	30.80
Bihar	341.42	30.99	2188.00	11.01	12.82	67.10	62.90	61.40	32.70
Gujarat	424.47	29.07	2027.00	10.83	8.96	49.90	58.40	54.90	57.90
Haryana	442.50	28.35	2140 00	9.56	10.46	55.45	53.90	63.60	49.40
Karnataka	418.95	31.83	2026.00	11.55	10.87	61.39	55.70	53.10	37.60
Kerala	472.11	34.37	1966.00	13.15	9.46	55.34	53.90	52.40	37.00
Madhya Pradesh	433.18	33.06	2082.00	9.52	11.32	62.01	52.90	59.80	40.30
Maharashtra	479.89	35.73	1989.00	9.69	9.37	53.53	53.00	57.20	47.90
Orissa	384.84	30.69	2261.00	9.37	13.36	67.84	57.80	61.80	28.10
Punjab	480.91	28.05	2069.00	10.27	8.92	48.86	53.00	66.50	53.70
Rajasthan	411.56	29.34	2184.00	8.73	11.52	59.73	56.70	48.70	51.60
Tamil Nadu	445.42	34.78	1922.00	13.14	10.05	60.15	54.60	63.20	33.90
Uttar Pradesh	426.50	32.63	2114.00	10.68	11.08	59.37	56.00	56.60	41.20
West Bengal	461.72	33.79	2131.00	9.45	11.64	62.40	55.90	57.20	34.20
All-India	458.04	34.42	2071.00	10.51	10.63	58.53	54.70	57	42.00

Note: Author's estimates based on Minhas, Jain and Saluja (1990) and NSSO (1996 & 1997b).

TABLE 10. MEASURES OF CALORIE DEFICIENCY ACROSS STATES: URBAN SECTOR (1993–94)

State	*Incidence of calorie deficiency* (C_0)	*Calorie Gap index* (C_1)	*Severity of calorie deficiency* (C_2)
Andhra Pradesh	63.31	10.11	2.31
Assam	54.11	6.27	1.15
Bihar	44.27	5.94	1.24
Gujarat	58.67	9.29	2.24
Haryana	44.90	5.69	1.33
Karnataka	56.91	9.81	2.57
Kerala	66.74	12.33	3.42
Madhya Pradesh	54.32	7.14	1.38
Maharashtra	68.30	9.68	1.94
Orissa	30.91	3.87	0.84
Punjab	52.18	7.61	1.61
Rajasthan	38.12	4.75	1.06
Tamil Nadu	69.30	13.50	4.01
Uttar Pradesh	54.72	6.94	1.39
West Bengal	47.24	6.04	1.26
All-India	53.88	8.03	1.76

Note: Author's estimates based on NSSO (1996 & 1997b).

terms of the nutritional status of its population though not in terms of nutrient consumption.

The diet of the Indian population is also deficient in micro-nutrients. Three important micro-nutrients which are important for public health are iron, iodine and vitamin A (DeRose and Millman, 1998). Iron is the most common micro-nutrient deficiency among pregnant women whose requirements are higher than those of the rest. During 1975–91, about 88 per cent of women aged 15–49 years were suffering from anaemia (UNDP, 1997b). Among the seven states surveyed by the NNMB in 1993–4, the average iron intake exceeded the recommended dietary intake (RDI) only in Karnataka and Maharashtra (NNMB, 1996; p. 15). Its long-term consequence would be chronic poverty resulting from reduced physical and cognitive development and function. The mean intake of Vitamin A fell short of the RDI norm in all the seven states (NNMB, 1996; p. 15). Deficiency of Vitamin A causes blindness mainly in childhood and increases vulnerability to diseases.

5. CONCLUSION

Much has been made out of the estimates indicating reduction in poverty for the last two decades and their budgetary implications for targeted welfare programmes. The emphasis during the ongoing reform era is on efficiency in resource use. But there is little appreciation of the possibilities for improving efficiency of labour use through improvement in human capital via education and adequate nutrition. This paper attempt to examine and quantify the degree of nutrition security (particularly with reference to calorie intake) across states and in all-India.

Poverty declined between 1983 and 1993–4, as per the estimates by the Expert Group method, in both rural and urban sectors across states in India except Assam and Haryana, where rural poverty had increased. Poverty in India as a whole was 35.97 per cent in 1993–4. It was less than 50 per cent in both rural and urban sectors in all the states of the Indian Union. The proportion of households reporting adequate food availability had increased. Contrary to what one would expect in such a scenario, average calorie intake declined in both rural and urban sectors in the majority of the states and in India as a whole. As a result, incidence of calorie deficiency stood at 75 per cent in rural all-India and 54 per cent in urban all-India in 1993–4.

Thus, hunger had disappeared but not malnutrition. This was because cereal consumption, a major determinant of calorie intake, had declined. The decline was due to increase in costs of cereals as a result of the changes in production conditions, cropping patterns and exchange entitlement of the rural poor, in particular, and also changes in consumer preferences. Accordingly, foodgrain production and cost of cereals emerged as major determinants of calorie intake across states. From this perspective, policy instruments like the PDS have a major role to play in ensuring enough cereal availability and calorie intake in food deficit states like Kerala. Serious attention needs to be paid in almost all states except Haryana, Punjab and Rajasthan where the rural aggregate calorie shortfall was less than 10 per cent of the required amount. The urban aggregate calorie shortfall exceeded 10 per cent in the states of Andhra Pradesh, Kerala and Tamil Nadu. In almost all the states, incidence of calorie deficiency was much higher than that of poverty both in rural and urban areas. If so, poverty alleviation programmes may not ensure nutrition security. Other policies like consumer education programmes may be needed to guide consumer choices. In fact, educating households to improve their diets within the available budget may be the most cost-effective way to improve nutritional status and hence, could prove an effective strategy for growth.

ENDNOTES

1. The term 'nutrition' means utilising food to promote growth, maintenance and the day-to-day functioning of mind and body. Inadequate nutrition imposes costs in terms of productivity and quality of life. An individual is called undernourished if he or she is deficit with respect to all the essential nutrients; and malnourished if he or she suffers from inefficient allocation of nutrients due to incorrect dietary choices or inefficient processing and use of food due to illness or poor hygiene. Diets should be adequate with respect to both protein and energy. An individual is said to suffer from protein-energy malnutrition if his diet is deficient in either or both these components. Two important indicators of protein-energy malnutrition are (i) stunting (low height for age) for children of ages 24 to 59 months; and (ii) wasting (low weight for height) for children of ages 12 to 23 months. While the former indicates chronic (protein-energy) malnutrition, the latter results from acute or short-term malnutrition. Estimates of these two measures for India for the period 1980 to 1990 are 65 per cent and 27 per cent respectively (World Bank, 1993; p. 204).
2. Of course, per capita income has more than doubled during these fifty years; yet the levels of income are abysmally low (GOI, 1997a). Increase in foodgrains production along with effective public intervention has virtually eliminated famine and starvation. Macro estimates, derived from national food balance sheets, show significant improvement in calorie intake as resulting from economic growth in India (Dawson and Tiffin, 1998). Life expectancy doubled from 32.1 years in 1951 to 60.8 years in 1992. Infant mortality declined by more than 50 per cent from 146 in 1951 to 74 deaths per 1,000 live births in 1995 (UNDP, 1997a).
3. Between 1972–3 and 1993–4 average calorie intake declined in all states except in both the rural and urban sectors of Kerala, Maharashtra and West Bengal, the rural sector of Orissa and the urban sectors of Bihar, Karnataka and Tamil Nadu (see Tables 1).
4. This is quite important because during the current era of reforms, the emphasis in discussions on instruments for poverty alleviation and their cost effectiveness is on income transfers and not on its final impact on

nutrition security. This is so in spite of the fact that the poor are identified as those with incomes less than a subsistence minimum, defined with respect to a normative calorie intake level.

5. See Suryanarayana (1997a).
6. This realisation depends upon adequate care, adequate water and sanitation (Haddad *et al.*, 1996).
7. The question of nutrition security is examined with reference to intake of calories. This is because (i) undernourishment in India has to do more with calorie deficiency than with protein deficiency (Sengupta and Joshi, 1978; Sukhatme, 1973 and Sukhatme and Margen, 1978); and (ii) diets that are adequate with respect to calories contain enough protein also (Dasgupta, 1998; DeRose and Millman, 1998; and Lipton and Ravallion, 1995). The estimates of protein intake by decile groups for rural and urban all-India for 1983 (Suryanarayana, 1995) show that protein intake of even the poorest decile group exceeded the normative dosage of 37 gms per capita per day (Panikar, 1980).
8. The per capita estimates are derived by the author based on the population and net foodgrains production estimates (GOI, 1997a; pp. S-24–S-25)
9. The discussion is confined largely to the pre-reform era, that is, the period before 1991 so as to keep the discussion insulated from liberalisation and its consequences.
10. Between 1954–5 and 1989–90, the shares of rice in the cereal (physical) consumption basket increased from 25.00 to 48.10, 32.30 to 52.13 and 41.40 to 53.31 per cent for the poorest three decile groups respectively. The share of wheat increased and that of coarse cereals decreased gradually until 1977–8; the decline was quite pronounced thereafter. The experience of other poor decile groups was no different. The urban sector's experience was similar to that of the rural sector with the difference that the pattern and magnitude of changes are not as striking as for the rural sector. In sum, the share of wheat in the cereal basket increased and that of coarse cereals decreased for the entire population (Suryanarayana, 1995; p. 214).
11. The NSS estimates are corroborated by the findings of the National Nutrition Monitoring Bureau (NNMB) diet and nutrition surveys based on clinical and anthropometric measures. The NNMB surveys covered the seven states of Andhra Pradesh, Gujarat, Karnataka, Kerala, Madhya Pradesh, Maharashtra and Tamil Nadu for 1975–9 and 1988–90.
12. This is a serious issue given the macro evidence for India that calorie intake is caused by income and that income is not constrained by calorie intake (Dawson and Tiffin, 1998).
13. The increase in per capita availability of cereals at the national level was from 334.2 gms per day in 1950–1 to 464 gms per day in 1995–6 (GOI, 1997a; p. S-24).

14. The coefficient of variation in per capita cereal production across states increased form 0.54 in 1970–1 to 0.84 in 1989–90. Per capita cereal output during the post-green revolution period increased only in the states of Punjab, Haryana and Uttar Pradesh (Krishnan, 1992; p. 2,485).
15. The results for 1993–4 are subject to the limitation that the corrections for inter-state price variations were made assuming that the state specific price indices with all-India as base for the year 1970–1 (Minhas and Jain, 1990) are valid for 1993–4. This is a restrictive assumption, as it does not take care of inter-state variations in temporal price movements for want of appropriate price indices.
16. Similar to the regression estimates for the rural sector, for the urban sector too the state-wise estimates of per capita consumer expenditure and non-agricultural income were adjusted for inter-state price variations assuming that the state specific price indices with all-India as base for the year 1970–1 (Minhas, Jain and Saluja, 1990) are valid for 1993–4. As already noted, this can be a restrictive assumption.
17. The proportion of households reporting non-availability of adequate food in different months is more and the problem acute in rural and urban areas of Kerala, Orissa and West Bengal and in the rural areas of Assam and Bihar (NSSO, 1998).
18. For more details, see Datt (1994).
19. Our estimates of poverty tally with those of the Expert Group (PPD, 1993; p. 39) even though the methods of estimation are different.
20. The elasticity estimates are not reported here to save space. Those interested can get them from the author.
21. The estimates for 1993–4 show that the average rural cereal consumption across states in the country fell short of the quantity consumed by the expenditure group with the normative calorie intake level in 1983 (NSSO, 1989b, c and 1996).
22. For urban India, the published estimates of maximum level of cereal consumption for the year 1993–4 was less than the observed levels corresponding to the expenditure group with the normative calorie levels for 1983 (NSSO, 1989c,d & 1996).
23. The eight states are Andhra Pradesh, Gujarat, Karnataka, Kerala, Madhya Pradesh, Maharashtra, Orissa, and Tamil Nadu. The percentage varied from 31.40 per cent in Andhra Pradesh, 38.70 in Kerala to 70.30 per cent in Tamil Nadu (NNMB, 1996; p. 17).
24. The Body Mass Index is measured as the ratio of weight in kg to height in meters^2 (NNMB, 1996; p. 8).
25. The NNMB survey for 1991–2 showed that CED tended to be more in women than in men in Andhra Pradesh, Karnataka, Maharashtra, Orissa, Tamil Nadu and West Bengal; it was the reverse in Kerala and Gujarat (NNMB, 1993; p. 22).

REFERENCES

Adelman, Irma and Peter Berck, 1991. 'Food Security Policy in a Stochastic World', *Journal of Development Economics*, 34 (1–2): 25–55.

Bhargava, Alok, 1996. *Econometric Analysis of Psychometric Data: A Model for Kenyan Schools*, World Bank, Policy Research Department, Washington, D.C.

Bhattacharya, Nikhilesh, Dipankar Coondoo, Pradip Maiti and Robin Mukherjee, 1991. *Poverty, Inequality and Prices in India*, Sage Publications, New Delhi.

Centre for Development Studies (CDS), 1975. *Poverty, Unemployment and Development Policy—A Case Study of Selected Issues with Reference to Kerala*, United Nations, New York.

Chai, C.P., 1995. *Rural Human Capital and Economic Growth in Developing Countries*, senior honours thesis, Department of Economics, Harvard University, Cambridge, MA.

Dasgupta, Partha, 1998. 'The Economics of Poverty in Poor Countries', *Scandinavian Journal of Economics*, 100 (1): 41–68.

Datt, Gaurav, 1994. 'Computational Tools for Poverty Measurement and Analysis', *Sarvekshana*, 61st Issue, XVIII(2): 1–10, National Sample Survey Organisation (NSSO), Department of Statistics, Government of India, New Delhi.

Dawson, Philip J. and Richard Tiffin, 1998. 'Estimating the Demand for Calories in India', *American Journal of Agricultural Economics*, 80(3): 474–81.

DeRose, Laurie F. and Sara R. Millman, 1998. 'Introduction', in DeRose, Laurie, Ellen Messer and Sara Millman (eds.), *Who's Hungry? And How Do We Know?*, United Nations University Press, Tokyo, pp. 1–19.

EPW Research Foundation, 1998. *National Accounts Statistics of India 1950–1 to 1996–7* (Third Edition), Mumbai.

Fogel, R.W., 1991. 'The Conquest of High Mortality and Hunger in Europe and America: Timing and Mechanisms', in Higonnet, P., D.S. Landes and H. Rosovsky (eds.), *Favourites of Fortune: Technology, Growth and Economic Development Since the Industrial Revolution*, Harvard University Press, MA, pp. 35–71.

Foster, James, Joel Greer and Eirk Thorbecke, 1984. 'A Class of Decomposable Poverty Measures', *Econometrica*, 52(3): 761–66.

Glewwe, Paul, Hanan Jacoby and Elizabeth King, 1996. *An Economic Model of Nutrition and Learning: Evidence from Longitudinal Data*, World Bank, Policy Research Department, Washington, D.C.

Government of India (GOI), 1985. *Seventh Five Year Plan*, Planning Commission, New Delhi.

______, 1992. *Bulletin on Food Statistics: 1991*, Ministry of Agriculture, New Delhi.

______, 1997a. *Economic Survey 1996–7*, Economic Division, Ministry of Finance, New Delhi.

———, 1997b. *Focus on the Poor: Guidelines for the Implementation of the Targeted Public Distribution System*, Department of Consumer Affairs and Public Distribution, Ministry of Civil Supplies, New Delhi.

Haddad, Lawrence, Saroj Bhattarai, Maarten Immink and Shubh Kumar, 1996. *Managing Interactions between Household Food Security and Pre-schooler Health, Food, Agriculture and the Environment*, Discussion paper 16, International Food Policy Research Institute, Washington, D.C.

Kakwani, N., 1980. 'On a Class of Poverty Measures', *Econometrica*, 48: 437–46.

Krishnan, T.N., 1992. 'Population, Poverty and Employment in India', *Economic and Political Weekly*, XXVII(46): 2479–97.

Kumar, Gopalakrishna and Frances Stewart, 1992. 'Tackling Malnutrition: What can Targeted Nutritional Interventions Achieve?', in Harriss, Barbara, S. Guhan and R.H. Cassen (eds.), *Poverty in India: Research and Policy*, Oxford University Press, Mumbai, pp. 259–81.

Lipton, Michael and Martin Ravallion, 1995. 'Poverty and Policy', in Behrman, J. and T.N. Srinivasan (eds.), *Handbook of Development Economics*, III: 2553–7, Elsevier Science, B.V.

Jain, L.R. and B.S. Minhas, 1991. 'Rural and Urban Consumer Price Indices by Commodity Groups (States and All India: 1970–1 to 1983)', *Sarvekshana*, XIII(1): 1–21.

Minhas, B.S. and L.R. Jain, 1990. 'Incidence of Rural Poverty in Different States and All-India: 1970/1 to 1983', in Indian Society of Agricultural Economics (ed.), *Agricultural Development Policy: Adjustments and Reorientation*, Oxford & IBH Publishing Co. Pvt. Ltd., New Delhi, pp. 342–81.

———, L.R. Jain and M.R. Saluja, 1990. 'State Specific Urban Consumer Price Differentials Relative to All-India for Middle Fractiles and Total Population: 1961–1983', *Indian Economic Review*, XXV(2): 207–39.

———, L.R. Jain and S.D. Tendulkar, 1991. 'Declining Incidence of Poverty in the 1980s: Evidence versus Artefact', *Economic and Political Weekly*, XXVI(27 & 28): 1673–82.

National Nutrition Monitoring Bureau (NNMB), 1991. *Report of Repeat Surveys (1988–90)*, National Institute of Nutrition, Indian Council of Medical Research, Hyderabad.

———, 1993. *Nutritional Status of Rural Population, Report of NNMB Surveys (1991–2)*, National Institute of Nutrition, Indian Council of Medical Research, Hyderabad.

———, 1996. *Nutritional Status of Rural Population*, National Institute of Nutrition, Indian Council of Medical Research, Hyderabad.

National Sample Survey Organization (NASSO), 1986. 'A Report on the Third Quinquennial Survey on Consumer Expenditure: National Sample Survey. 38th Round (January–December 1983)', Sarvekshana, IX(4): S-1–S-102.

———, 1989a. 'Per Capita and Per Consumer Unit Per Diem Intake of Calorie, Protein and Fat and Perception of the People on Adequacy of Food', *Sarvekshana*, XIII(2): 27–37.

______, 1989b. 'Results on Per Capita Consumption of Cereals for Various Sections of Population: National Sample Survey. 38th Round (1983)', *Sarvekshana*, XIII(2): S-1–S-176.

______, 1989c. 'Results on Per Capita and Per Consumer Unit Per Diem Intake of Calorie, Protein and Fat and Perception of the People on Adequacy of Food: National Sample Survey. 38th Round (1983)', *Sarvekshana*, XIII(2): S-177–S-258.

______, 1996. 'Level and Pattern of Consumer Expenditure, 5th Quinquennial Survey 1993–4', Report No. 402, Central Statistical Organisation, New Delhi.

______, 1997a. 'A Note on Operational Land Holdings in India, 1991–2—National Sample Survey 48th Round (January–December)', *Sarvekshana*, 70th Issue XX(3): 1–44.

______, 1997b. 'Survey Results on Nutritional Intake in India—National Sample Survey, 59th Round (July 1993–June 1994), *Sarvekshana*, XXI(2): S-1–S-214.

______, 1998. 'A Note on Reported Adequacy of Food Intake in India: National Sample Survey, 50th Round (1993–4)', *Sarvekshana*, XXI(3): 61–8.

Panikar, P.G.K., 1980. 'Inter-regional Variation in Calorie Intake', *Economic and Political Weekly*, XV(41, 42, & 43): 1803–14.

Perspective Planning Division (PPD), 1979. *Report of the Task Force on Projections of Minimum Needs and Effective Consumption Demand*, Planning Commission, New Delhi.

______, 1993. *Report of the Expert Group on Estimation of Proportion and Number of Poor*, Planning Commission, New Delhi.

Radhakrishna, R., 1991. 'Food and Nutrition: Challenges for Policy', *Journal of the Indian Society of Agricultural Statistics*, XLIII(3): 211–27.

______, and C. Ravi, 1992. 'Effects of Growth, Relative Price and Preferences on Food and Nutrition', *Indian Economic Review*, Special Number, XVII: 303–23.

Rao, C.H. Hanumantha, 1994. *Agricultural Growth, Rural Poverty and Environmental Degradation in India*, Oxford University Press, New Delhi.

Reutlinger, S. and K. Knapp, 1980. *Food Security in Food Deficit Countries*, World Bank Staff Working Paper No. 393, World Bank, Washington, D.C.

Schultz, T.P., 1993. *Sources of Fertility Decline in Modern Economic Growth: Is Aggregate Evidence on the Demographic Transition Credible?*, Economics Department, Yale University, New Haven, CT.

Sengupta, S. and P.D. Joshi, 1978. 'Consumption of Cereals and Energy Content of Food Consumed', Sarvekshana, II(1): 1–11.

Sukhatme, P.V., 1973. 'The Calorie Gap', *The Indian Journal of Nutrition and Dietics*, cited in Sengupta and Joshi, op cit.

______, and Sheldon Margen, 1978. 'Models for Protein Deficiency', *The American Journal of Clinical Nutrition*, 31: 1237–56.

Suryanarayana, M.H., 1995. 'Growth, Poverty and Levels of Living: Hypotheses, Methods and Polices', *Journal of Indian School of Political Economy*, VII(2): 203–55.

______, 1996. 'Food Security and Calorie Adequacy Across States: Implications for Reform', *Journal of Indian School of Political Economy*, VIII(2): 203–65.

______, 1997a. 'Food Security in India: Measures, Norms and Issues', *Development and Change*, 28(4): 771–89.

______, 1997b. 'Food Policies: Need for an Integrated Perspective', *Productivity*, 38(2): 207–17.

Tendulkar, Suresh D., K. Sundaram and L.R. Jain, 1993. *Poverty in India: 1970–71 to 1988–9*, Asian Regional Team for Employment Promotion, International Labour Organisation, New Delhi.

Tyagi, D.S., 1990. 'Increasing Access to Food through Interaction of Price and Technology Policies—The Indian Experience', in Tyagi, D.S. and Vijay Shankar Vyas, (eds.), *Increasing Access to Food: The Asian Experience*, Sage Publications, New Delhi, pp. 55–98.

United Nations Development Programme (UNDP), 1997a. *India: The Road to Human Development*, Document of the United Nations Development Programme, New Delhi.

______, 1997b. 'Human Development Report 1997', Oxford University Press, New York.

Vaidyanathan, A., 1994. 'Employment Situation: Some Emerging Perspectives', *Economic and Political Weekly*, XXIX(50): 3147–56.

Villasenor, J. and B.C. Arnold, 1984. *The General Quadratic Lorenz Curve*, Technical Report, Colegio de Postgraduados, Mexico.

______, 1989. 'Elliptical Lorenz Curves', *Journal of Econometrics*, 40: 327–38.

World Bank, 1986. *Poverty and Hunger: Issues and Options for Food Security in Developing Countries*, World Bank, Washington, D.C.

______, 1993. *World Development Report 1993*, World Bank, Washington, D.C.

part three

Health

chapter 8

Social Objectives of Health Care Services: Regulating the Private Sector

• *Amar Jesani*

1. INTRODUCTION

There are two major issues which usually vie for attention in understanding problems of health and health care in India. The first is about giving preventive health priority over medical or curative care. It is correctly argued that improvement of preventive health and social and economic conditions would improve the health status of people. There is clinching evidence available to prove that much before scientific medicine discovered drugs to cure many common diseases, they were brought under control in the developed countries by public health measures and by improving the general living standards of people. Indeed, the contribution of curative medical care in improving people's health status is very little. This perspective thus correctly identifies preventive health and socio-economic intervention and strategy as the primary need for tackling our health problems. Virchow came to this conclusion one and a quarter century back when he coined the slogan, 'Medicine is a social science, and politics nothing but medicine on a grand scale' (Rather, 1983: xiii).

The second issue is an expressed or underlying assumption of many discussions that health care services in India are underdeveloped. This assumption flows from the understanding that since India is an underdeveloped country and there are millions of people having no physical access to health care, such care, therefore, must be underdeveloped. Thus, the attention is more on the *stated* policies of the government, the number of Primary Health Centres (PHCs), public sector hospitals and beds etc.; and the operational problems therein. Much of the debate on decentralisation of health care under the panchayati raj system is also about health care in the government sector.

Although these two issues appear to be unconnected, we feel that it need not be so. In this paper, an attempt is made to explain the inadequacy of the narrow public health perspective, for it fails to take into account the medical power structure existing and acting as a great bulwark against public health reforms. It attempts to show that health care services in India are not as underdeveloped as assumed, for the major part of health care does not exist in the public sector but in the private sector. Health care services in the private sector are almost exclusively curative. The power acquired by the private sector in curative health care is so great that unless a strategy for public health reforms are combined with reforms in the entire curative medical care sector (both government and private), we may not be able to achieve the desired results.

The health care delivery sector in general, and the private sector in health in particular, is virtually not regulated in India. There is hardly any license-permit raj in health care delivery. Given the great inequity in distribution of health care and the great chaos therein, it is relatively easy to make a case for regulating the private sector. However, as it is argued in this paper, the kind of strategy adopted and its social objectives are of crucial importance.

The following section sets out the social objectives of health care services. This is followed by Section 3, that provides an overview of health care services in India. Section 4 discusses the regulations governing the health care sector in India. The last section outlines the strategy for regulation.

2. SOCIAL OBJECTIVES OF HEALTH CARE SERVICES

What are the social objectives of health care services and to what extent do the present health care services fulfil them? Undoubtedly, the exercise in listing social objectives would generate some differences, particularly because it would primarily reflect one's expectation and perspective. If we start with the basics that were narrated in the very first paragraph of this essay, one could safely say that health care, in so far as it is within the medical care paradigm, could at best aid in achieving desired health status. Achievement of health is thus a result of the complex interplay of socio-economic, political and medical care developments.

Having said this, the specific objectives of services or medical care become obvious, that is aiding in the achievement of health by making available basic health care services (curative, preventive and promotive) to all who need it. Just as universal access to basic resources of society for achieving health for all is the objective of socio-economic and political development, universal access to health care is the chief objective of health services or health care development. In essence, health care is a part of the broad development process and therefore, shaped by it. From here, one can fine-tune the argument. It is not simply universal access to any health care services, but to the services that could actually aid in achieving health. Thus, the services made available must be appropriate, adequate and rational in order to be effective. Besides, the services must be in dynamic in nature in order to meet the changing epidemiological needs.

In order to understand the extent to which the existing health care is geared to achieving social goals, it is necessary to look at the size and distribution of health care services, and the system within which it is operating.

3. HEALTH CARE IN INDIA

In several papers in the past, we have indicated that the total size of health care services in India is large enough to make it universally accessible to all people in the country (Jesani and Anantharam, 1993; Jesani and Nandraj, 1994; Jesani, 1998). It was repeatedly pointed out that the actual size of the private health sector is kept hidden by policy makers who have hardly made any attempt to study it. Similarly, official health data reporting agencies like the Central Bureau of Health Intelligence (CBHI) have grossly under-reported information on the private sector as they have no means to collect data in the absence of proper registration laws for private hospitals. However, from the findings of various field studies conducted in last the fifteen years, it has become now clear that the private health sector has an overwhelming presence in health care services.

Tables 1, 2 and 3 reveal the size of the health care sector in India. The data presented is taken from CBHI, and Census reports. Along with that, we have also provided our estimates based on findings of various surveys and reports. Clearly, the government has shown a great amount of political will in developing or allowing the unfettered development of the curative health care sector in India, and that much of it is due to the expansion of the private sector.

TABLE 1: HEALTH HUMAN POWER

Doctors	CBHI (1994)	Total Number (1992)	9,49,722
		Population Per Doctor	889
	Our Estimates	Percentage of all Doctors in Private Sector	85
		Population Per Private Doctor	1,048
		Population Per Govt. Doctor	5,924
	CBHI (1993)	Number of Doctors at the PHCs	23,490
		Doctor Per PHC	1.12
		Rural Population Per PHC Doctor	24,938
	Census (1981)	Percentage of Doctors in Rural Areas (1981)	41
	Our Estimates	Urban Population Per Urban Doctor	387
		Rural Population Per Rural Doctor	1,611
Dentists		Total Number (1993)	19,523
		Population Per Dentist	43,228
Nurses		Total Number (1993)	6,74,946
		Population Per Nurse	1,250
		Doctors Per Nurse	1.4

Notes: (1) Our estimation of proportion of doctors in the private sector is an under-estimation.
(2) In order to calculate Doctor-Population ratio for rural and urban areas, the proportion found in the 1981 Census has been applied, as the 1991 Census data on this are still not available. (3) 1991 Census population (rural, urban, total) figures are used for calculating ratios.

Sources: (1) Central Bureau of Health Intelligence (CBHI), *'Health Information of India'*, 1991, 1992, 1993, 1994.
(2) Census (1981).

TABLE 2: HEALTH CARE INSTITUTIONS (HOSPITALS, BEDS, PHCs)

Hospitals	CBHI, 1994	Total Number (1993)	13,692
		Population Per Hospital	61,637
		% of Hospitals in Private Sector	67
		Population Per Private Hospital	92,607
		Population Per Govt. Hospital	1,84,305
	Our Estimates	Total Number	71,860
		Population Per Hospital	11,744
		% of Hospitals in Private Sector	93
		Population Per Private Hospital	12,628
Hospital Beds	CBHI, 1994	Total Number (1993)	5,96,203
		Population Per Hospital Bed	1,416
		% of Beds in Rural Areas	21

(Table 2. contd...)

		Rural Population Per Rural Bed	5,136
		Urban Population Per Urban Bed	457
		% of Beds in Private Sector	35
		Population Per Private Bed	4,000
		Population Per Govt. Bed	2,191
	Our Estimates	Total Number	12,17,427
		Population Per Bed	693
		% of Beds in Private Sector	64
		Population Per Private Bed	1,083
		Population Per Govt. Bed	1,926
PHCs	CBHI (1996)	Total Number	21,854
		Rural Population Per PHC	28,768

Notes: (1) Our estimations of number of hospitals and beds are based on the extent of under-estimation in government (CBHI) data found in Andhra Pradesh in 1993 Survey (census of all hospitals) by the Director of Health Services (Andhra Pradesh) and the Andhra Vaidya Vidhan Parishad. They found 2,802 hospitals and 42,192 hospital beds in the private sector in Andhra Pradesh as against only 266 hospitals and 11,103 beds officially reported by the CBHI in that year (Nandraj and Duggal, 1997). Thus, the Official (CBHI) data under-reported the private hospitals by 10.5 times and beds by 3.8 times. This indeed is a very rough and inaccurate estimation. However, the intention is only to show the trend.
(2) 1991 Census population (rural, urban, total) figures are used for calculating ratios.

Sources: CBHI, *'Health Information of India'*, 1994, 1996.

TABLE: 3: HEALTH EXPENDITURE, PUBLIC AND PRIVATE

Expenditure	*Estimates*	Total Health Expenditure as % of GNP	5 to 7
	Govt. (1995)	Health as % of total revenue expenditure	2.63
	Govt. (1995)	Per capita revenue expenditure on health	85.1
	CEHAT (1997)	Per capita household expenditure on health	624
	Our estimates	Private expenditure as % of total health expenditure	8 8

Sources: (1) Ravi Duggal, Nandraj Sunil, Vadair Asha (1995), 'Health expenditure across states' (Part I & II), in *Economic and Political Weekly*, 15 April 1995 and 22 April 1995, pp. 834–44 and 901–8. (2) CEHAT (1998), Health Sector Database, CEHAT, Mumbai. (3) Madhiwalla Neha, *et al.* (2000), *'Health, Households and Women's Lives: A Study of Illness and Child-bearing among Women in Nashik District, Maharashtra'*, CEHAT, Mumbai.

As against official attempts to provide a community based non-professional health worker per 1,000 rural population, we find that we already have one formally qualified and registered doctor for 889 people. Similarly, according to our estimates, there is one hospital for 11,744 persons and one hospital bed for 693 people. Availability of such abundant human resources and infrastructure does not give a picture of genuine under-development of health care services in India. Indeed, the real shortage shown by the data is of nurses, and not of doctors, hospitals or hospital beds. Since nurses cannot do 'independent' or private market based practice in the manner and to the extent as doctors, they have been paid scanty attention. This has precluded the market driven expansion of nursing education. Medical education, on the other hand, is increasingly driven by market demand, and thus we have one-fourth of allopathic and two-thirds of non-allopathic medical colleges in the private sector. As a consequence, and contrary to the genuine needs of people, the doctor-nurse ratio in our country is in favour of doctors. The prevailing ratio is 1.4 doctors for 1 nurse when it should be two or three nurses for one doctor.

While in absolute terms the size of the health care sector appears to be 'good enough'; its distribution is very lopsided. As shown in the tables, there is an overwhelming dominance of the private sector in all categories. In fact, on examining data from the 1961, 1971 and 1981 census, we find that there is a progressive de-ruralisation in the location of doctors. In 1961, 49.65 per cent of all doctors were in rural areas, but in 1981, only 41.2 per cent were located there. As a consequence, for urban areas, the doctor-population ratio (1 urban doctor for 387 urban persons) is better than many of the developed countries. The ratio for rural areas (1 rural doctor for 1,611 rural persons), is bad, but the ratio of doctors at the PHCs (1 PHC doctor for 24,938 rural persons), is the worst. Thus, the real under-development is related to government services and not to the whole health care sector.

Similar issues emerge while examining data on hospital infrastructure. The quality of data on human power are better simply because there are laws for the registration of doctors from various systems of medicine. However, in the absence of uniform laws for the registration of hospitals, the data provided by official agencies are greatly underestimated. We have tried to correct this underestimation by using the findings of the survey done in Andhra Pradesh. This survey of 1993 (census of all hospitals) by the Director of Health Services (Andhra Pradesh) and the Andhra Vaidya Vidhan Parishad, found 2,802 hospitals and 42,192 hospital beds in the private sector as against only 266 hospitals and 11,103 beds officially reported by the CBHI in that year (Nandraj and Duggal, 1997, p. 23). Thus, the official (CBHI) data under-reported private hospitals by 10.5 times and beds by 3.8 times.

We had a similar experience in Maharashtra. In 1991, as a result of the High Court order in the Public Interest Litigation filed by the Medico Friend Circle, the Bombay Municipal Corporation did a rigorous listing and registration of private hospitals in the city. They found 907 hospitals and nursing homes. However, CBHI (1992) data for that year provided a total of only 1,174 private hospitals and nursing homes for the entire state of Maharashtra, thus showing the gross underestimation of the private sector in official data (Nandraj and Duggal, 1997, p. 23). Interestingly, official data show that there is one urban hospital bed for 457 urban persons in urban areas. If we are able to make our own estimation, the finding may be that there is actually one hospital bed for less than 300 persons in the urban areas. Indeed, there are problems in our estimates, which are based on the reported underestimation in Andhra Pradesh. However, even if one applies finer statistical correction to the data, that would reduce the size of the private sector by only a few percentage points. In any case, the health sector needs the attention of competent statisticians and economists to put its data system in order. While conceding the possibility that our estimates might be over-estimating the number of hospitals and beds in the private sector, it is indisputable that the private sector has a dominant presence in the hospital sector.

Lastly, similar trends are visible when we look at the data on health care financing. While the government was spending, in 1995, only Rs 85.10 per capita per annum from its revenue expenditure on health, people were spending from their own pockets over Rs 600 per capita per annum in 1997. Over the years, private spending on health care has increased while the increase in government spending has slowed down. In the situation of extreme poverty of a large proportion of population, this only makes health care inaccessible to a large mass of people.

It is easy to conclude from this account that in terms of absolute numbers, India has a very large health care sector. This size is also largely due to the dominant presence of the private sector. Further, the growth of the private sector is unplanned. It is not promoted as part of a larger system of national health services. It is allowed or is encouraged to grow within the unfettered market forces in health care. Private sector domination has made health care a commodity. This has created a strong medical business class, which acts in league with companies manufacturing drugs, instruments, equipment and other essential items for health care services. Besides, the unfettered market in health care delivery has attracted powerful corporate business groups. This trend in the corporatisation of health care is growing very fast, and as soon as the health sector is opened up to the private insurance companies, the power of medical business classes would only get stronger. Thus, the large size of the health sector and private sector dominance has created a powerful social force which needs to be taken into account in any planning for public health and in achieving the social objective of making health care universally accessible.

4. REGULATING HEALTH CARE SERVICES

As stated earlier, health care is one sector where the neo-liberal criticism of the license and permit raj is the least applicable. This is simply because health care laws and regulations are prominent due to their absence and not due to their preponderance.

It is interesting to note that the much of the government health sector under the ministry of health and family planning was created through policy pronouncements, without translating such policies into laws. While the Bhore Committee made a recommendation for enacting a uniform and comprehensive Public Health Act to streamline and promote efficient administration (Bhore Committee, 1946, p. 502–7), it was not followed up. As a consequence, unlike in Canada and many Western European developed countries, there is no comprehensive framework or system created for health care delivery in India. Thus, the Primary Health Centres (PHCs) catering to health care needs of the rural masses have been established without enacting any comprehensive laws for their governance. While the laws for local government bodies such as panchayati raj institutions, municipalities and municipal corporations stipulate that they should be involved in the provision of health care, they do not specify any basic minimum provision as their responsibility. As a consequence, there is a large public sector in health care with minimum legislative framework. In the absence of law making it mandatory to provide the stipulated minimum health care, citizens are not able to exercise any right over the quantity and quality of health care provided. The only options available to citizens are to either not use the services or find a political solution by supporting one set of politicians against another. While people have been adopting the former strategy by gradually abandoning government services, the latter is not as yet a major issue as health care is still not a priority political issue for people. This has helped in the proliferation of the medical market and irrational care.

While government health care services are not established and run under any comprehensive law, they are highly bureaucratised. One aspect of this bureaucracy is the existence of too many procedures, regulations and orders. These regulations and orders do specify, at least on paper, the standards for basic minimum infrastructure and services, though they do not provide a justiciable right to minimum quantity of health care. These regulatory standards are often used to create public outcry and to show that the services are failing. As a result, government health care services usually come under closer public scrutiny.

It is even more interesting to note that in the fifty years since independence, not a single committee has looked at the role and functioning of the private sector in health care. The government has also not undertaken or commissioned any national level study of the private sector. It is normally assumed that since people are using the private sector, the services provided by it must be of good quality and the providers must be behaving rationally and ethically. It is also assumed that the market itself is a good regulator for both quality of care as well as ethical behaviour of the providers. To what extent are these assumptions true?

While the market mechanism in general has its own problems, its operation in the health care sector is a problem that even the most market-friendly societies have failed to solve. There are severe limitations to the notion of the sovereign, rational and informed consumer in health care. In the health care sector, the provider decides on behalf of the consumer what the consumer should buy. As a result, consumer autonomy is greatly limited. When there is a fusion of consumer and supplier in the health care professional and institution, market failure becomes an inevitable reality. Any regulatory mechanism devised for market regulation, therefore, becomes counter-productive as the provider finds newer ways to take decisions on behalf of the consumer. There is a sizeable body of literature in health economics to show that when the number of health care providers increases, there is neither a drop in the quantity of care supplied, nor in the average income of the providers. On the contrary, the trends indicate that with an increase in the number of providers, the total quantity of services provided also increases with the concomitant increase in health care expenditure and the income of providers (Auster and Oaxaca, 1981;

Fuchs, 1978). The 'supplier induced demand' is the most commonly encountered phenomenon in health care.

The expansion of the health care market also depends upon people's perception about health and illness. The market treats everything, including the body and its parts as commodities in order to expand its operation. Normality is in no time converted into perceived ill-health and the body is made an object. What the services provide in response to such demand is also not always rational or good for the body.

The assumption that competing providers and the existence of rational consumers leads to provision of better quality of health care has also been proved incorrect. On the contrary, one observes an increasing supply and consumption of irrational care, which is both of low quality and high price. (Illich, 1975, Uplekar and Rokle, 1987, Phadke *et al.*, 1995). There is sufficient evidence to show that market expansion in health is often related to increase in irrational and harmful medication, investigations and surgeries. As stated earlier, there is a high concentration of private health care in urban areas, so much so that in some respects, the urban health service indicators appear as good as in any developed country. However, the fast accumulating evidence from India suggests that a situation contrary to such an assumption exists. The glitter that goes with the private hospital's attempts to attract more patients hides the fact that the medical quality of care provided in these institutions is not as good as it is made out to be. Patient satisfaction is a very vague operational concept for the real medical quality of care. In most studies of poor patients in public hospitals, it was found that patient satisfaction was of a high order. This is not always due to high quality of medical care, but largely due to the fact that the facilities provided are much better than what such poor patients actually have at their own homes. The same is often true for the patients using 'five star' hospitals. Here too, they get facilities which are as good as or better than what they normally have.

However, when all these institutions are studied by using the objective minimum criteria for standards of medical quality, different results come out. In a district level study of private hospitals and clinics, it was found that a large majority of private hospitals did not confirm to the minimum standards of medical care (Nandraj and Duggal, 1997). Not only were they of low quality; some of the measures taken to circumvent quality standards were dangerous for the safety and well-being of patients. A committee appointed by the Mumbai High Court in 1993 to assess the situation in private nursing homes and hospitals in Mumbai City encountered a similar situation. Thus, neither in rural areas, nor in over-supplied urban areas, did the market on its own create conditions for improving the quality of health care in the private sector.

4.1 Where are our Health Laws?

In the absence of any comprehensive planning or laws governing the entire health care sector, health care in India can hardly be called a system. In this regard, the Indian system resembles the health care services in the USA. Scholars have shown great reluctance to call the US health care service a system because of its fragmented, overlapping, unplanned nature and diverse delivery pattern (Morgan Capron, 1989, p. 503). All these characteristics are present in India too. However, there is a crucial difference in that the market based private supplier dominated health care in the USA has the highest number of laws and regulations governing it. In India, laws and regulations are prominent for their absence.

In the USA, laws and regulations have been an integral part of the market friendly health care provision. There is neither a comprehensive law to plan and systematise health care, nor a fundamental constitutional right to health care. Instead, the country has numerous laws and regulations to reduce market failure, to regulate expenditure and financing, ensure better quality of health care, make information available so that patients could become more informed, confer confidentiality of medical information, and so on. Interestingly, serious efforts to deregulate the US health care system have always failed and led to the enactment of new regulations. A classic example of this phenomenon was observed during the presidency of Ronald Reagan. His administration, in its zeal to deregulate health care, made serious attempts to do so. But much before his term got over, he was forced to put in place a number of newer regulations (David, 1988). In essence, the US example shows that market friendly health care inevitably leads to a plethora of laws and regulations. For without them, it is neither possible to sustain market friendliness, nor people's political support for the market in health care.

As against this, in India, we have hardly any laws or regulations in the field of health. The only law that could be called somewhat complete is related to the education, registration and monitoring of doctors. The laws which have created three medical councils (Allopathic, Indian System and Homeopathic), the Indian and State Medical

Council Acts, lay down some standards for education, registration and disciplining of unethical medical practices. Despite these laws being the best among health laws, they are grossly deficient. There is absolutely no standard for continuing medical education and competency of medical practitioners. The medical councils are virtually defunct and normally biased on the question of disciplining unethical medical practitioners.

The scenario is absolutely dismal with regard to hospitals. There are only two states in India (Maharashtra and Delhi) where longstanding hospital and nursing home registration laws exist. In the rest of the states, only very recently were efforts made to enact registration laws. As far as we know, only three more states have succeeded in enacting such laws in recent times. It is still not clear whether the laws have been notified and thus implemented in even these states.

Besides, the registration laws enacted are merely for registration, they do not contain even basic rules defining the minimum physical and medical quality standards for the establishment of hospitals and nursing homes. The Maharashtra Act, the oldest one passed in 1949 and the Delhi Act of 1952, do not specify standards, nor have newer laws paid attention to this aspect. The only law on hospitals, which not only specified concrete standards but also laid down certain ceiling on the cost of each aspect of hospital care, was passed as an ordinance in Karnataka during the Emergency. But it was never ratified as a law and thus lapsed, and nobody seems to ever remember it simply because it happened to be a part of the bitter memory of the Emergency.

The last but most talked about law is the Consumer Protection Act of 1986. This law, which covers doctors and hospitals, simplifies the operation of tort laws as applicable in the civil courts and cuts down the waiting time for cases to be decided. While many high profile cases of negligence tried under the Consumer Protection Act have been reported in the media, the fact remains that malpractice litigation is neither as common nor as pernicious as found in developed countries. In a country with nearly a million doctors, cases of malpractice are still counted in hundreds, showing that patients in India are not very litigation oriented and that the legal forums created for them are not functioning as efficiently as made out to be. Besides, the compensation awarded is not so spectacular as to make people make greater use of such legal provisions. While one can always discuss the pros and cons of malpractice litigation, it must be kept in mind that such litigation has a very limited role to play in regulating the market and providers. For as witnessed in recent times, much before many cases get filed, providers over-react and try to create their own defences. This behaviour of providers only perpetuates the existing market mechanism, that if services are charged for, then one must be prepared to pay when one goes wrong.

5. STRATEGY FOR REGULATION

It is not necessary to stress any more the need for regulating the market and health care providers. There is enough evidence to prove that without basic laws and regulations, the market succeeds neither in fulfilling its own promises, nor in fulfilling the social objective of making health care universally accessible. What is more important to understand in the Indian context is the kind of regulations needed and how these regulations would be a part of the larger strategy for health sector reforms.

If the issue is tackled as merely regulations for the private sector, one inevitably gets pushed on the path taken by the US. More so when the structure of health care in India is very similar to that in the US. In that case, what is required is only to enumerate various areas of health care in which new laws and regulations are required. There is no doubt that one needs to regulate the market, safeguard interests of consumers and provide them with information, but all this still does not add up to making health care universally accessible to the masses of poor in our country. Thus, while the preceding measures are absolutely essential in any system, to keep the structure of health care intact, they would only perpetuate the market which is responsible for reducing access for the poor. There is no historical example in any country showing that the market with some or more regulatory laws would on its own solve the social problem of access. The US is again a classic example. Despite the highest number of laws and regulations for the market and for controlling the behaviour of providers, the highest amount of resources spent on health care, and over 40 per cent of health care financed by the government, the US has miserably failed in providing health care to all citizens. There are still 40 to 50 million US citizens who are neither covered under government health schemes (Medicare and Medicaid) nor have the resources to buy private health insurance. Interestingly, a simple study of US laws on health would show that only criminals and psychiatric patients involuntarily institutionalised have the basic right to health care from the government. For the rest, there is no such right available (Curran and Shapiro, 1982; Morgan Capron, 1989; Fuenzalida-Puelma and Scholl,

1989). The situation in India is identical, the only difference being that even our prisons and mental asylums do not the offer the right to basic health care services. Hence, enacting new laws and regulations, though necessary, is not going to be adequate in creating a radically different situation.

Thus, the point is not just to regulate the private sector, but to go beyond it. The regulation of the private sector needs to be articulated within the context of fundamental reforms aimed at making health care universally accessible. This has been achieved in many developed capitalist and democratic countries. Most parts of Western Europe and Canada are classic examples of such reforms within market economies. This path raises a different set of questions. What are the overall aims of regulations and reforms? Is the aim universal access to basic health care? Is it to keep the cost of health care at an affordable level? Is it to put the system under the democratic and participatory control of people? In this context it should be remembered that the failure of the community health movement in India had a lot to do with the fact that it existed within the market set up, and did not raise the political demand for creating universal access by reforming the entire health sector. The same fate awaits all efforts to bring health care under the control of the panchayati raj system. This is not because the concept of putting health care in people's hands is incorrect. But unless the panchayats are also given the right to reorganise both public and private health care, and unless both of them are brought under one umbrella of plan and regulation for meeting social objectives of health care, such decentralisation would fail to achieve universal access. In the worst case, the situation would only help the state to reduce its expenditure and the private sector and health care market to expand.

Thus, structural and planned reforms with the basic aim of making health care universally accessible is indicated for the simple reason that it is only such a strategy that would bring under control the powerful medical business interests in health care provision. Medical interests in the public system as well as in private health care are not only powerful, but also work in tandem to defeat organised public health reforms. At this stage in the history of health care development in India (more so when the medical care sector is so vast), the public health movement cannot think in terms of bypassing medical power. The basic reorganisation of medical care would create greater space for both the public health as well as community health movements to succeed.

REFERENCES

Auster Richard D. and Ronald L. Oaxaca, 1981. 'Identification of Supplier Induced Demand in the Health Care Sector', *The Journal of Human Resources*, XVI (3): 327–42 Summer 1981.

Bhore Committee, 1946. *Report of the Health Survey and Development Committee: Recommendations*, II, GOI, New Delhi.

Committee, *Recomendations*, II; 901, New Delhi.

Centre for Enquiry into Health and Allied Themes (CEHAT), 1998. *Health Sector Database*, Mumbai. This is a computerised time-series state-wise database on India.

Central Bureau of Health Intelligence (CBHI), *Health Information of India*, 1981, 1993, 1994, 1996.

Curran William, Shapiro E. Donald, 1982. *Law, Medicine and Forensic Science*, Third Edition, Little, Brown and Company, Boston.

David, Kinzer, 1988. 'The Decline and Fall of Deregulation', *The New England Journal of Medicine*, 14 January 1988: 112–16.

Duggal Ravi, Sunil Nandraj and Asha Vadair, 1995. 'Health Expenditure Across States' (Part I & II), *Economic and Political Weekly*, 15 April 1995 and 22 April 1995, pp. 834–44 and 901–8.

Fuenzalida-Puelma, H.L., Conner S. Scholl (eds.), 1989. '*Right to Health in the Americas: A Comparative Constitutional Study*', Pan American Health Organisation, Washington D.C.

Funchs, Victor R., 1978. 'The Supply of Surgeons and Demand for Operations', *The Journal of Human Resources*, (Supp): 35–56.

Illich, Ivan, 1975. *Medical Nemesis*, Rupa and Co., Mumbai.

Jesani, Amar, 1998. 'From Philanthropy to Human Rights: A Perspective for Activism in the field of Health Care', *The Indian Journal of Social Work*, 59(1): 291–320 Mumbai. TISS, (Special Issue: Towards People-Centred Development, Part 2), January 1998.

______, and Anantharam Saraswathy, 1993. *Private Sector and Privatisation in Health Care Services*, A review paper for the ICSSR-ICMR joint panel on health, p. 97, Foundation for Research in Community Health, Mumbai.

______, and Sunil Nandraj, 1994. 'The Unregulated Private Health Sector', *Health for the Millions*, 2(2): 25–8, February 1994.

Madhiwalla, Neha, Sunil Nandraj, and Roopashri Sinha, 2000. '*Health, Households and Women's Lives: A Study of Illness and Child-bearing among Women in Nashik District, Maharashtra*', CEHAT, Mumbai.

Morgan, Capron Alexander, 1989. 'United States of America' (National Studies on the Constitution and Right to Health), in H. L. Fuendzalida-Puelma, Scholl Conner, S. (eds.), *Right to Health in The Americas: A Comparative Constitutional Study*, Pan American Health Organisation, Washington D.C.

Nandraj, Sunil, and Ravi Duggal, 1997. *Physical Standards in the Private Health Sector*, Mumbai: CEHAT, 1997, p. 23.

Quotes the data of 1993 Survey (census of all hospitals) by the Director of Health Services (Andhra Pradesh) and the Andhra Vaidya Vidhan Parishad, supplied to them by those agencies.

Phadke, Anant, Audrey Fernandes, L. Sharda, Pratibha Mane and Amar Jesani, 1995. *A Study of Supply and Use of Pharmaceuticals in Satara District*, FRCH, Mumbai, June, p. 152.

Rather L.J., 1983. 'Forward to the English Edition' in Virchow Rudolf (ed.), *Collected Essays on Public Health and Epidemiology*, Amerind Publishing Co., New Delhi.

Uplekar, Mukund, and Madhu Rokle, 1987. 'Aren't We Being Dangerously Overdrugged?' *FRCH Newsletter*, I(4), May–June 1987:2.

chapter 9

Primary Health Care: From Adjustment to Reforms

• *Imrana Qadeer*

1. STATUS OF PRIMARY HEALTH CARE

If primary health care is to be saved from becoming yet another cliché in the health service vocabulary, it is necessary to know the reasons for which it originally acquired its undisputed status in public health debates. Primary health care, as defined in the Alma Ata Declaration (World Health Organisation (WHO) 1978), had some distinctive features because of which it emerged a historical winner over the previous forms of ideas in public health practices ranging from sanitary measures to mass therapeutic interventions and immunisations and the organised provision of medical care (clinical services). While each of these modes of practice contributed to the containment of suffering, it was evident that these strategies by themselves were limited in their impact.

The role of therapeutics was questioned by the European and American experiences. The decline of mortality rates in these economies began much before the discovery of antibacterial drugs, which are now considered to be the main instruments for the success of medical intervention. The power of mass therapeutics and immunisation programmes, that emerged as the key interventions in the early twentieth century, was questioned by the experiences of the Third World. These strategies of basic health care very often showed limited success when implemented through weak infrastructure amidst populations living under conditions of extreme deprivation. Except for the eradication of small pox, none of the other programmes could achieve the expected results. Thus, the need to tackle poverty, which was at the root of constraints such as poor nutritional status, sanitation, and the availability of drinking water, housing and transportation emerged as one of the major thrusts in public health debates. Historically, the decline of mortality from malaria in Punjab over 1860–1930, after the introduction of famine relief measures in British India (Zurbrigg, 1992), was a clear indication of the importance of socio-economic interventions for health.

The importance of providing subsistence and welfare infrastructure along with basic health services and the critical role of people's participation, control, and self-sufficiency had been undeniable in the experience of countries such as China, Cuba, Nicaragua, and Zimbabwe. Primary health care thus reflected this dream of Third World nations striving to stand on their own feet. Its distinctive features were that it a) considered developmental inputs, other than health, as necessary for health, b) included secondary and tertiary care as elements of primary health care and c) understood that people's health needs, participation, and affordability of care were basic to primary health care.

The following section discusses the transformation of primary health care. Section 3 provides the reasons for such a transformation. The last section deals with prerequisites for primary health care.

2. TRANSFORMATION OF PRIMARY HEALTH CARE

This extremely political concept of public health was difficult to reject in the late 1970s, when a large number of newly emerging national democracies were asserting themselves, and the value of investment in 'human capital' had been widely accepted. Consequently, though at Alma Ata primary health care was accepted as a basic right, its intrinsic political nature, one that questioned the direction of development, was used as a means to dilute it. Thus, the Alma Ata Declaration, instead of highlighting the importance of achieving equity in development, accepted that the implementation of primary health care would depend on the nature of governments. In other words, due to the constraints of a UN organisation, it was not clearly stated that primary health care, devoid of its comprehensive approach, would remain the same as the basic health care that was being practised earlier. Except being mentioned in the definition, the notions of a community's development, its self-reliance and self-determination, were not elaborated. The Declaration professed to recognise the importance of 'political will' but did not spell out the consequent prerequisites for primary health care.

The inability of the Declaration to centrally locate the developmental issue in the debate on public health, in contrast to the importance given to technology and its organisation, set the stage for the transformation of primary health care at its inception. The concept of equity in development and self-reliance was lost and mere reorganisation of health services remained the focus of primary health care. This obscured the distinction between *basic health care* and *comprehensive primary health care*. The term primary health care thus got automatically diluted into basic health care for all practical purposes. But for the dominant paradigm in public health, even this was not enough. Hence, it was argued that selective interventions based on technology could give quick results without investing in less 'efficient' strategies (both technological and socio-economic). Thus, even the basic components of primary health care were dropped in favour of selective primary health care, which depended upon effective technology and its availability and not on people's needs. Selective primary health care also ignored the relevance of self-sufficiency and emphasised transfer of technology and the use of international experts.

For the South Asian countries, the 1990s have been a significant period in which the concept of primary health care regressed one step closer to its extinction. The acceptance of Structural Adjustment policies brought along with them a new notion of reforms, very different from the reforms of the 1970s. In the health sector, it meant cutbacks in the role of the public sector, privatisation, and cost recoveries. In the social arena, it meant cutbacks on all other welfare inputs, undermining of food security systems, and increasing the burden of unemployment for the poor. 'Reforms' then, was a mere euphemism for 'adjustments'. To give these reforms a human face, a veil of a 'safety net' was drawn to protect the vulnerable, but this veil remained invisible.

The reforms, in other words, were antithetical to primary health care. Yet some analysts chose to create a convergence between them and, in the process, undermined the concept of primary health care. A good example of this was the effort of the World Bank to plan for India's primary health care. On one hand, it advanced notions of cost reduction, cost recovery through privatisation of public hospitals and medical education, and opening up of medical care to the private sector. At the same time, it claimed to protect primary health care since, despite overall cuts, once hospital and educational costs were reduced, the health service infrastructure and communicable disease control programmes could be strengthened (World Bank, 1992). The proposed package of services emphasised reproductive health as a key component of primary health care. It, however, chose to ignore that devoid of intra-sectoral development, adequate support from the secondary and tertiary level medical care, an epidemiological basis for prioritisation of problems and strategies, and an integrated approach, primary health care simply could not exist.

In 1995, the Bank came out with a second report that explored policy and finance strategies for strengthening primary health care (World Bank, 1995). On the basis of its analysis, it proposed the following:

1. Primary health care should be provided by both the private and public sectors. While the former should focus on preventive and promotive services, the latter should provide curative care. This was despite the fact that the public sector was found to achieve higher levels of equity and cost-containment.

2. Preventive and promotive services are the primary needs of the poor. However, this was proposed without actually defining these needs or the notion of prevention itself. Theoretically, the latter includes social sector investment such as drinking water, housing, public distribution system for food, and medical inputs such as immunisation, communicable disease control, and health education. The report thus ignored the logic that major disease control programmes are largely based on curative interventions that call for coverage of total populations (including the rich and the middle classes) with standardised therapeutic strategies in an organised, monitored and consistent way over a period of time. Hence, breaking primary health care into curative and preventive domains destroyed disease control programmes central to such care as they required standardisation, epidemiological monitoring, and extensive population coverage, and not just a high proportion of private spending in 'curative care', as proposed by the Bank's investigators.

3. An 'environment' should be created to encourage the private sector to offer primary health care, even while it was known that the out-of-pocket expenses on serious illnesses were large and disproportionately affected the poor.

4. A package of public health called the 'basic package' was put forward without any epidemiological basis to it and cost-effective results were sought in the public sector. However, no mechanisms were visualised for the control and monitoring of the private sector.

5. Cost recovery from hospitals and medical education and means-tested user charges were proposed to enhance 'efficiency' of the public sector without any concern for the evidence that these are not only inefficient by themselves but that they also further marginalise the poor (Krishnan, 1994).

This truncated version of primary health care was tested out by the Bank in 1997 in four Indian states. The report revealed that primary health care was nothing but a cost-reducing exercise, which saves public sector resources and promotes uncontrolled proliferation of the private sector irrespective of its ability to provide primary health care (World Bank, 1997). In this final exercise, primary health care is converted into 'First Level Care' through Primary Health Centres. It was devoid of the integrated character and all principles of public health and was thus rendered meaningless. This exercise was not only unconvincing but also irrational and devoid of basic scientific principles. For example, it proposed the following:

1. Given the existence of private and NGO sectors, population-based norms for institutional coverage by the public sector need to be changed.

2. The epidemiological transition in disease patterns calls for changes in priorities and a shift towards chronic and non-communicable diseases.

3. Technological improvement should be introduced to improve efficiency of interventions.

Unfortunately, no evidence is provided by the Bank's report on the regional or class basis of access to services in public, private, or voluntary sectors. Independent evidence already exists that private institutions dominate in economically better areas (Baru, 1994). Promoting them further will only mean perpetuating inequalities. Similarly, instead of providing time series data to establish epidemiological transition, rural-urban differences in a point survey were used as evidence for epidemiological transformations. This was an obviously inadequate proof of their claim. The report also ignored the factor of population coverage along with effectiveness of technology while assessing efficiency. In other words, recommendations were made without paying any heed to the basic methodological requirements of evidence collection.

The preceding analysis indicates that there were a series of transformations from *comprehensive primary health care* to just *basic health care*, then to *selective health care*, and finally, to *primary level health care*, for the purposes of cost reduction. In the following section, we explore the reasons for this transformation by looking at the conceptual shifts that altered the process of prioritisation as well as the logic behind them.

3. THE REASONS FOR TRANSFORMATION OF PRIMARY HEALTH CARE

3.1 Conceptual Shifts

While in the original concept of primary health care, the effort was to emphasise people's perceptions of their illness, the Bank uses experts to decide priorities. The experts' tools and concepts are not necessarily in tune with reality as experienced by the majority, particularly the poor. The discrepancy between the experts' and the people's perception of needs and priorities are perceptibly wider if they come from totally different backgrounds as in the case of the World Bank's experts. For example, the Disability Adjusted Life Years (DALYs) was a favourite tool of these experts that not only incorporates expert biases but also treats diseases as discrete entities.[1] It fails to capture the distinction between mortality declines with or without increasing morbidity, and mortality declines in conjunction with morbidity declines. Second, instead of incorporating socio-economic strategies for disease control—such as clean water supply, strengthened food security systems, sanitation and housing—the strategy adopted by the World Bank depends purely upon medical technological interventions. It has consistently tried to reduce organisational structures in the name of efficiency. Economic costs thus become central and social costs peripheral to the Bank's plan. The plan acquires a retrogressive character when seen along with other elements of Structural Adjustment policies, such as cutbacks in subsidies and, therefore, subsistence of the poor. These policies take away people's control over their resources, push up prices in the 'free' market, and undermine all social security and welfare services including health services. They force open tertiary and secondary level medical care to private markets and this lethally hits the poorest.

3.2 The Logic behind the Shifts

The current use of these concepts in health has been largely derived from the sphere of neo-classical economics. The operative condition is that of a competitive market where individuals have the means to spend out of their pockets according to their needs for a utility or service. Thus, effectiveness of a good or service is its power to effect a certain impact (its utility), and efficiency relates to the optimisation of resources, both in production and purchase, in a manner that the outcome is maximised—be it the profit or the desired impact. Costs are assessed as the money spent for procuring services or producing them. The two underlying assumptions common to these concepts are the importance of individuals as units that are 'free' to act as they please, and the reduction of all 'costs' into money. In public health, both these assumptions are highly questionable.

3.3 The Logic of Public Health

These concepts fit very well into that clinical paradigm where individuals choose doctors and therapies depending upon their likes and dislikes or their disease. But in public health, where single diseases or individuals are not the focus of attention, these concepts have a different meaning. 'Effectiveness' has to be assessed not only for individuals but for groups and classes, not only of technological interventions but of socio-economic interventions as well, not only for single interventions but for multiple synergistic intervention strategies, as a number of interrelated problems are tackled simultaneously. Take, for example, the danger of isolated assessment of effectiveness of DDT for malaria, filaria, and as an agricultural pesticide. Singly, it may be found to be 'effective' in each instance but, when combined effects of its use in all three cases are considered, it becomes lethal for a population.

Similarly, the notion of 'efficiency' deals with maximisation of output through optimum use of resources. The output in public health, however, cannot be assessed in terms of technical effectiveness alone. It needs to take into account coverage of population. For example, in tuberculosis the new drug regime gives 95 per cent cure rates as against the standard drug regime where the cure rate is 85 per cent. The former, however, is six times more expensive. In a population of a hundred persons, therefore, while the standard regime will give eighty-five cured cases, the more effective new drug regime can be offered to only sixteen persons, of which fifteen (95 per cent) will be cured! In other words, technical effectiveness does not necessarily ensure efficiency. In public health terms—for the control of tuberculosis—both, acquiring cure in as many persons as possible and treating the resistant and chronic cases are critical. The latter constitutes about 20 per cent of the total cases. The present strategy of patient coverage with multi drug therapy uses criteria that neither ensure full coverage of chronic cases, nor succeed in providing for the most needy and vulnerable populations (Chakraborty, 2001)

In addition to these notions of 'effectiveness' and 'efficiency', the most crucial concept that is often ignored is of efficacy. Efficacy of an intervention contextualises it and places it in relation to other possible processes which might also produce similar results. Thus, 'efficacy' of oral rehydration for the control of diarhoeal diseases in children has to be measured in relation to the traditional practice of feeding cereal-based fluids, strategies to improve child nutrition, water supply, or provision of anti-diarhoeal drugs. The narrower the boundary of the conceived health system, the fewer are the efforts to assess the efficacy of technological strategies, as is evident in the World Bank's exercise in planning primary health care.

The notion of costs in public health also no more remains confined to money. It acquires the additional dimensions of social and political costs. Thus, it is not sufficient to say that there is a decline in infant mortality. If the evidence shows relatively higher infant mortality rates among the poor, or slower declines among female infants, then it indicates that these sections pay a higher social cost for the techno-centric strategies that are meant to reduce infant mortality. Similarly, the use of quinicrine as a contraceptive may be considered 'economical' and, therefore, 'efficient' within the cost-benefit framework, but the enormous costs paid by women in terms of ill-health and suffering have to be accounted for (Rao, 1997).

The use of technology-based clinical paradigms and market-based notions of effectiveness, efficiency, and costs have thus completely unhinged the original concept of primary health care. It has been transformed to an extent that it is unrecognisable, at least in the World Bank's strategies. If the Public Health basis of primary health care is to be restored and its basic tenets revitalised, then certain prerequisites need to be set up. Without them no claims to provide primary health care should be taken seriously.

4. PRE-REQUISITES FOR PRIMARY HEALTH CARE

The prerequisites for achieving primary health care begin with defining it as *comprehensive care* based on priorities evolved through common epidemiological and subjective priorities of experts and people, and supported by inter-sectoral developmental inputs and secondary and tertiary level medical care. This calls for the following:

1. Recognition of the urgency for investing in the welfare sector, particularly public distribution systems and food security systems.

In other words, the invisible net of social security must become visible.

2. Ensuring primary health care coverage of the most vulnerable, which requires that the state shoulder the full responsibility of providing comprehensive primary health care wherein secondary and tertiary level care is integrated. A system of rationalising these levels should be based on epidemiological data on major diseases, which can help assess the quantum of services required at these levels.

3. There is no doubt that curative care in certain sections of the population is amenable to cost recovery. If a system of payment must be introduced for cost recovery or for providing additional medical care, then the public sector should take advantage of this potential and not hand over the opportunity on a platter to the private sector. It should do so through running a certain proportion of public sector hospitals on the basis of full charges for consultation and treatment and not through the present uniform policy of 'means tested user charges' which only marginalises the poor. These public hospitals that could run on a full fee system can provide quality care at a reasonable cost and make profits to invest back into the public sector. The public sector can thus have two sets of hospitals, within which teaching hospitals providing tertiary care and district hospitals providing secondary care must always remain financially fully supported by the state. The quality of care must be standardised and monitored in both sets of hospitals. This can be ensured by a system of rotation in postings of personnel at all levels in the two sets of hospitals.

4. On no account should curative and promotive care be disaggregated. Instead, there is a need to encourage health systems research to develop adequate integrated strategies for interventions and organisational forms that can cut down costs and inefficiencies by reducing duplication, waste, and laxity (Qadeer, 1995).

5. The human power and infrastructure for rural areas and slums in the cities need to be rejuvenated by better training, support, and supervision. Motivated personnel with a good grasp of problems can do much more than unfit, untrained workers taken on a casual and temporary basis.

6. The list of basic drugs and minimum care needs to be worked out at each level and provided for, if people's participation is to be achieved.

7. An effective referral system is a basic necessity and can be created only if each level of health care performs its full function.

8. Decentralisation and involvement of local communities in decision making will make primary health care more community oriented. To achieve this, information dissemination in a form that

is accessible to people is necessary. The current information and educational communication strategies need to be transformed into more people-friendly strategies.

9. The role of non-governmental organisations (NGOs) cannot replace the public sector in provision of services. They can only provide specific services, keep vigil over local institutions, and take up in-depth experiments for innovative strategies. The use of NGOs as providers to reduce costs cannot by itself eliminate the inequity in the provision of primary health care, since they are not in a position to provide comprehensive or integrated health care and are largely being called upon to take up family planning or reproductive health care programmes.

10. For any coordination with the private sector in the provision of primary health care, standardisation of treatment, sharing of information, minimum quality of care, and rationalisation of costs is a must. A public sector that is itself under pressure to roll back and is unable to retain its own monitoring units, is hardly in a position to control or coordinate with the private sector unless adequate legislative and institutional reforms are introduced to monitor, check, and control the private sector. There is sufficient evidence to show that the public sector is already being exploited by the private sector and, when this trend is controlled, the performance of the public sector improves (*The Hindu*, 1998). Implementation machinery for such monitoring, therefore, is critical.

11. Epidemiological monitoring systems must be an integral component of primary health care if epidemics such as plague, cholera, gastroenteritis, and kala azar are to be controlled.

12. Medical education must remain oriented to creating basic doctors and not super-specialists. For this, not only is the content of basic medical education critical, but also the background of those who come for training. The state should not absolve itself from the responsibility of monitoring these key elements of primary health care. Private practice by doctors in public institutions needs to be abolished at all costs.

If these are the prerequisites for primary health care, then it is obvious that public sector investments and state monitoring will have to play a critical role. People's experiences need to be enriched to help them accept new responsibilities of looking after their own health. And for this we need a little bit of pride in what we have, a little confidence in our own abilities, and a little insight into the accumulated knowledge that lies uncared for, pointing to creative directions for a healthy future.

ENDNOTE

1 Disability Adjusted Life Years (DALY) was a concept introduced in the World Development Report (World Bank, 1993, p. 1) as a measure that combines healthy life years lost because of premature mortality with those lost as a result of disability. The burden of diseases measured in terms of DALY includes several assumptions. The key choices include the potential years of life lost due to death at a given age, the relative value of healthy life lived at different ages, the discount rate, or the extent of time preference for human life and health, and the disability weights used to convert life lived with a disability to a common measure with a premature death (World Bank, 1993, p. 213).

REFERENCES

Baru, Rama V., 1994. 'Structure and Utilisation of Health Services: An Inter-State Analysis', *Social Scientist*, 22(9–12): 98–111.

Chakraborty, A.K., 2001. 'Tuberculosis Programme in India: Current Operational Issue', pp. 339–60. In, 'Public Health and the Poverty of Reforms: The South Asian Predicament', Qadeer I., K. Sen and K.R. Nayar (eds.), Sage, New Delhi.

Krishnan, T.N., 1994. 'Access to Health and Burden of Treatment in India', UNDP Research Project, CDS, Thiruvananthapuram, Studies on Human Development in India, Series No. 2.

Qadeer, Imrana, 1995. 'Primary Health Care, A Paradise Lost', *IASSI Quarterly*, 14(1&2):1–20.

Rao, Mohan, 1997. 'Surreptitious Sterilisation: An Endangering Process', *Health for the Millions*, 23(4): 26–8.

The Hindu, 1998. 'A Boost to Medical Education in UP', 14 April, p. 20, Col. 4.

World Bank, 1992. *India, Health Sector Financing: Coping with Adjustment Opportunities for Reform*, Report No. 10859–N, p. i–v.

______, 1993. *World Development Report 1993: Investing in Health*, World Development Indicators, Published for the World Bank, Oxford University Press, New York.

______, 1995. *Policy and Finance Strategies for Strengthening Primary Health Care Services*, Report No. 13042-IN, p. i–xxii.

______, 1997. *New Directions in Health Sector Development at the State Level: An Operational Perspective*, Report No. 157530-IN.

World Health Organisation (WHO), 1978. '*Primary Health Care: Report of the International Conference on Primary Health Care*', Alma Ata, USSR, 6–12 September 1978, Geneva, WHO, p. 3.

Zurbrigg, Shiela, 1992. 'Hunger and Epidemic: Malaria in Punjab 1868–1940', *Economic and Political Weekly*, 25 January, pp. 2–25.

chapter 10

Building Coalitions: From Subsidies to Social Sector Spending

• *Ajit Karnik and Mala Lalvani*

1. INTRODUCTION

The initial macroeconomic stabilisation component of economic reforms often leads to severe curtailing of government expenditures. The axe generally falls on those expenditures which are not supported by strong interest groups and lobbies, specifically, basic health and education (Karnik, 1997a). Unfortunately, the beneficiaries of these facilities are the least well equipped to bear the burden of transition from a dirigiste regime to a market-oriented one. Interest groups, on the other hand, fearing a loss of government patronage in a less interventionist system, are more adept at protecting their turf, namely, subsidies, secure public sector employment and protection from national and international competition, among others. Examples of such behaviour abound and include large farmer lobbies, public sector trade unions (eg. banking and insurance sectors) and domestic businesses (the so-called Bombay Club, for instance).

If the reforms process has to be made secure and broad-based, then safety nets in the form of basic amenities have to be provided (Graham, 1994). For the poor, the arcane nitty-gritty of economic reforms has little relevance; what is of relevance to this section of the population is alleviation of poverty and availability of basic facilities. Even though the actual creation of these facilities will most likely

We would like to thank Professor Abhay Pethe for his comments on the paper. The usual disclaimer applies.

depend on the pursuit of reforms and a rapid rate of growth, the government will be judged by the poor only in terms of availability of basic amenities. While this is true, it is not automatically the case that the government will provide these safety nets to the poor. Governments generally derive their support from interest groups, which, being vocal, are able to appropriate disproportionate benefits and compel the government to continue the patronage that had become endemic under a dirigiste regime.

We take a public choice view here that political parties in power would like to remain in power. Consequently, any distancing from interest groups, which will lead to loss of political power, will be shunned by the government. Therefore, if a case has to be made for re-orienting government spending towards genuine welfare activities from subsidies to interest groups, one should be able to convince the government that such a re-orientation will not lead to a loss of political support for it. It should be possible to establish that the loss of political support from interest groups could be made up by the gain in support from the beneficiaries of welfare oriented spending. It is this that we propose to do in this paper.

The paper is divided into five sections including this one. The following section looks more closely at the process of coalition building and economic reforms. Section 3 seeks to estimate the cost of providing primary health care to a unit of population (where one unit is understood as 100,000 persons); this is an important task since such estimates are not easily available. Section 4 looks at re-allocating interest group oriented subsidies to primary health care and seeks to indicate the kind of political support that would be forthcoming to the government as a consequence. Section 5 concludes.

2. REFORMS AND COALITION BUILDING

It is well known that the process of reforms puts in jeopardy networks and nexuses that have been built up over a number of years under a dirigiste regime. The power of interest groups as well as the discretionary powers of politicians and bureaucrats tends to come under strain, provoking strong anti-reform attitudes and positions. Political opposition to reform (and possibly support for it) comes from interest group leaders and other political entrepreneurs who react to the programmes' anticipated effects on their constituents. (Haggard and Webb, 1994). Newly reforming economies can often be overwhelmed by the demands of interest groups, many of whom may be very vocal and well organised and possibly eager to maintain the pre-reform system. Examples come easily to mind in the Indian context—banking and insurance sectors, farming lobbies, etc. Witness the difficulties that have been experienced in re-structuring the banking sector as well as in opening the insurance sector; equally instructive has been the appeasement, in the form of free electric power, of large farmers by politicians in various Indian states. The demands of such groups usually outweigh those of the poor and vulnerable, especially under a democratic system, which responds to the loudest and best organised groups (Graham, 1994). Graham, however, also points out that governments in transition do have alternatives and it is possible to break with common practice and focus efforts on the poor. This, however, requires concentrating not on the political obstacles to economic reforms but on the political opportunities created by the reform process for re-directing public resources to the poor.

The process of pushing through reforms over the long term involves a battle of attrition against the status quo and must often be seen as a process of coalition building (Waterbury, 1989). The process basically involves building encompassing coalitions so that the pool of beneficiaries of the reform process widens to counter those who are opposed to the reforms process. Thus, essentially what must happen is that the configuration of interest groups has to change as the economy undergoes stabilisation and structural adjustment. This has to happen if the status quo is ever to be transcended (Haggard and Webb, 1994). It is this simple idea of building encompassing coalitions that we pursue in this paper. It is not at all our claim that the process is simple; quite the contrary it is likely to prove enormously difficult to get the government to move away from narrow sectarian interest group politics to building encompassing coalitions.

The basic obstacle to an elected government is the danger of forsaking established interest groups for coalitions, which may not vote it back to power. Even if the aggregate benefits of such a strategy are widespread, politicians may not be able to capture these gains politically if institutional arrangements weaken or dissipate support from beneficiaries and strengthen anti-reform forces (Geddes, 1992). The dilemma that most elected governments face is that they must remain in power long enough for reforms to take hold and yield tangible benefits; at the same time they cannot forsake groups which can least afford the negative effects of economic reforms. The first part of the dilemma forces the government to rely on interest groups to muster support for re-election. However, if the disadvantaged groups are persistently neglected, then that too leads to disaster. One form of the disaster is that the relatively disadvantaged suffer the adverse effects of reforms, at least in the initial stages, disproportionately. In the initial stages, the macro aspects of market oriented reform (Graham, 1994) are aimed at eliminating macroeconomic distortions and curtailing extensive state intervention. The axe often falls on those government expenditures which do not have strong political support i.e., health and education for the poor. A second kind of disaster awaits governments which persistently neglect issues related to the welfare of the poor. Political opposition is then able to create a critical mass to dislodge the reforming government from power.

In the context of this paper we are concerned with two kinds of government intervention, the first is in the form of subsidies to strong lobbies, such as large farmers. These are subsidies on what are called 'non-merit' goods by the Government of India Discussion Paper (1997) on subsidies. This is not the place to critically examine the approach of GOI (1997) nor to disagree with its use of the terms 'merit' and 'non-merit' goods (Karnik, 1997b). The other kind of government intervention is in the area of genuine welfare enhancing measures, such as basic health and education. These areas of intervention have strong public goods characteristics with important positive externalities and make the process of subsidisation justifiable; public expenditures which benefit interest groups on the other hand, rarely involve externalities and subsidisation of such governmental activities is unjustified.

We argue in the following discussion that a re-allocation of government expenditures from subsidies (to interest groups) towards health will be a means by which the benefits of the reforms process become available to a large mass of people. From the perspective of vast sections of the population, the tangible benefits come in the form of basic amenities; it is this availability of amenities that might enable the government to reap popular support for the reforms process. Such an approach will mean that the government will be able to make its support base broader through a process of coalition building—the beneficiaries of health facilities become a part of this coalition which develops a stake in these 'reforms with a human face'.

On the other side, those who no longer receive subsidies and largesse from the government will necessarily withdraw support. The question that will trouble the government is whether this withdrawal of support will be compensated by the gain in support from those who benefit from the provision of health facilities. If the answer to that question is yes, then government intervention can be re-oriented towards genuine welfare enhancement. If the answer is in the negative, then the status quo will prevail.

As stated in the forgoing, it is not at all our contention that this re-orientation will be easy; quite the contrary, in fact. The object of the exercises in this paper is to try to answer the question raised in the previous paragraph. However, before we do so we need to have, at least, a rough idea about how much it would cost to deliver health benefits to a unit of population. Unfortunately, no estimates for this are easily available. It is towards this estimation that we turn to in the next section.

3. ESTIMATING THE COST OF PRIMARY HEALTH CARE FACILITIES

3.1 Primary Health Care Facilities Available

The Bhore Committee Report (1946) was the first plan for an Indian National Health Service. It envisaged the construction of a massive publicly managed health infrastructure that would have required substantial increases in the government's allocation to health as a proportion of GDP. Two concepts of the Bhore Committee Report were pursued in the initial Five-Year Plans, viz. Primary Health Centres (PHCs) and special disease control programmes.

PHCs were initially to have three or four emergency beds with one or two doctors. At the same time one PHC was planned for every 100,000 to 200,000 population; this was subsequently scaled down to one PHC per 30,000 population. Further, each PHC was to support six sub-centres (SUBCs), with each sub-centre serving a population of 5,000 people. Over and above this, there was to be a community Health Centre (CHC) for every 100,000 population. CHCs are mainly multi-functional outpatient facilities though they were planned to include thirty inpatient beds and a minimal cohort of specialist medical personnel.

The norms that have been laid down during the Sixth Plan for population coverage and staffing of CHCs, PHCs and SUBCs are as in Table 1. Further, the norms given in Table 1 suggest that for a population of 100,000 the facilities listed in Table 2 should be available.

3.2 Estimating the Cost of Primary Health Care Facilities

Our objective is first to compute the cost of setting up one CHC, one PHC and one SUBC. Unfortunately, no direct estimates are available and some rough estimates will have to be derived. Given a rough

TABLE 1. NORMS FOR PRIMARY HEALTH FACILITIES

Facility	*Norm*
CHCs	1/100,000 population
PHCs	1/30,000 population*
SUBCs	1/5,000 population **
Staffing In:	Norm
CHCs	Doctors: 4
	Paramedical: 13
	Administrative: 8
PHCs	Doctors: 2
	Paramedical: 7
	Administrative: 7
SUBCs	Paramedical: 2

Notes: *20,000 for hilly/tribal areas.
**3,000 for hilly/tribal areas.
Source: World Bank (1995).

TABLE 2. FACILITIES REQUIRED AS PER NORMS FOR 100,000 POPULATION

Facility/Personnel	*Numbers*
CHCs	1
PHCs	3.3
SUBCs	20
Doctors	11
Paramedics	36
Administrative	71

Source: Table 1.

estimate of a set of primary health care facilities, that is one CHC, one PHC and one SUBC, we will be able to compute the cost of covering 100,000 persons by these facilities as per the norms laid down by the Government of India. Given the cost estimate of improving the welfare of 100,000 people, we will be able to argue the case for re-allocating interest group-directed government spending towards welfare enhancing government spending.

One clarification is in order here. Even though the relevant government macropolicy variable is subsidy we often use the expenditure concept. What allows us to do this is the fact that rate of recovery for a majority of such government activities is so low as to make entire government expenditure no different from a subsidy. Thus, in some cases, the rate of subsidy will be assumed to be 100 per cent or equivalently the rate of recovery to be 0 per cent. (GOI, 1997).

World Bank (1995) has estimated for nine districts across four states (Gujarat, Tamil Nadu, West Bengal and Uttar Pradesh), the shortfall or gaps in inputs or resources for public sector health programmes at the primary level. Resource gaps in public facilities were estimated by comparing the actual inputs available for primary health care services in districts and municipalities with the levels of provision already sanctioned and with the available norms. The gap between actual and 'sanctioned ' resources represents a shortfall in the provision of facilities. This gap or shortfall has been categorised into three components: facilities (non-recurring capital expenditure), staff and drugs, and supplies (the last three being recurring expenditure). The estimates of World Bank (1995) indicate the following shortfall along with attendant monetary implications (Table 3).

Since information on salaries of doctors, paramedics and administrative staff are not available, and moreover, since this is likely to vary across states, we estimate average cost per individual employed in a CHC, PHC or SUBC. This simplifying procedure implies that we are assuming the emoluments of doctors, paramedics and adminis-

TABLE 3. MISSING HEALTH CARE FACILITIES IN FOUR SAMPLE STATES

Facility/Item Of Expenditure	*Numbers/Amount*
CHCs	178
PHCs	178
SUBCs	605
Doctors	1,068
Paramedics	4,770
Administration	2,670
Total personnel	8,508
Annual recurrent cost	Rs 332 million
Salary cost	Rs 255.38 million
Non-salary cost	Rs 76.62 million
Annual capital cost	Rs 2,082.25 million

Notes: 1. Number of personnel estimated using norms given in Table 1.
2. Non-salary cost estimated at 30 per cent of salary cost.
3. Capital costs: Rs 7.5 million per CHC; Rs 2.5 million per PHC; Rs 0.5 million per SUBC.

Source: World Bank (1995) p. 174.

trative staff to be the same. A more disaggregated study will be able to obtain better-cost estimates; however, in an aggregative study such as ours, this has not been possible.

Bearing this in mind we have the following estimate of costs for setting up primary health care facilities (Table 4).

On the basis of our computations in Table 4 we then estimate the

TABLE 4: ESTIMATED COST OF PRIMARY HEALTH CARE

	Cost per facility (Rs)		
	CHC	*PHC*	*SUBC*
Salary cost	750,425	480,272	60,034
Non-salary cost	225,128	144,082	18,010
Total recurrent cost	975,553	624,354	78,044
Initial capital cost	7,500,000	250,0000	500,000

Notes: 1. Salary cost computed for twenty-five personnel in a CHC; sixteen in a PHC; and two in SUBC.
2. Average salary cost computed as follows:
Total number of personnel = 8,508 (Table 3).
Total salary cost = Rs 255.38 million (Table 3).
Therefore, cost per personnel = Rs 30,017.
3. Non-salary cost computed at 30 per cent of salary cost.

cost of providing health care to one unit of population, where one unit has been taken to be 100,000 persons. Bearing in mind the norms for provision of CHC, PHC and SUBC (see Table 1), we obtain the estimates given in Table 5.

TABLE 5. ESTIMATED COST OF PROVIDING PRIMARY HEALTH CARE TO 100,000 PERSONS.

(Rs million)

	CHC	*PHC*	*SUBC*
No. of facilities required	1	3.3	20
Recurrent cost	0.975	2.060	1.561
Capital cost	7.500	8.250	10.000
Total cost in first year (Recurrent + Capital)	8.475	10.310	11.561

Notes: 1. Number of facilities required estimated from norms (Table 1).
2. Recurrent cost estimated from Table 4.
3. Capital cost estimated from assumption (see note 3 of Table 3).
4. Total cost in first year will include recurrent plus capital costs; in subsequent years only recurrent costs have to be incurred.

4. REALLOCATING GOVERNMENT EXPENDITURES / SUBSIDIES TOWARDS WELFARE ENHANCING ACTIVITIES

The Government of India Discussion Paper (1997) on 'Government Subsidies in India' has, as stated earlier, provided estimates of subsidies on 'Merit' and 'Non-Merit' goods and services at both the central and state government levels. A few estimates of GOI (1997) are reported in Table 6.

TABLE 6. ESTIMATES OF SUBSIDIES IN INDIA (1994–95)

(Rs million)

	Central Government	*State Government*
I. Merit Goods (Total)	69,229.9 (2.41%)	209,974.1 (1.07%)
1. Elementary Education	16,293.8 (1.45%)	93,777.8 (0.94%)
2. Public Health	972.7 (0.21%)	9,967.2 (1.90%)
II. Non-Merit Goods (Total)	361,248.3 (12.13%)	311,227.4 (12.87%)
1. Agriculture and allied activities	336,275.8 (4.53%)	43,815.9 (32.86%)
2. Irrigation and flood control	1,327.2 (3.83%)	124,207.6 (4.23%)
3. Power	39,289.4 (36.77%)	59,571.9 (14.99%)

Note: Figures in brackets are recovery rates.
Source: GOI (1997) Annex 1 and 2.

GOI (1997) states that a reduction in the subsidy rate to 50 per cent will shrink the fiscal deficits of the centre, states and union territories from 6.5 per cent of GDP to less than 2 per cent of GDP. However, if one were considering a re-allocation of expenditures from 'non-merit' subsidies to, say, public health, the level of fiscal deficit would remain unchanged, especially if one assumed no change in the recovery rates in the social sector. It is our feeling that assuming a reduction in the subsidy rate to 50 per cent (or equivalently pegging the recovery rate at 50 per cent) is too drastic a change, which no government amenable to interest group pressures will be able to undertake. We look at certain milder scenarios:

One, where the recovery rate rises 1 percentage point over current rates and

Two, where the recovery rate rises 5 percentage points over current rates.

Table 7 looks at the savings in subsidy that will be available at both the centre and states under these two scenarios.

TABLE 7. SAVINGS IN SUBSIDIES

(Rs million)

	Hike in Recovery Rates Over Existing Rates By:	
	1 Percentage Point	*5 Percentage Points*
I. Central Government		
1. Agriculture and allied activities	856	4298
2. Irrigation and flood control	13	69
II. State Governments		
1. Agriculture and allied activities	654	3265
2. Irrigation	1298	6480
3. Power	698	3502
III. *Total Savings* (I+II)	3513	17614

Source: GOI (1997) Annex 1 and 2.

It may be noted that the subsidies considered for savings in Table 7 account for less than half the estimated 'non-merit' subsidies. They account for 23 per cent of central government non-merit subsidies and 44 per cent of state government non-merit subsidies.

The savings in subsidies that have been made by hiking recovery rates (Table 7) may be re-distributed by the government towards welfare enhancing activities, such as health. The dilemma that the government faces is that the hike in recovery rates hurts interest groups which are strong supporters of the government; on the other hand by re-allocating the savings in subsidies towards health, the government bestows benefits on a diffused mass of people, which may not translate into votes. It is quite likely that the government will have to spend a substantial amount of money for publicising its welfare-oriented activities so as to claim credit for them. This publicity will enable the government to translate the increase in welfare into votes at election times. As a working assumption we suppose that about 10 per cent of the savings in subsidies will have to be allocated for information dissemination and publicity. In order to be conservative in our estimates of available savings in subsidies, we permit a further 5 per cent of these savings to be consumed in leakages, which are endemic in government activities. In Table 8, we estimate the number of persons who will benefit by re-orienting net savings in subsidies to welfare-enhancing activities.

The results of Table 8 are striking to say the least. A hike of 1

TABLE 8. BENEFITS FROM RE-ALLOCATION OF SUBSIDIES

(in Rs Million)	*Hike in Recovery Rates Over Existing Rates By:* 1 Percentage Point	5 Percentage Points
Total savings[1]	3,513	1,764
Expenditure on publicity	351	1,761
Other leakages	176	881
Net savings	2,986	14,972
Cost of primary health care set[2]	30.35	30.35
No. of primary health care sets available from net savings	98.39	493.31
No. of beneficiaries	9.8	49.33

Notes: 1.Total savings taken from Table 7.
2. Primary health care set consists of 1 CHC, 3.3 PHCs and 20 SUBCs and the cost includes capital plus recurrent costs (Table 5).

percentage point over existing recovery rates can yield benefits to 9.8 million persons; if the hike in recovery rates is 5 percentage points, the number of beneficiaries shoots up to 49.33 million.

It may be mentioned here that the cost of the primary health care set in Table 8 includes capital plus recurrent costs. Capital costs need to be borne only in the initial year of setting up the facility. In subsequent years only recurrent costs will have to be met. A further qualification needs to be made to the results of Table 8. The gain in the number of beneficiaries from health facilities has to be set off against the loss in the number of beneficiaries of interest group subsidies. The latter will lead to a loss of political support, while the former will probably lead to a gain in political support. The exact quantum of political support, either gained or lost, is difficult to measure precisely. For instance, among the beneficiaries of health care there will be non-voting individuals; also, the loss of political support from say, the farming lobby (since agriculture subsidies are being reduced as per Table 7) cannot be estimated merely by counting the number of large farmers (who receive interest group oriented subsidies). The loss of support would spread to the kith and kin of large farmers as well. Consequently it is very difficult to quantify the exact change in political support that will occur after subsidies are re-allocated. To get a very rough idea of the possible loss of support from the large farmers lobby, consider the following: in 1990–1, there were 1.67 million large holdings (Centre for Monitoring the Indian Economy, 1995). It is safe to presume that it is these large holdings that would be receiving government subsidies. Therefore, there is a clear loss of 1.67 million votes here; however, the loss of votes will not be confined to only the owners of these holdings but will cover their extended kith and kin and the number 1.67 million will have to be augmented. The question is what the augmentation factor should be. Possibly, the gain in the number of beneficiaries from a 1 percentage point hike in recovery rates (Table 8) will be nullified by the loss of political support of the farming lobby. However, it seems inconceivable that the gain in support from a 5 percentage point hike will be wiped out by the loss in support from the farming lobby.

In spite of the caution and difficulties indicated in the previous paragraph, the numbers in Table 8 are rather persuasive. A government which manages its publicity well, could well be able to win over the political support of beneficiaries of genuine welfare activities to counter-balance the decline in support of interest groups.

6. CONCLUSION

This paper was concerned with a re-orientation of government intervention from mere distribution of subsidies to interest groups towards genuine welfare improving interventions, such as in basic health. As stated in the introduction, we take a public choice view here that the government will not introduce policy changes which adversely affect its popularity and diminish its chances of re-election. It is our belief that most studies, which call for more focused government intervention in the social sector, do so without recognising the political economy considerations involved. Non-recognition of these political considerations makes the recommendations of such studies operationally vacuous.

This study placed political economy considerations in sharp focus while recommending diversion of government expenditures from subsidies to spending on basic health. The results that we have obtained in this paper, and which are encapsulated in Table 8, are revealing. A mere 1 percentage point hike in the recovery rates will yield enough savings to provide health benefits to approximately 10 million persons. Even if some of these beneficiaries will be non-voting, these numbers could compensate for the loss of political support arising out of curtailment of subsidies. A hike in the recovery rates of 5 percentage points or more will lead to a net increase in political support to the government. However, it needs to be borne in mind that since the beneficiaries of health facilities are a diffused mass of people, the building of such coalitions may not translate into votes, which re-elect the government. This is where the real danger lies. Getting the newly formed coalitions to vote for the incumbent political party will require active publicity and information dissemination on the part of the government. In spite of this caution, however, the results of the paper suggest that even within the existing political economy framework, it is possible to transcend the status quo and improve the quality of government intervention.

ENDNOTE

1. Professor Pethe has pointed out that we are implicitly assuming that the beneficiaries of health facilities are all floating voters, without loyalty to any political party. We would like to believe that the beneficiaries of health facilities, who come from the deprived stratum of society, would most likely cut across party loyalties. Where this does not happen, we will have to account for some additional leakage of political support. Of course, party loyalty is a double-edged criticism: can one assume that members of interest groups who lose subsidies will continue to support the party in power?

REFERENCES

Centre for Monitoring the Indian Economy (CMIE), 1995. *India's Agricultural Sector: A Compendium of Statistics*, September, CMIE, Mumbai.

Geddes, B., 1992. *The Effect of Political Institutions on Feasibility of Structural Adjustment*, Background paper prepared for the World Bank project on the Political Economy of Structural Adjustment in New Democracies, World Bank, Washington D.C.

Government of India, 1997. *Government Subsidies in India*, Department of Economic Affairs, Ministry of Finance, New Delhi.

Graham, C., 1994. *Safety Nets, Politics and the Poor: Transitions to Market Economies*, Brookings Institutions, Washington D.C.

Haggard, S. and S.B. Webb, 1994. 'Introduction', in S. Haggard and S.B. Webb (eds.), *Voting For Reform: Democracy, Political Liberalization and Economic Adjustment*, Oxford University Press, New York.

Karnik A.V., 1997a. 'Budget 1997–8 and the Role of the State', *Economic and Political Weekly*, 31 May 1997.

———, 1997b. 'White Paper on Subsidies: Vexing Aspects of Targeting', in *The Hindu Business Line*, 2 September 1997.

Waterbury, J., 1989. 'The Political Management of Economic Management and Reform', in Joan Nelson (ed.), *Fragile Coalitions: The Politics of Economic Adjustment*, Transaction Books, New Brunswick, N.J.

World Bank, 1995. *India: Policy and Finance Strategies for Strengthening Primary Health Care Services*, World Bank, Washington D.C.

chapter 11

Health Care Services in Rural India: Implications for Reproductive Health

• *Abusaleh Shariff and Anil Gumber*

1. INTRODUCTION

Access to basic health services, especially reproductive care, has continued to remain poor in developing countries due to several reasons, including supply-side factors. Despite substantial public investment in health infrastructure in India, both access to and use of services varies considerably across population groups, regions and settlements. A comprehensive review of the health care system in India clearly suggests that these variations persist partly due to differences in health-seeking behaviour, which is guided by economic, social and cultural factors. An additional factor is the type of policies, programmes and investments, especially in the health sector, pursued by the government over the last five decades. As a result of these factors, the present health care system suffers from several biases such as over-emphasis on secondary and tertiary hospitals, skewed distribution of health services in favour of urban and large settlements, stress on physicians rather than paramedics, and importance on services that have large private rather than social returns. More importantly, it has failed to adequately address the reproductive health needs of women living in diverse socio-economic conditions.

It is appropriate to recall in this context the guiding principles suggested by the Bhore Committee as early as 1946 in regard to the provision of health care to the citizens of India:

(a) No individual should fail to secure adequate medical care because of inability to pay for it.

(b) The health programme, must, from the very beginning, lay special emphasis on preventive work with consequential development of environmental hygiene.
(c) Health services should be placed as close to the people as possible in order to ensure maximum benefit to the communities to be served.
(d) The doctor, the leader of the health team, should be a 'Social Physician', who should combine remedial and preventive measures as to confer the maximum benefit on the community, and future doctors should be trained to equip them for all such duties.

One would find echoes of these principles emphasised by this Committee even in the Alma Ata declaration of 1978 and the later emphasis of the UNICEF on 'economic reforms with a human face' (Cornia *et al.*, 1987). In India, organised efforts of the last fifty years have failed to achieve the above mentioned targets and quality in the provision of health care. More recently, however, the International Conference on Population and Development in 1994 underscored the importance of reproductive health.[1]

It is against this scenario that the present paper examines the use of health care services and treatment facilities for men and women according to socio-economic status in different population settings. The study has utilised data from two nationwide household surveys collected by the National Council of Applied Economic Research (NCAER) in 1993 and 1994. The 1993 survey with primary focus on health care use and spending elicited information from 18,693 households (6,354 rural and 12,339 urban) on type and nature of illness, source of treatment and expenditure on treatment. The latter survey with a much broader focus of creating a human development profile of population, however, limited its coverage to rural areas. The survey of nearly 33,000 rural households not only collected information on morbidity and curative care but also included preventive care and reproductive details of married women in the age group 15–49 years. To explore the determinants of variations in health care use and spending by men and women, both the surveys collected data on socio-economic characteristics of the households. The objectives of the paper are as follows:

1. To examine health care utilisation patterns by gender, especially seeking inpatient and outpatient services at public and private facilities,
2. To examine differentials in the use of immunisation, ante-natal,

post-natal and other preventive services which have a direct bearing on reproductive health of rural women by socio-economic status; and

3. To suggest policy prescriptions and reforms to enhance the outreach of women in seeking both preventive and curative care services.

The following section discusses the pattern of health care utilisation. Section 3 deals with various aspects of reproductive health care pertaining to maternal care. This is followed by a discussion on child immunisation in Section 4. The last section sets out the main ingredients of overall health care reforms.

2. PATTERN OF HEALTH CARE UTILISATION

Estimating morbidity and disease burden is severely affected by a number of factors including perception and recall errors on the part of those reporting morbidity during household surveys (Gumber and Berman, 1995). In the recent past, however, the National Sample Survey (NSS) and the NCAER have made efforts to estimate morbidity rates through carefully designed sample surveys. The data points to considerable inter-state differentials in the prevalence of morbidity. Incidentally, Kerala, considered to be in the advanced stage of demographic and health transition, had recorded the highest level of morbidity in all the surveys reviewed. Generally speaking, incidence of morbidity was higher in rural than in urban areas. In terms of incidence of morbidity, as compared to males, the rate was marginally higher for females, but the difference was larger in urban than in rural India. Both the NSS and NCAER data revealed that the incidence of morbidity for women in the reproductive age group 15–49 was considerably higher than those for men. According to the NCAER survey, the rate was 89 and 136 per month per thousand population for women aged 15–24 and 25–34; the morbidity rates for men were 79 and 116, respectively. The NSS data suggested that the incidence of both illness and hospitalisation increases with Monthly Per Capita Expenditure (MPCE) class. The NCAER data, on the other hand, indicated that the decision to hospitalise was not significantly related to income levels. However, both the surveys have confirmed that the Scheduled Castes (SCs) and Scheduled Tribes (STs) reported lower levels of hospitalisation, which was largely due to their inaccessibility to health care facilities on the one hand and lack of resources on the other (see more on this issue in Gumber, 1996 and Shariff, 1995).

About 10 to 15 per cent of all those reporting sickness may not seek treatment at all; the proportion tends to be higher in rural than in urban areas. It is apparent from the data that the probability of not seeking treatment was higher among females, the elderly (aged 60 years and above), and the never married individuals. This probability was also higher among the SCs and STs, and those belonging to the lower MPCE quintile (Gumber, 1996). Accessibility, physical proximity and financial constraints were extremely important for taking decisions to seek treatment. Of those having received treatment, 93 per cent had received outpatient care without much inter-state variation.

Both the NSS and NCAER data have confirmed that the patients from rural as well as urban areas had overwhelmingly chosen public facilities such as government hospitals and Community Health Centres (CHCs) for inpatient care. The reliance on public hospitals for inpatient care was found to be much greater in hilly and backward states, among the SCs and STs and those belonging to the lower MPCE quintile. Private facilities were used largely for outpatient care, particularly in urban parts of India. Unlike public facilities, which were centrally located, private practitioners were found even in remote and backward areas. For instance, 70 per cent of hospitals and 85 per cent of hospital beds in the public sector were located in urban areas. The private practitioners were usually contacted first for day-to-day health care needs before availing the distantly located public facility. It was also observed that public facilities were used more often in cases of severe and catastrophic illnesses, which the private practitioners were reluctant to deal with.

The estimates of medical and total cost of treatment, by type of facility in rural and urban areas separately for inpatient and outpatient care, were also available. According to the NCAER data, the average medical expenditure for inpatient care in rural and urban areas on fees, medicines, clinical and diagnostic tests, surgery, and hospital bed charges per episode in 1993 were Rs 850 and Rs 1,065, respectively. The respective figures for outpatient care were Rs 70 and Rs 97. There were large inter-state and rural-urban variations in the cost of treatment. As expected, the cost of treatment was higher in urban than in rural areas, in the private than in the public sector and for inpatient than for outpatient care. Private sector agencies, on an average, charged three to four times higher as compared to public sector agencies for both inpatient and outpatient care. Overall, medical expenditure constituted 84 per cent of the total cost of treatment, which also included indirect costs such as expenses on transport, special diet, rituals, gifts, tips and other miscellaneous expenses. In most states, the proportion of indirect cost (mainly transportation) was higher in rural than in urban areas thus reflecting poor distribution of health care facilities in rural areas, particularly in hilly states.

An average Indian household spends Rs 250 per capita per annum on the use of health services; the figure for urban households was about 40 per cent higher than their rural counterparts (Table 1). The earlier estimates provided by the World Bank (1995, p. 20) for 1990–1 was Rs 240, which was based on the 1991 household survey of the NCAER using two weeks reference period for illness reporting.[2] Overall, 80.2 per cent of the total health expenditure by the households was for receiving health care from private sources. This was largely because private health care expenditures, both for inpatient and outpatient care, were considerably higher in terms of out-of-pocket payments by the households. This was despite the fact that public health care services were not free and people do incur considerable out-of-pocket expenditure to realise public health care. The NSS data, for instance, clearly highlighted that more than two-fifths of inpatients and one-third of outpatients who availed public facilities had to pay for the services. Public facilities nevertheless were relatively cheap as compared to the private facilities.

A perusal of Table 1 indicates that there were large inter-state variations in both government and household spending on health care whether expressed in per capita terms or as percentage of state domestic product (SDP). While hilly states of Jammu and Kashmir and Himachal Pradesh, and the state of Kerala spend more than nine per cent of their SDP on health, in the relatively developed states of Punjab, Haryana and Maharashtra this share is only around three per cent. The percentage share of government health expenditure of NSDP, in nine out of seventeen states ranged between two and five per cent. It appears from selected health care indicators across major states, except for the hilly states, that government spending on health among the poorer states was low and, therefore, the out-of-pocket expenditure by households in these states as relatively higher. Also, high level of morbidity raises the share of household expenditure in total health spending. The utilisation rates of public health services ranged between a low of 24 per cent (West Bengal) to a high of 70 per cent (Orissa). As many as eleven states recorded less than 50 per cent utilisation of public health facilities. This included states that incurred relatively high government expenditure on health (eg. Kerala) as well as those recording lower levels (eg. West Bengal) of expenditure.

TABLE 1. SELECTED HEALTH CARE INDICATORS FOR MAJOR STATES IN INDIA (1993)

States Ranked by Col. 6	*Per Capita Annual Health Exp. (Rs)*			*Share of Household Health Exp. (2 or % of 3)*	*Household Health Exp. as % of Household Income*	*Total Health Exp. as % of NSDP/NNP*	*Annual Morbidity rate/1,000 Population*	*% Use of Public Facilities*
	Govt.	*Household*	*Total*					
(1)	*(2)*	*(3)*	*(4)*	*(5)*	*(6)*	*(7)*	*(8)*	*(9)*
Jammu & Kashmir*	238	325	563	57.7	NE	10.7	2,130	NE
Kerala	111	482	593	81.3	11.9	9.5	2,171	37.6
Himachal Pradesh	209	370	279	63.9	6.7	8.9	1,785	56.4
Bihar	51	223	274	81.4	6.1	7.5	1,182	37.2
Orissa	74	276	350	78.9	8.2	7.4	2,102	70.1
Andhra Pradesh	66	421	487	86.4	7.8	7.4	1,504	36.0
Karnataka	93	360	453	79.5	8.8	6.5	1,306	55.9
Rajasthan	83	196	279	70.3	4.2	5.4	1,421	62.8
Uttar Pradesh	55	175	230	76.1	4.5	4.9	1,217	30.5
Gujarat	78	259	337	76.9	4.7	4.4	938	35.0
Madhya Pradesh	63	168	231	72.7	6.9	4.32	1,340	36.3
Tamil Nadu	100	202	302	66.9	6.5	4.2	924	45.0
West Bengal	73	154	227	67.8	3.4	3.8	841	24.4
Haryana	83	267	350	76.3	4.1	3.4	927	39.6
Punjab	110	282	392	71.9	6.2	3.2	1,606	40.6
Maharashtra	85	259	344	75.3	5.4	3.2	848	40.5
Assam	66	96	162	59.3	2.4	2.8	994	64.0
All India	84	250	334	74.9	6.0	5.5	1253	41.3

Notes: (1) *Estimates for Jammu & Kashmir are based on the NCAER survey of 1990.
(2) NE—Not Estimated.

3. REPRODUCTIVE HEALTH CARE UTILISATION

The 1994 survey of the NCAER collected data on pre-natal care, medical interventions during birth and post-natal care for all women in the sample who were either currently pregnant or had delivered a child during the year preceding the date of the survey. Some of the salient features of the data collected are as follows:

3.1 Ante-natal Care (ANC)

The survey revealed that ANC received by currently pregnant women varied remarkably across different states (with the coefficient of variation across states being as high as 89.7 per cent).[3] This rate was low in the southern states (viz., Andhra Pradesh, Karnataka, Kerala and Tamil Nadu) but high in the north-eastern region and states falling in the northern (viz., Haryana, Himachal Pradesh and Punjab) and lower central regions (viz., Madhya Pradesh, Orissa, and Rajasthan) of the country. The proportion was as high as 46.8 per cent in Tamil Nadu though it was much lower in the other states—22.5 per cent in Himachal Pradesh, 20.5 per cent in Karnataka, 18 per cent Punjab and 17 per cent in West Bengal. However, in developed states such as Haryana, Gujarat and Maharashtra, where health care infrastructure was generally expected to be better, only a very small percentage of expectant mothers were beneficiaries of ANC services. The percentage of those who had received these services was also very low in the upper and lower central regions. Further information on the type of ANC received revealed that about 90 per cent of beneficiaries were immunised against tetanus, but few had check-ups for blood pressure.

In rural India, about 7 per cent of Ever Married Women (EMW) had received ANC during the reference period. Inter-population group comparison does not correspond with poverty line groups and household income groups for mothers who receive ANC. When data on immunisation was collected from mothers rather than pregnant women, the findings were similar.[4] There was a clear association of ANC services with levels of household income. Land holding categories and occupational groups, however, did not show much correspondence (Table 2). The level of ANC services among STs (42 per cent) and Muslims (52 per cent) was relatively low, while it was 82 per cent among Christians. The wide variation may be related to differences in levels of education among these categories. Expectant mothers who were literate also received better ANC. A similar

TABLE 2. DISTRIBUTION OF CURRENTLY PREGNANT WOMEN RECEIVING ANTE-NATAL CARE BY POPULATION GROUP IN RURAL INDIA

(Per cent)

Population Group	*Received Ante-natal Care*	*Type of Ante-natal Care*		
		TT immunisation	*Iron Tablets*	*BP Checks*
(1)	*(2)*	*(3)*	*(4)*	*(5)*
Household Income Groups				
Upto 20,000	55.9	51.5	33.4	24.5
20,001–40,000	57.9	53.5	34.3	27.9
40,001–62,000	61.4	57.3	34.5	27.2
62,001–86,000	60.1	55.4	39.8	34.4
Above 86,000	68.1	60.1	39.8	42.8
Poverty Line Groups				
Lower Segment below	52.2	47.8	29.8	19.9
Upper Segment below	54.3	50.6	32.0	23.4
Lower Segment above	60.9	55.7	37.2	30.2
Upper Segment above	63.9	60.1	38.1	35.6
Land Holding Groups				
Landless Wage Earners	61.5	57.5	41.1	30.6
Marginal	56.5	51.4	32.0	24.0
Small	54.9	51.0	31.7	22.8
Medium	51.5	46.5	31.7	24.8
Large	55.8	51.4	36.0	27.9
Landless Others	62.6	58.5	34.5	32.8
Land Owners	55.3	50.5	32.2	24.2
Landless	62.0	58.0	38.1	31.6
Occupation Groups				
Cultivators	55.8	50.9	32.3	23.3
Salaried+Prof.+Empl.	61.2	57.5	37.6	31.0
Wage Earners	58.7	54.8	38.5	29.7
All Others	57.1	52.1	29.5	26.9
Social Groups				
Caste				
STs	42.2	39.4	29.6	12.8
SCs	57.6	52.5	35.0	24.3

(Table 2 contd...)

Religion				
Hindus	57.8	53.3	35.1	26.7
Muslims	51.7	46.4	24.5	20.8
Christians	81.9	81.3	54.6	68.0
Other Minorities	65.4	60.3	39.6	34.2
Households Size Groups				
Upto 4	63.8	59.9	41.8	35.8
5–7	57.6	54.0	35.2	24.9
8 and above	54.9	49.2	30.0	24.8
Adult Literacy Groups				
None Literate	47.3	42.4	24.5	16.3
Female Literate	75.6	73.0	55.1	46.6
Male Literate	49.0	44.1	28.6	18.7
Both Literate	72.9	69.1	46.3	41.6
Village Development				
Low	40.6	36.0	21.0	13.1
Medium	59.6	54.9	33.0	26.8
High	76.8	72.8	53.5	44.3
All Groups	57.5	53.0	34.2	26.2

Source: NCEAR/HDI Survey, 1994.

positive association of ANC with village development was evident in the survey suggesting that better provision of health care infrastructure had a bearing on the use of ANC facilities.

Data regarding three types of ANC services, namely, tetanus toxoid immunisation, prophylaxis through iron and folic acid tablets and blood pressure check-ups across fifteen major states indicated that overall, 58 per cent of women who had delivered during the year preceding the survey received some type of ANC. There were high inter-state variations, with almost all women receiving services in Kerala (94 per cent) and Tamil Nadu (90 per cent) but very few in Rajasthan (32 per cent), Madhya Pradesh (39 per cent), the North-east, Bihar and Uttar Pradesh (between 43 and 53 per cent). The utilisation of iron and folic acid tablets was relatively lower. It is interesting to note data on blood pressure checks since it has become available for the first time through a nationally representative sample survey. Overall, about 27 per cent of all women had undergone such checks, with 93 per cent of these in Kerala, 72 per cent in Tamil Nadu and 66 per cent in Andhra Pradesh. However, the percentages are very low in all the five upper central and lower central states.

3.2 Deliveries Conducted by Trained Personnel

Data regarding total deliveries in hospitals, CHCs and primary health centres (PHCs) and at home attended by trained or untrained personnel are presented in Table 3. At the all-India level, of the total deliveries (during the one-year reference period), about 18 per cent

TABLE 3. PERCENTAGE OF EVER MARRIED WOMEN (EMW) WHO DELIVERED IN YEAR PRIOR TO THE SURVEY ATTENDED BY TRAINED PERSONNEL AND BY PLACE OF DELIVERY IN RURAL INDIA

Region/State	*Attended by Trained Personnel*	*Place of Delivery*		
		Hospital	*CHC / PHC*	*Home*
(1)	*(2)*	*(3)*	*(4)*	*(5)*
NORTH				
Haryana	61.7	8.7	5.2	86.2
Himachal Pradesh	31.6	12.5	1.5	86.0
Punjab	71.3	15.3	6.3	78.5
UPPER CENTRAL				
Bihar	15.7	6.7	8.8	84.5
Uttar Pradesh	30.4	8.1	6.0	85.9
LOWER CENTRAL				
Madhya Pradesh	47.8	3.0	3.0	94.1
Orissa	20.5	8.2	3.6	88.2
Rajasthan	20.3	4.3	2.9	92.8
EAST				
North-eastern region	41.5	16.4	3.7	79.8
West Bengal	28.1	19.9	4.6	75.4
WEST				
Gujarat	55.9	23.2	5.5	71.4
Maharashtra	48.2	23.0	5.3	71.7
SOUTH				
Andhra Pradesh	71.9	37.8	8.5	53.7
Karnataka	56.8	28.1	6.4	65.5
Kerala	96.5	92.4	0.7	6.9
Tamil Nadu	82.6	69.7	4.9	25.4
Rural India	40.0	17.9	5.5	76.6
C.V	47.4	101.2	44.7	34.1

Source: NCAER/ HDI Survey, 1994.

took place in hospitals while 6 per cent deliveries were in CHCs and primary health centres while over 77 per cent deliveries were conducted at home. A scrutiny across fifteen major states indicated that deliveries at hospitals and CHCs/PHCs were the highest among the southern states (ranging between 92 per cent in Kerala to 57 per cent in Karnataka) followed by the north eastern states (80 per cent) and the states in the western region (viz., 56 per cent and 48 per cent in Gujarat and Maharashtra respectively). The highest percentage deliveries at home was recorded in the lower central states of Madhya Pradesh (94 per cent), Orissa (88 per cent) and Rajasthan (93 per cent).

About 60 per cent of total births were attended by untrained health personnel in rural India.[5] The upper central states, lower central states and states in the eastern region had relatively higher untrained personnel deliveries as compared to the states in the southern, northern and western region. Instances across specific states such as Haryana, Punjab, Madhya Pradesh, the north-eastern states, Gujarat, Maharashtra Andhra Pradesh and Karnataka, indicated that while over 60 per cent of the deliveries were at home, they were conducted by trained personnel. Kerala was the only exception, with a negligible percentage of deliveries taking place at home and by untrained personnel. Such instances have also had an impact on the quality of deliveries and consequentially greater complications during childbirth. About 11 per cent of all deliveries reported had complications; this incidence was high in Andhra Pradesh (3 per cent), in the North-east (22 per cent), and in Himachal Pradesh, Kerala and Tamil Nadu (15 per cent).[6]

3.3 *Post-natal Care (PNC)*

Type of PNC among women who had delivered a child during the year preceding the survey indicated that about one-fourth of rural women had received post-natal care. The use of PNC was highest in Maharashtra followed by the southern states of Tamil Nadu, Andhra Pradesh, Karnataka, Gujarat and Punjab. Post-natal care among women was almost absent in Bihar and West Bengal (8 per cent), Rajasthan (11 per cent) and Uttar Pradesh (16 per cent).

Overall, less than one-third of the women received post-natal care across various income categories (Table 4). There seemed to be a strong association between utilisation of PNC and income levels. Thus, less than one-fourth of women belonging to the lower income households had received PNC as against over one-third of women belonging to higher income households.[7] A comparison across different

FIGURE 1. PERCENTAGE OF BIRTHS ATTENDED BY UNTRAINED PERSONS AND WOMEN UNDERGOING COMPLICATED DELIVERIES BY STATE IN RURAL INDIA

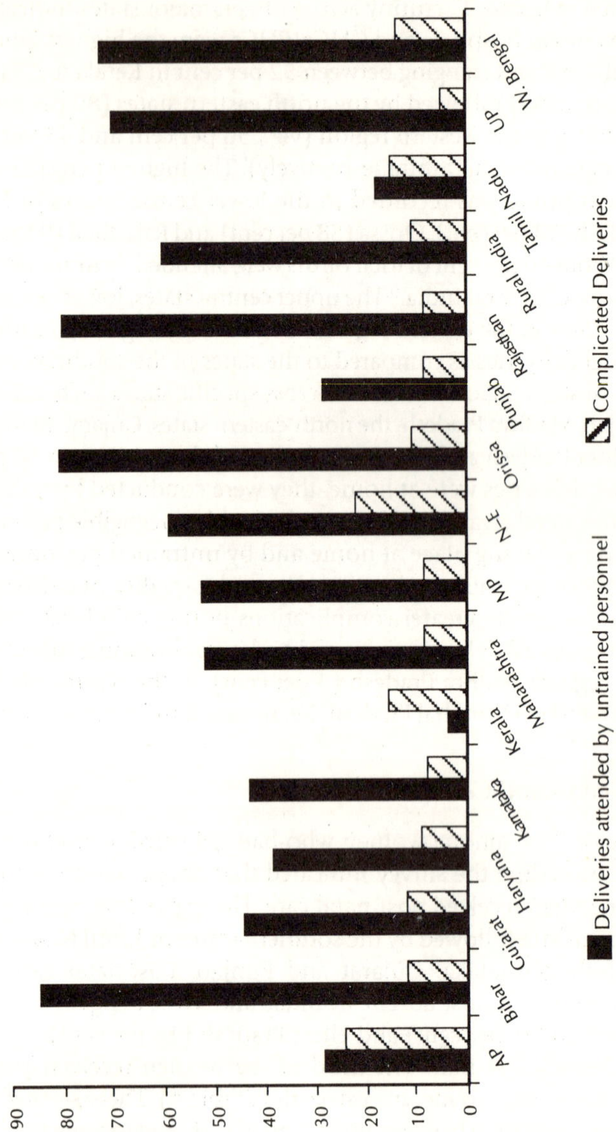

TABLE 4. POST-NATAL CARE RECEIVED BY WOMEN WHO HAD DELIVERED IN THE PREVIOUS YEAR BY VARIOUS GROUPS FOR RURAL INDIA

Groups	*EMW having delivery last year*	*Still Births*	*Received post-natal care*	*One check-up*	*Two or more check-ups*
(1)	(2)	(3)	(4)	(5)	(6)
Household Income Groups					
Upto 20000	17.6	4.8	22.0	56.5	41.1
20001–40000	16.7	6.1	26.5	53.8	44.9
40001–62000	16.9	8.4	24.5	56.4	4.06
62001–86000	16.9	7.6	36.1	50.5	48.8
Above 86000	17.5	4.1	30.7	54.1	45.7
Occupation Groups					
Cultivators	16.7	6.4	21.9	54.5	43.0
Salaried+Prof.+Empl.	16.7	5.5	27.9	51.8	47.0
Wage Earners	18.0	4.2	25.8	58.7	40.0
All Others	18.4	5.3	22.3	55.2	42.5
Social Groups					
Caste					
STs	18.7	6.0	23.3	43.0	57.0
SCs	18.2	4.6	21.3	61.2	36.0
Religion					
Hindus	16.9	5.2	24.8	56.3	41.7
Muslims	22.6	7.7	13.5	50.4	47.2
Christians	10.6	3.3	39.3	57.8	39.4
Other Minorities	16.5	6.5	34.6	41.1	58.1
Adult Literacy Groups					
Non-Literate	19.9	4.2	17.5	64.1	33.8
Female Literate	12.9	3.3	39.4	62.1	37.9
Male Literate	17.6	5.3	18.2	58.6	38.6
Both Literate	15.5	7.0	33.4	49.5	48.9
All Groups	17.3	5.5	23.8	55.4	42.7

Source: NCAER/ HDI Survey.

occupational categories indicated that utilisation of PNC was influenced by the nature of occupation. The lowest proportion of PNC use was among women in the cultivators group (22 per cent) while those from the regular/salaried class recorded the highest proportion (28 per cent). About one-fifth of women from the SCs and STs received PNC. Of the various religious groups, PNC utilisation was lowest among Muslim women (14 per cent). Further, the survey also indicated that literacy influenced the nature of health seeking behaviour of women. The highest proportion of PNC utilisation was among female literates (39 per cent).

Information about 'still births', identified as babies born dead during the reference period, across states indicated that in rural India about 6 per cent of all births were still born during 1993[8] (Table 4). These rates varied remarkably across states. While still births comprised about 14 per cent of total births in Bihar and 15 per cent in West Bengal, these rates were comparatively lower in Orissa and Himachal Pradesh, at 8 and 7 per cent respectively. Such high rates of still births are usually associated with low age of mother, poor nutritional levels of women, and low utilisation of primary health care in these particular states. Still birth rates also varied across various economic and social groups.[9]

3.4 Contraceptive Prevalence

Prevailing trends and patterns of 'ever use' of modern contraceptives among all currently married women aged 13–49 collected in this survey are comparable with the National Family Health Survey (NFHS) estimates (Table 5). Overall, 36 per cent of eligible women reported having used some method of contraception. The survey gave a relatively higher CPR for spacing methods as compared with NFHS estimates. A disaggregation according to methods used suggested that about 30 per cent of EMW were using terminal methods such as tubectomy and laparoscopy or their husbands had undergone vasectomy. The proportion of males who had undergone vasectomy to those who had used permanent methods was about 8 per cent. CPR for spacing through the use of intra-uterine devices (IUDs), oral pills and conventional contraceptives was 6 per cent.

There were wide variations in CPRs between states. CPR was generally higher than the national average in all the southern and western states and in the northern states. The use of family planning methods was extremely low in Bihar (18 per cent), Uttar Pradesh (22 per cent)

TABLE 5. CONTRACEPTION PREVALENCE RATES (CPRS) FOR EVER MARRIED WOMEN IN RURAL INDIA

Region / State	*Termination method*				*Spacing method*				*All Methods*	
	All		*Vasectomy as % of All*		*All*		*Loop/Copper T as % of All*			
	HDI (1993–94)	*(NFHS) (1992–93)*	*HDI (1993–94)*	*(NFHS) (1992–93)*	*HDI (1993–94)*	*(NFHS) (1992–93)*	*HDI (1993–94)*	*(NFHS) (1992–93)*	*HDI (1993–94)*	*(NFHS) (1992–93)*
(1)	*(2)*	*(3)*	*(4)*	*(5)*	*(6)*	*(7)*	*(8)*	*(9)*	*(10)*	*(11)*
NORTH										
Haryana	36.3	37.0	4.2	13.5	6.9	5.8	20.7	41.4	43.3	46.7
Himachal Pradesh	50.5	46.6	27.3	29.2	5.4	6.9	29.7	30.0	55.9	57.1
Punjab	30.1	35.4	8.6	6.8	15.4	14.8	39.6	38.5	45.5	57.2
UPPER CENTRAL										
Bihar	15.6	16.6	1.5	6.0	2.2	2.0	13.0	20.0	17.8	19.8
Uttar Pradesh	13.7	12.4	9.5	9.7	8.6	3.4	25.8	17.6	22.3	16.7
LOWER CENTRAL										
Madhya Pradesh	32.0	30.7	10.2	17.3	4.9	1.8	11.1	22.2	36.0	33.4
Orissa	31.4	30.6	13.5	10.8	2.4	2.1	33.8	57.1	33.8	34.2
Rajasthan	24.4	25.1	1.9	8.4	1.9	2.0	37.5	45.0	26.4	28.2
EAST										
North-eastern region	12.1	15.6	18.2	7.9	15.5	6.5	18.7	43.0	27.6	31.9
West Bengal	23.2	32.5	5.7	15.7	9.6	5.0	29.0	22.0	32.5	55.7

(Table 5 contd...)

(Table 5 continued)

Region / State	*Termination method*				*Spacing method*				*All Methods*	
	All		*Vasectomy as % of All*		*All*		*Loop/Copper T as % of All*			
	HDI (1993–94)	*(NFHS) (1992–93)*	*HDI (1993–94)*	*(NFHS) (1992–93)*	*HDI (1993–94)*	*(NFHS) (1992–93)*	*HDI (1993–94)*	*(NFHS) (1992–93)*	*HDI (1993–94)*	*(NFHS) (1992–93)*
(1)	*(2)*	*(3)*	*(4)*	*(5)*	*(6)*	*(7)*	*(8)*	*(9)*	*(10)*	*(11)*
WEST										
Gujarat	44.3	42.6	3.3	8.7	6.2	3.2	33.0	53.1	50.6	47.5
Maharashtra	50.1	50.8	10.5	16.7	4.1	2.9	27.3	37.9	54.2	54.3
SOUTH										
Andhra Pradesh	44.9	42.4	14.2	15.1	3.3	0.9	31.3	44.4	48.2	43.6
Karnataka	49.5	43.5	1.3	4.1	2.2	2.9	63.6	79.3	51.7	47.7
Kerala	49.3	47.5	14.5	12.6	9.2	5.8	48.4	50.0	58.5	61.4
Tamil Nadu	38.8	42.2	3.5	5.5	2.6	3.4	56.0	64.7	41.4	49.2
Rural India	30.1	29.8	8.3	11.7	5.6	3.4	28.5	35.3	35.7	36.9
C.V	39.5	34.7	92.3	53.2	70.2	76.9	44.4	41.0	31.4	32.3

Source: NCAER/ HDI Survey.

and Rajasthan (26 per cent). In India, family planning programmes had consistently been criticised for excessive dependence on terminal methods, which was evident across states. States with a higher proportion of spacing methods even with low prevalence levels were Uttar Pradesh and Madhya Pradesh. The estimates of this survey generally conform to NFHS and NSSO (1986–7) estimates.

The use of contraceptives was influenced more by the social group to which people belonged than to income groups or type of occupation. Among different social groups, the data indicated that the CPR was highest among the Christian community (48 per cent), followed by Hindus (36 per cent), STs (34 per cent), SCs (31 per cent) and Muslims (25 per cent). The use of family planning measures shows a positive and significant association with adult literacy. Households with female literates had the highest CPR (43 per cent).

The data on proportion of non-users along with dominant reasons for non-use of contraceptives suggested that the most frequent reasons were demand related and included current pregnancy and desire for children of unspecified sex. However, 14 per cent of all non-users expressed a desire for more sons. Thus, demand factors account for 54 per cent of total responses. One-fourth of non-users expressed lack of knowledge of contraceptives, another 14 per cent gave cultural reasons including opposition from family members as reasons for non-use. The non-availability of contraceptives or supply factors did not seem to be a dominant reason for non-adoption of family planning methods.[10]

States that cited demand factors were Andhra Pradesh, Madhya Pradesh and Karnataka. The desire for another son was mentioned more often in Karnataka, Rajasthan, Haryana, Maharashtra and Orissa. Supply factors were major impediments in Bihar, Himachal Pradesh, Rajasthan and the North-eastern states. It was surprising to note that in Kerala, of the non-users comprising 39 per cent (possibly in the younger age group) 41.3 per cent expressed lack of knowledge. In Punjab, too, lack of knowledge as a reason for non-acceptance was high (39.5 per cent), as also in Bihar (34.1 per cent), and Karnataka (31.0 per cent).

The cross-classification of data according to population groups indicated that there was hardly any variation according to household income, land holding, occupation, poverty groups and the level of village development. But there was variation in the case of desire for another son. For example, this was a common reason among the high-income category, large landholders and the illiterate. However, there were variations according to social groups and household size. It needs to be noted that notwithstanding the need for standardisation, that desire for a son was relatively less common among the Muslims. The reasons cited by about 36 per cent of the Muslim respondents were related to household factors such as elders and husband's approval, and religious reasons. Appropriate information, education and communication strategies could help in promoting contraception among the Muslims.

The study broadly indicated that the nature of reproductive health care behaviour with respect to ante-natal care, post-natal care and utilisation of family planning measures were strongly influenced by female literacy rates, economic conditions, and religious and cultural norms. Among these factors, literacy levels were critical as is evident from the high proportion of mothers who gave birth during 1993 who were illiterate and fell in the lower segment of the poverty line. It was also high among Muslims. In addition, high proportion of deliveries at home without trained personnel also influenced the outcomes considerably with such deliveries being associated with a higher incidence of complications during childbirth. Thus, better availability of health care facilities and female literacy levels were the most important factors that had a bearing on utilisation of reproductive health care facilities.

4. CHILD IMMUNISATION

Immunisation of infants and children against infectious and degenerative diseases is one of the most effective strategies for ensuring child survival and child health. Recommended vaccinations for children during the first year of their lives are BCG, Polio, Diphtheria-Pertussis-Tetanus (DPT) and measles. Booster doses were then administered at different stages of childhood.

The survey provided information regarding the percentage of immunised children in the 1 to 2 years age group and the 0 to 2 years age group against DPT, Polio, BCG and Measles and also of those who were immunised against all six diseases. About 49 per cent of the children (between one to two years of age) were fully immunised in rural India although the proportion of partly immunised children (i.e. immunisation against Polio or BCG or Measles) was relatively higher at 64 per cent.

Chart 1 provides a diagrammatic representation of percentage children aged 12–23 months who were immunised. The proportion of both fully immunised and partly immunised children was higher among the economically developed states of Haryana, Gujarat, Maharashtra and Punjab and among the southern states of Kerala, Tamil Nadu and Andhra Pradesh. Immunisation (full and part) was low in Rajasthan (only 21 per cent of the total) followed by the states in the North-eastern region and Bihar. Thus, better health care facilities and infrastructure played a dominant role in higher levels of immunisation among children.

Although the immunisation rate improved marginally across income categories and was high among the salaried, professionals, self-employed, and the better educated, the variation was found only among social groups and between villages at different levels of development. The survey also indicated that the percentage of fully immunised and partly immunised children was higher among households with literate parents and more particularly female literates, as compared to households where none were literate. Similarly, the village development index also revealed a significant association with levels of immunisation or health care of children. In developed villages, about two-thirds of the children in the referred age-group were fully immunised and about 75 per cent were partly immunised as compared to the situation in less developed villages where only one-third received vaccinations for all major infectious diseases. As far as caste and religion are concerned, the data indicated that the levels of immunisation were low among Muslims, followed by ST households but were highest among Christians. Better education levels among Christians seemed to have the contributed to this factor. About 50 per cent of Hindu children were immunised.

4.1 Source of Immunisation

An important point to be noted was that public facilities were the dominant source of immunisation in India. About 85 per cent of all DPT and 83 per cent of measles immunisations were conducted through government facilities located at the village, SUBCs, PHCs or other government dispensaries. It may be inferred that easy availability of government primary health care services through the extension approach played an important role in determining levels of immunisation. Kerala was the only exception where about one-third of total immunised children had received vaccination from private sources. It may be noted that in Kerala, levels of immunisation were also quite high. Hence, it could be inferred that better awareness impels

FIGURE 2. PERCENTAGE CHILDREN (12–23 MONTHS) FULLY IMMUNISED AND GENDER DISPARITY IN RURAL INDIA

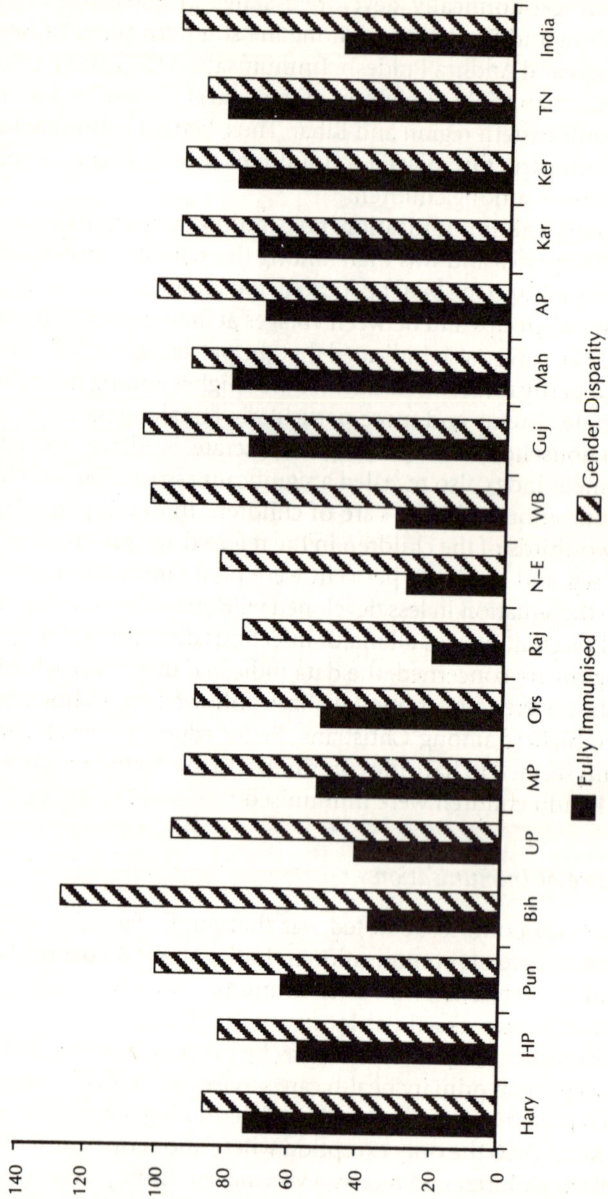

people to get their children immunised even if they have to go to private clinics.

Levels of immunisation also indicated a clear correspondence with household income. Thus, the higher the income of the household, the better was the level of children's immunisation. Similar patterns existed among different poverty groups, where significant development in the levels of child health care was evident with better economic status. Adult literacy and village development too revealed a correspondence with levels of children's immunisation. Hence, villages which were relatively developed, and where the levels of literacy were high reported better care of children. However, occupational and social categories did not show much correspondence with children's immunisation. Overall, it may be said that levels of immunisation were relatively low among Muslims and relatively high among Christians and both tended to depend more on private sources for immunisation. Almost all the social groups preferred public health care services to get their children immunised. However, among high-income groups there was a tendency to go to private sources or doctors as well.

4.2 Reasons for Non-immunisation

In developing countries, non-availability of health care facilities and lack of awareness constitute the main reasons for non-immunisation of children. The statistics presented here indicate that in the case of both DPT and measles vaccinations, about 50 per cent of respondents stated non-availability of vaccinations as the main reason for non-immunisation. Another important reason seemed to be wrong beliefs, i.e., lack of awareness about its effects and existing cultural norms or practices. About 7 to 10 per cent of non-users who had a positive attitude towards immunisation stated that they had taken the child/children for vaccination, but did not receive it due to illness at the time of vaccination. Hence, levels of immunisation could be increased with better supply of vaccines and health awareness programmes.

There were wide inter-state variations among non-users. In the case of developed states such as Haryana, Punjab, Karnataka and Kerala, the major reason for non-immunisation seemed to be wrong beliefs. Though Gujarat and Maharashtra were among the better provided states in terms of availability of health care facilities, they continued to experience wide gaps in the rural areas. In the central states of India namely Bihar, Rajasthan, Madhya Pradesh and Orissa, as well as in Himachal Pradesh and Tamil Nadu, the non-availability of vaccines was a major reason for not immunising children against DPT and measles and also reflected the lack of target oriented camps in these states. Thus, the goal of 'immunisation for all' by 2000 seems to be yet a distant dream as the non-availability of vaccines and wrong beliefs were reported by 25 per cent of households in the country.

The proportion of immunised children was higher among households belonging to higher income levels (i.e. above Rs 86,000). As expected, non-availability was not a major reason among such households for non-immunisation of children, because they could choose to access health care facilities even outside the village due to their better economic status. However, wrong beliefs and existing social norms came out as major reasons for non-immunisation. Since household income groups overlap the poverty line categories, the picture was similar in both categories. Development of villages has governed the level of immunisation of children in most villages. Highly developed villages generally enjoyed better infrastructure to deal with health problems and therefore had a lower percentage of non-immunised children. Poorly developed villages, on the other hand, had either no provision or had poor health facilities that led to an increasing number of non-immunised children.

5. HEALTH-CARE REFORMS

In view of the main findings of the preceding survey, we may identify a few aspects on which health sector reforms could be centred.

5.1 Expanded Definition of Primary Health Care

The role and commitment of government in delivering quality primary health care delivery should be increased. Primary Health Care (PHC), which is normally associated with immunisation and maternal and child health services should include outpatient services, day care surgeries and treatment, basic diagnostics, ophthalmic care and dental services. PHCs and SUBCs, which are the focal points, should be strengthened for delivery of basic curative, preventive and promotive services.

Since many of the health problems faced by pregnant women and children have their roots in under-nutrition and malnutrition, a cost efficient strategy to ensure the health status of future citizens in India should aim at nutritional deficiencies and morbidity among expectant women and lactating mothers. This strategy is essential to minimise low-weight births and improve child survival. Financing programmes aiming to eliminate malnutrition among women of reproductive age in general, and pregnant women in particular, will go a long way in improving the morbidity and mortality situation in India. This can be achieved through (a) enhancing public expenditures on primary health care and nutrition supplement programmes; (b) integrating public nutrition supplement programmes such as the ICDS and the primary health care programme at the grass roots with increasing the role of community level institutions including non-governmental organisations (NGOs); and (c) introducing innovative community health insurance systems to insure pregnant women through non-governmental regulatory institutions.

5.2 Private Providers and the Involvement of NGOs in Delivery of Essential Health Services

Besides strengthening the role of the public sector, the new approach would be to set up an organised public-private mix to provide universal and comprehensive health care to all. In other words, the public providers, NGOs and private practitioners should not compete with each other. The need of the hour is to look at the entire health care delivery system in unison and evolve a comprehensive and integrated national system. This approach would help considerably in avoiding wastage and duplication, achieving optimum utilisation of health humanpower and financial resources, and improving efficiency and quality.

In this regard, private providers and NGOs need to be encouraged through information, training, incentives and finance schemes to identify public health related diseases such as tuberculosis, acute respiratory infections, diarrhoea and dysentery, malaria, leprosy and so on and in providing diagnostic, referral and treatment for such priority diseases. The government can persuade them through incentive schemes to deliver both preventive and promotive health services particularly in remote and under-served regions. NGOs are other potential partners in the delivery of these essential services to the community. State governments can be asked to set up district level co-ordination committees to identify priority diseases and interventions and to facilitate interaction between private providers, NGOs and government PHCs, CHCs and secondary level hospitals in order to cut costs, increase efficiency and ensure quality.

5.3 Improvement of Reproductive and Child Health Services

Despite achievements in reducing infant mortality from a level of 146 in 1951 to 72 in 1994 and the substantial gain in life expectancy from about 40 to 60 years during the same period, the government has failed to improve delivery and outreach facilities of reproductive and child health (RCH) services. Given the current scenario of insufficient reduction in MMR (which is about 437), ante- and post-natal coverage is poor, and institutional deliveries and those attended by trained professionals are low. The government has to readdress these issues in a more integrated manner. The new RCH programme on the anvil with the help of the World Bank introduces some of these concepts. The programme aims at: (a) integrating all interventions of fertility regulation, maternal and child health with reproductive health of both men and women; (b) providing client-centred, demand driven and high quality services based on community needs through decentralised participatory planning; (c) upgrading the level of facilities by setting up First Referral Units (FRUs) at sub-district level and basic RCH facilities (obstetric care, MTP and IUD insertion) at all PHCs, and (d) involving NGOs, panchayat raj institutions, private doctors and practitioners of ISM in planning and delivery of services. However, all these initiatives require additional training, guidelines, local management and monitoring controls, mechanisms of flow of funds to local institutions, medical supplies and other logistics for which serious thought needs to be given. It remains to be seen how effectively the programme would be implemented at the grassroots level.

ENDNOTES

1. For a recent review of the state of reproductive health in India, see Srinivasan and Shariff, 1997.
2. It appears that the estimate of Rs 250 from the 1993 survey of NCAER was an underestimate because of the thirty day reference period for morbidity reporting.
3. This information was collected from those who were pregnant on the date of survey (irrespective of duration of pregnancy). Percentage of women who receive ANC is computed from women who had already delivered.
4. Overall, only about 10 per cent of all those who reported pregnancies had received ANC in rural India. Among various social groups pregnant mothers from the SCs had received twice as much ANC as compared to those from the STs group. Women belonging to salaried and profes-

sionally employed households had received higher ANC as compared to other working classes. However, adult literacy groups more specifically female literacy groups and also groups where both partners were literate had more expectant mothers who had received ANC. A much more significant correspondence is seen with village development categories. In highly developed villages, expectant mothers who had received ANC were about three times higher than those in low developed villages. In developed villages, the quality of ANC was better with periodic checks to monitor intake of iron tablets and blood pressure.

5. Since fertility rate was high in the states of Rajasthan, Bihar and Uttar Pradesh the proportion of mothers who delivered a child was also high in these states ranging from 20 to 25 per cent.
6. Only 2.2 per cent of all births or 22 per cent of complicated births were by Caesarean section. The highest number of so-called complicated births were in Kerala (78 per cent) and 51 per cent of all Caesarean births were in Punjab and Tamil Nadu. An equal number of births classified as 'bleeding' were high in the North-east, West Bengal, Gujarat and Orissa. About 4 per cent of all and 37 per cent of complicated deliveries were reported to have taken place after prolonged labour and 1.5 and 14 per cent reported convulsions and fever during deliveries. Less than one per cent of all births were with the aid of forceps.
7. Women belonging to 'upto Rs 20,000 income' households received the lowest PNC viz., 22 per cent, as against 36 per cent women belonging to '40,001–62,000 income' households.
8. These rates varied remarkably across states. While still births comprised about 14 per cent in Bihar and 15 per cent in West Bengal, these rates were comparatively lower in Orissa and Himachal Pradesh, which were 8 and 9 per cent respectively.
9. Of the total births in the cultivator occupation group, 6.4 per cent were still births. Still birth rates were particularly high among the backwards groups, especially the STs (6 per cent) and in the Muslims (8 per cent).
10. It needs to be reiterated that the reasons for non-adoption of family planning methods should be standardised according to duration of marriage and the number of surviving children. In the absence of such data, the analysis here presents only the frequency distribution for various states.

REFERENCES

Alam, Moneer, 1996. 'India's Health Scenario: An Overview', Background paper, *Sub-group on Health Care Financing and Insurance: Strategies for the Ninth Five Year Plan*, constituted by the Planning Commission and the Ministry of Health and Family Welfare, Government of India.

Duggal, Ravi, 1996. 'A Note on Health Care and Financing Strategies for the

Ninth Five Year Plan', Background paper, *Sub-group on Health Care Financing and Insurance: Strategies for the Ninth Five Year Plan*, constituted by the Planning Commission and the Ministry of Health and Family Welfare, Government of India.

_____, Nandraj, Sunil and Vadair Asha, 1995. 'Health Expenditure Across States—Part I & II—Regional Disparity in Expenditure', *Economic and Political Weekly*, XXX (15 & 16): 834–44 and 901–8.

Gumber, Anil and Berman, Peter, 1995. *Measurement and Pattern of Morbidity and Utilisation of Health Services: A Review of Recent Health Interview Surveys in India*, Working Paper No. 65, Gujarat Institute of Development Research, Ahmedabad.

Gumber, Anil, 1996. 'Burden of Disease and Cost of Ill-Health in India: Setting Priorities for Health Interventions During the Ninth Plan', Background paper, *Sub-group on Health Care Financing and Insurance: Strategies for the Ninth Five Year Plan*, constituted by the Planning Commission and the Ministry of Health and Family Welfare, Government of India.

National Sample Survey (NSS), 1980. 'Notes on Morbidity: NSS 28th Round (October 1973–June 1974)', *Sarvekshana*, 4 (1 & 2): pp. 17–21 and S137–80, July–October.

_____, 1992. 'Morbidity and Utilisation of Medical Services: NSS 42nd Round (1986–7)', *Sarvekshana*, 15 (4): 50–75, April–June.

Cornia, G.A., R. Jolly and Frances Stewart (eds.), 1987. *Adjustment with a Human Face: Protecting the Vulnerable and Promoting Growth*, Vol. I, Oxford University Press, Oxford.

Krishnan, T.N., 1996. 'Hospitalisation Insurance—A Proposal', Background paper, *Sub-group on Health Care Financing and Insurance: Strategies for the Ninth Five Year Plan*, constituted by the Planning Commission and the Ministry of Health and Family Welfare, Government of India, also published in *Economic and Political Weekly*, XXXI (15): pp. 944–9.

National Council of Applied Economic Research (NCEAR), 1992. *Household Survey of Medical Care*, NCAER, New Delhi.

Shariff, Abusaleh, 1997. 'Indian Budget 1997–8—Poverty Alleviation and Social Sectors', mimeo, National Council of Applied Economic Research, New Delhi.

_____, 1995. *Health Transition in India*, Working Paper No. 57, National Council of Applied Economic Research, New Delhi.

_____, 1994. 'Employee's State Insurance Scheme in Gujarat: Key Results of a Survey', Gujarat Institute of Development Research, Ahmedabad, mimeo.

_____, Gumber, Anil, Duggal, Ravi and Alam, Moneer, 1996. *Health Care Financing and Insurance Perspective for the Ninth Plan (1997–2002)**, proceedings of a sub-group on Health Care Financing and Insurance, constituted by the Planning Commission in consultation with the Ministry of Health and Family Welfare, Government of India, March 1996.

Srinivasan K. and Shariff A.,1997. *India: Towards Population and Development Goals*, Oxford University Press, Delhi.

Sundar, Ramamani, 1992. 'Household Survey of Medical Care', *Margin*, 24(2): 169–75, January–March.

Tulasidhar, V.B., 1993, 'Expenditure Compression and Health Sector Outlays', *Economic and Political Weekly*, XXVIII(45): 2473–7.

Visaria, Pravin and Gumber, Anil, 1994, *Utilisation of and Expenditure on Health Care in India, 1986–7 (A Study of Five States)* Gujarat Institute of Development Research, Ahmedabad.

______, and Jacob, Paul, 1996. *Morbidity, Health Care Utilisation and Expenditure Pattern in Andhra Pradesh, Kerala, Madhya Pradesh and Punjab, 1986–7*, Gujarat Institute of Development Research, Ahmedabad.

______, 1997. *Level and Pattern of Morbidity, Health Care Utilisation and Expenditure in India, 1986–7*, Gujarat Institute of Development Research, Ahmedabad.

World Bank, 1993. *World Development Report 1993: Investing in Health*, Oxford University Press, New York.

______, 1995. *India: Policy and Finance Strategies for Strengthening Primary Health Care Services*, Population and Human Resources Operations Division, Report No. 13042-IN, Washington D.C.

part four

Education

chapter 12

Parental Motivation and Private Schooling

• *Anuradha De and Claire Noronha*

1. INTRODUCTION

It is often assumed both by laypersons and in official circles that many parents need to be coaxed, bullied or threatened into sending their children to school. To illustrate, in its golden-jubilee analysis of India's failure to achieve Universal Elementary Education (UEE), *The Times of India* (15 August 1997, p. 37), confidently asserted that 'illiterate and semi-literate parents see no reason to send their children to school'. On the same day, a similar article in the *Indian Express* (written by a leading expert on the sociology of education) stated that, 'Although there is general awareness that literacy is a basic need and right of every person, it is not perceived as such by every individual. The vast majority of adult illiterates belonging to the poor economic stratum are not convinced of it.' The then Prime Minister Narasimha Rao, while speaking to the press about the release of the new book, bemoaned the fact that laws were never implemented in this country. In spite of compulsory education laws on the statute book, he had never heard of a single parent being punished for not sending their child to school. The chief barrier to achieving elementary education goals is, then, assumed to be the reluctant, irresponsible or unmotivated parent. The findings from a recent field survey (hereafter the PROBE survey)[1] contradict this assumption.

This paper is the outcome of work on PROBE survey data, most from discussions between the authors, Meera Samson and Jean Dreze. We are grateful for the useful suggestions given by K. Seeta Prabhu and V.K. Ramachandran.

In this paper, which is based on the survey, we focus on the interplay between high parental motivation and low quality of government schools resulting in the rapid spread of private schools, even in the rural areas. The following section provides a brief outline about the details of the survey. Section 3 looks closely at parental motivation for education—its nature and its determinants. Section 4 explores parental response to the schooling system to understand why their motivation for education is not necessarily translated into demand for government schooling and how this relates to the emergence of private schools. Section 5 deals with the types and features of private schools available in the PROBE villages. Section 6 explores the schooling alternatives available to parents in these villages and the background of the children attending private schools. After this follows a discussion on the opportunities and challenges of the current scenario, briefly touching on implications for the goal of universalising elementary education.

2. DETAILS OF THE SURVEY

A sample of 188 villages from the states of Uttar Pradesh, Bihar, Rajasthan and Madhya Pradesh was surveyed between September and December 1996. These states accounted for 40 per cent of India's population and more than half of out-of-school children.

The villages surveyed were a sub-sample of a random sample of villages studied in 1994 by the National Council for Applied Economic Research (NCAER, 1996).[2] For each state, the districts were first grouped according to female literacy. From each group, the sample districts were selected at random and from them villages within the 300–3,000 population range were selected at random. Thus, all the villages surveyed were large enough for a primary school to be viable, but not so big as to make the survey exercise unmanageable.

The selected NCAER sub-sample (122 villages in all) was extended by surveying one 'neighbouring village' for every other sub-sample village, i.e. the nearest village within the same 300–3,000 population range. This procedure was adopted to increase the sample size at relatively low cost. Taken together, the NCAER sub-sample and neighbouring villages constitute our 'sample villages' (188 in all).

In each village, the investigators surveyed all schools with a primary section. In the 188 sample villages, 236 such schools were identified—195 government schools and 41 private schools. This possibly would be an underestimation of private schools since the unrecognised private schools were difficult to identify, and even when identified, could not always be surveyed due to time constraints. The respondents were usually the head teachers and, in his or her absence, the senior-most teachers were interviewed. In addition, one teacher, usually the teacher teaching at class I, was interviewed. The questionnaire for private and government schools was similar, with the exception that some additional information of specific relevance to private schools was also collected.

For each of the 'NCAER sub-sample' villages, twelve households with at least one child in the 6–12 age group were selected through circular random sampling. The respondent was usually an adult in the household, but preference was given to the mother of a child in the 6–12 age group. General information about the respondent's background and perception was collected. Further, all children in that age group were grouped according to their school-going status—never-enrolled, drop-out and currently-enrolled children. Detailed information was collected about one child, randomly selected, from each group. Wherever possible, the selected school-going child was also interviewed.

3. PARENTAL MOTIVATION FOR EDUCATION

3.1. The Myth of Parental Indifference

Common perception suggests that since the survey villages were in the four lowest literacy states, parental indifference to education would be endemic. Yet, results of the survey revealed that parents were fully aware of the value of educating their children. Further, in response to the question 'is it important for a boy to be educated?' the proportion of parents who answered 'yes' was as high as 98 per cent. This was true for *all* families, irrespective of caste, class, gender, religion and literacy status. At least for boys, parents were convinced of the importance of education. The situation was indeed different for girls, in the sense that a significant minority (10 per cent) did feel that it was not important to educate girls. But the general pattern was not one of parental indifference. On the contrary, as Table 1 indicates, the 'typical' father and mother are very aware of the importance of education.

The high motivation of the parents was also reflected in their responses on compulsory education. A large portion (80 per cent) said that they would approve of making primary education compulsory for all children, only 3 per cent were opposed to it and the remaining 17 per cent were undecided; that too, for reasons such as whether such a law would be implemented seriously.

TABLE 1. PARENT'S ATTITUDE TOWARDS EDUCATION

(per cent)

'Is it important to be educated?'		*'Is it important for a girl to be educated?'*	
Yes	98	Yes	89
No	1	No	10
No response	1	No response	1

'Should primary education be made compulsory for all children?'	
Yes	80
No	3
Undecided	17

Source: PROBE survey (1999).

The survey results also indicated that an increasing number of children were being sent to school. In the age group of six to fourteen years, the proportion of children who have never been enrolled came down sharply from more than over 50 per cent (according to NSSO, 1986–7), to around 20 per cent. This trend was also supported by the NCAER Survey (1994). A part of this enrolment may be nominal, as a response to incentives like dry rations and enrolment drive by the teachers, but it cannot account for the improvement as a whole, specially since the trend was not location specific.

However, it is true that there were as yet many children out of school, thus contradicting the apparently high parental motivation for education. However, prior to looking into the possible reasons for this contradiction, it would be relevant to examine the nature of demand for education.

3.2. *Differentiated Demand*

(a) Gender Bias

As pointed out earlier, though the motivation for education was generally high, motivation for the education of girls was much lower than that for boys. In particular, the motivation for girls' education was lower among the disadvantaged: the illiterate, landless labourers and backward castes (Table 2).

Moreover, even among parents who had an enrolled girl child, most had (mothers no less than fathers) expressed much stronger interest in their sons' education than in their daughter's. Many other indications

TABLE 2. PARENTAL MOTIVATION AND SOCIAL BACKGROUND

Respondents' characteristics	*Proportion (%) who consider it 'important to educate a boy'*	*Proportion (%) who consider it 'important to educate a girl'*
Gender		
Male	99	91
Female	100	87
Literacy status		
Illiterate	99	84
Literate	100	95
Occupation		
Casual labour	99	81
Other occupations	100	93
Caste		
SC/ST	99	87
OBC	100	89
Other	100	94

Source: PROBE survey (1999).

of the gender bias were found in the survey, both from the quantitative and the qualitative data. Responses to the question 'How far would you like your son/daughter to study?' for instance, clearly revealed that parents had much higher expectations for their sons than for their daughters. Even among those who positively wanted their daughters to be educated, the level of education desired was quite low (Table 3).

TABLE 3. EDUCATIONAL ASPIRATIONS: HOW FAR WOULD YOU LIKE YOUR SON/DAUGHTER TO STUDY?

(percentage of responses)

	Son	*Daughter*
Not at all	1	7
Below grade 5	0	2
Up to grade 5	1	10
Up to grade 8	2	18
Up to grade 10	11	20
Beyond grade 10	28	15
As far as possible	57	28

Note: The percentages for 'sons' are based on the responses of parents who have currently-enrolled son (and similarly with daughters).

Source: PROBE survey (1999).

An overwhelming majority of parents wanted their sons to study beyond (often well beyond) grade eight, but many parents had no such expectations for their daughters. A substantial minority did not even expect their daughters to study beyond grade five.

(b) What Motivates Parents?

For most parents, rural as well as urban, education is an investment for the future. The level of motivation depends on the future role of the children in the family, as perceived by the parents. So, while most parents looked upon a boy's education as an investment for the family's future, educational needs of a girl were considered against her marriage prospects (Table 4).

TABLE 4. REASONS WHY PARENTS WANT TO EDUCATE THEIR CHILDREN

(most frequently cited reasons)

Reason	*Per cent*
Sons [a]	
1. Improves employment and income opportunities	87
2. Improves social status	29
3. Improves self-confidence or self-esteem	24
Daughters [a]	
1. Helps to write letters and keep accounts	50
2. Improves employment and income opportunities	40
3. Improves marriage prospects	35

Note: [a]Percentage of respondents who mentioned the stated reasons. The responses are not mutually exclusive.
Source: PROBE survey (1999).

(i) The 'naukree' *or employment motive*—About 87 per cent of parents felt that education of boys was important as it gave access to better employment and higher income opportunities. This included increased potential for self-employment. Further, parents in rural areas perceived a number of non-economic benefits as well. Chief among these was the role of education in improving one's self-esteem and social status. It was evident that, according to the parents' perceptions, education of boys directly benefits the family.

(ii) *The marriage perspective*—Socio-cultural factors play a predominant role in the decision-making of most parents. These factors played a major role in the north Indian states. Most parents in north India think of their daughter's upbringing mainly from the point of view of her marriage. One reason could be that at the time of marriage, a north Indian daughter typically leaves her family and joins her husband's family in his village. From then on, her relationship with her parents is given low priority.

One implication of this outlook would be that it is quite possible for parents to be simply indifferent to a daughter's educational achievements. From their own point of view, it doesn't really make much difference, since she is going to leave them anyway, possibly quite soon. This sentiment transpires in many of the comments made by parents who stated that it is 'not important' for a girl to be educated.

It is interesting that the most frequently cited reasons for educating girls are the ability to write letters and keep accounts (50 per cent). This possibly could be a reflection of the parent's concern about their daughters' well-being in their marital households. Their daughters would need to write letters to keep in touch with their parents and also to inform the parents if they have any problems. Again, the ability to keep accounts will be useful later for running her household. Other common motives for female education, again linked to marriage, include an increase in prospects of getting a better alliance, and that it would help a daughter to look after her own household and help her children with their studies.

But it is not that parents are unable to think of the employment potential of girls. Forty per cent of parents did mention this. Similarly, many parents (73 per cent) did feel that educated girls, but not too educated, are easier to marry off. Among the parents who felt that it was difficult to arrange the marriage of an educated girl, some mentioned that in it was due to a dearth of educated boys.

Since parents did not perceive their family benefiting directly from sending daughters to school, they often gave up trying to do so. In other words, they did not mind educating their daughters if the investment involved, whether in money or in energy, was not too much.

3.3. Changing Patterns

The findings of the survey suggested that parental motivation for education has constantly been evolving in response to circumstances. Increasing parental motivation for the education of girls, and among disadvantaged castes, was one such aspect. The negative attitude to women's education was much stronger earlier; it was only at the turn of the century, for example, that the first girl's school was opened in

Delhi. With the inspiration of adequate role models and the availability of more jobs for women, there has been a change in parental attitudes to female education. In addition, during earlier periods, families with land did not feel so much need for education. With increasing land fragmentation, we find respondents explaining that they have to think beyond land in order to survive. Caste-based reservation for employment has also motivated very poor parents to continue to educate their children. The Total Literacy Campaign (TLC) programme has also enhanced parental motivation for education.

More recently, incentives like food rations, mid-day meals, and free textbooks have attracted more children to school. Parental motivation is likely to continue to rise in the future, perhaps more rapidly than most observers expect today. To visualise parental motivation as the major constraint to the achievement of UEE does not seem to have a sound basis.

4. THE EMERGENCE OF PRIVATE SCHOOLING AND PARENTAL DEMAND

Parents were highly motivated as far as the education of boys is concerned. As regards the motivation to educate girls, though it is lower, there seems to be a rapid change towards educating girls. Yet the demand for education may not always translate into a demand for schooling. Parents could be highly frustrated in their search for schooling. This may due to various reasons,[3] but two obstacles are most important, a) high cost of schooling and b) absence of quality schooling. There could also be the absence of any school at all.

4.1. The Cost Factor

It is interesting to note that inspite of 'free' schooling offered by government schools, 'schooling is too expensive' came first (just ahead of the need for child labour) among the reasons cited by PROBE respondents to explain why a child had never been to school. Parents openly quoted poverty as a major constraint to sending their children to school.[4] Similar reasons for depriving a child of education include the need of elder siblings (especially girls) to look after the younger ones and the need for children to help with farm or household work. Wage labour related reasons did not work out to be a significant factor for non-enrolment in the PROBE findings (Table 5).

Expenditure data confirmed that the cash costs of sending a child to a government school were far from negligible. The average cost

TABLE 5. NEVER-ENROLLED CHILDREN

1. 'WHY HAS THIS CHILD NEVER BEEN ENROLLED IN ANY SCHOOL?'

(percentage of respondents who cited alternative reasons) *

Item	*Sons*	*Daughters*
1. Child is needed for other activities	26	49
2. Schooling is too expensive	43	44
3. School is too far	15	8
4. Poor teaching standards in local school	6	1
5. Hostile environment at school	2	1
6. Child is disabled	3	1
7. Child is not bright enough	6	4
8. Child is not interested in studying	32	18
9. Parents are not interested	37	31
10. Other reasons	29	23
11. Total responses	65	161

Notes: (1) *The listed responses are not mutually exclusive (hence column totals add up to more than 100 per cent).
(2) Random sub-sample of 226 never-enrolled children, currently in the 6–12 age group. The numbers in brackets in the column headings indicate the number of responses on which the percentages are based.

Source: PROBE survey (1999).

of sending a child to government primary school worked out to be Rs 318 per year (Table 6). This may not sound very high, but it is a substantial burden for a poor family, especially with several children. Even with this amount of money, children do attend school, though poorly dressed and equipped in terms of textbooks, stationery and so on.

This could be one of the major reasons why some parents do not

TABLE 6. COSTS OF SCHOOLING: GOVERNMENT VS PRIVATE SCHOOLS

Item	*Average cost of sending a child to primary school (Rs/year)*	
	Government school	*Private school*
1. Fees	16	296
2. Non-fees	302	644
Total	318	940

Note: These expenses are estimates provided by the parents.

Source: PROBE survey.

send their children to school, even when they are keen to educate them. Constrained by limited resources, parents often have to choose carefully and might decide to invest in the education of a few children, and deprive the rest.

4.2. The Quality Factor

Parents send their children to school to be educated. If that were not achieved, then there would be little motivation for schooling. In the surveyed villages, this seemed to be a common problem. Though no systematic tests were taken, the investigators often found while interacting with the children, that they were unable to read, even after three to four years of schooling. Their notebooks were full of scribbles, and were mostly not checked.

Parents were naturally angered about the lack of output from the schooling system. Their anger was fuelled by the indifference of the government schooling system to their problems. The school infrastructure was usually poor with a dilapidated and dirty building and a shortage of teaching aids. This was more so in Uttar Pradesh and Bihar where there was also a massive shortage of usable classrooms.

It should be noted that many parents, who are illiterate or barely literate, could not help their children at home. So the entire teaching depends on the teachers. But often, the pupil-teacher ratio was found to be very adverse, because of vacant teaching posts and teacher absenteeism. In fact the average pupil-teacher ratio was as bad as 50:1 (the implication is that some were much worse). What is even worse than this was that in 50 per cent of the schools visited there was no teaching activity going on at all at the time of the investigator's visit. So for these parents, often, enrolling their children in government schools turned out to be a frustrating experience.

The main reason for the emergence of private schools in the surveyed villages was the failure of government schools to satisfy parental expectations from schooling. Parents who are able to spend more on their children's schooling, looked out for other expensive options. About 18 per cent of the sample of currently enrolled children were sent to private schools. Many parents of the children enrolled in government schools also stated that if the costs of sending a child to a government and private school were the same, they would rather send their children to a private school. The reason, almost invariably, was that they were dissatisfied with the functioning of the local government school. Parents who could not afford this escape route thought about it wistfully—or sent the child / children whose education is of the highest priority. Even the principals from private school usually mentioned either the absence of a government school or its malfunctioning when asked why the school had been opened in the village.

5. PRIVATE SCHOOLS IN PROBE VILLAGES

5.1. *Types of Private Schools*

Private schools in the PROBE villages were of three different kinds:

1. Aided private schools, which were privately managed but heavily regulated and largely state-funded,
2. Unaided 'recognised' private schools, which received no state support and were effectively fee-charging schools (even though school fees are prohibited in many states). These recognised schools had to maintain a minimum level of infrastructure and were allowed to issue their own transfer certificates,
3. Unaided unrecognised private schools, over which the state has no control, that charged fees. These were not even considered as schools by the government.

In the 228 sample villages, 41 private schools were surveyed. Of these 26 were unrecognised, 13 were recognised but unaided and only 2 were aided. Uttar Pradesh had the largest number of private schools. There are possibilities that these figures have been some undercounted (especially of unrecognised schools).

5.2. *Quality of Private Schools*

The preceding figures for recognised and unrecognised schools indicate that private schools were not homogeneous in nature. Recognised schools tended to have better infrastructure, both in terms of school buildings and facilities as well as in terms of teaching staff. They were obliged to follow norms laid down by the state and are allowed to issue their own certificates when their pupils wish to leave the school, or graduate from the school. The unrecognised schools were at a considerable disadvantage because they could not issue these certificates and most unrecognised schools did make the effort to acquire recognition. On the other hand, the unrecognised schools were not bound to any standard infrastructure nor did they have to pay their teachers the officially laid down salary scales or recruit teachers who were qualified and trained. These advantages were also attractive for the school management. Hence, many schools were content to remain unrecognised and build up a 'relationship' with the local government school to overcome the transfer certificate problem.

As far as parents were concerned, almost all private schools scored heavily on the following points:

(i) Serious Teaching Activity

On the whole, parents perceived private schools as having high levels of teaching activity. This was confirmed by the PROBE survey: in most of the private schools visited, there was active teaching (more than 80 per cent) in the classrooms, and even in the remaining few, the teachers were in the class. Thus, in about four-fifths of the schools, class I students (the most neglected lot in government schools), were actually studying when the PROBE investigators arrived and the rest were at least sitting in their classrooms. Only two of the 41 schools had no teaching activity going on.

(ii) Discipline

As a rule, schools seemed disciplined and serious. This was in stark contrast to most government schools and highly appreciated by parents. There seemed in fact a deliberate attempt to give the impression of order and discipline, as even if teachers were absent, the teacher who was present was careful to supervise the whole set of pupils.

However, there have been both positive and negative features of private schooling. Some of these are:

(i) Infrastructure

Interestingly, infrastructure in the PROBE village private schools was somewhat better but not very different from that found in government schools (see Table 7) in terms of availability of various facilities (e.g. classrooms and blackboards). Private schools, however, maintained these facilities better. But this did not change the general picture—private schools, like government schools, lacked a satisfactory level of infrastructure. Many private schools managed to create some kind of learning environment with the simple means available to them because of the serious teaching activity. However, it needs to be mentioned that the simplest 'unrecognised' private schools would have an even worse environment than most government schools, with poky rooms, plenty of filth and no teaching aids. In five cases there was not a single blackboard.

In terms of teacher-student ratio, however, private schools had a

TABLE 7. PRIVATE SCHOOLS VS GOVERNMENT SCHOOLS
PART I: SCHOOL ENVIRONMENT

Item	*Government schools*[a]	*Private schools*	
		Recognised	*Unrecognised*
Infrastructure			
Proportion of schools with:			
1. Pre-primary facility	5	37	42
2. Pucca building	54	57	50
3. Lockable building	61	73	65
4. Waterproof building	44	59	65
5. Drinking water	41	78	65
6. Toilet	11	34	31
7. Electricity	3	27	23
8. Playground	49	51	50
9. Blackboard in each room	73	85	85
10. Library	24	32	23
11. Maps and charts	38	58	50
Teachers			
1. Teacher/pupil ratio	46	25	23
2. Proportion of female teachers	21	13	11
3. Proportion of 'interviewed' teachers who are:			
i. SC/ST	20	13	12
ii. Living in village	27	73	65
iii. Doing other work	47	76	77
iv. Giving tuition	3	27	19
v. Graduates	45	57	44
vi. Trained (pre-service)	69	20	4
Attendance			
1. Recorded attendance as % of recorded enrolment	69	84	79
2. Observed attendance as % of recorded attendance	81	96	98

Note: [a]Based on surveyed government schools with primary section.
Source: PROBE survey (1999).

definite edge over government schools (except for the two private aided schools where the ratio was 1: 42, almost like the average for the government schools). There was only one single-teacher private school, which was relatively new. Though multi-grade teaching was common, the groups were smaller and so was the range of classes being taught together.

Teaching methods like those employed in government schools

relied heavily on writing and rote learning with some recitation thrown in. Investigators did not report the use of teaching aids, though the teachers did claim that they used teaching aids.

The teachers themselves, generally, were young upper caste males. Ninety per cent of them were below 35 years (Table 8). Their formal educational qualifications were similar to those of government teachers, but only few of them had any pre-service training. Thus, teacher effort was not supplemented by special competence for teaching primary level children. The unrecognised schools often hired 'teachers' with only the bare minimum of qualifications. Two teachers had only studied up to class 8. Private school teachers also received very low salaries—sometimes as little as one-tenth of the salary of a government teacher at a similar level.

TABLE 8. PRIVATE SCHOOLS VS GOVERNMENT SCHOOLS
PART II: PUPIL CHARACTERISTICS

Item	*Government schools*[a]	*Private Schools*[b]
1. Proportion of female pupils	34	27
2. Proportion of SC/ST pupils	32	14
3. Proportion of pupils who go to schools outside the village	11	49
Proportion of pupils coming from a household with the following as one of the main occupations:		
1. Farming	73	79
2. Agricultural labour	20	10
3. Non-agricultural labour	13	9
4. Temporary wage employment	8	8
5. Permanent wage employment	8	15
6. Self-employment	14	24
7. Other	5	9

Note: The figures relate to all schools with primary sections. The figures on 'pupil characteristics' are based on household data.
Source: PROBE survey (1999).

(ii) English Medium

English-medium instruction has been the main factor that has attracted students to private schools. Among the forty-one private schools surveyed, seventeen were English-medium schools, and most of the others had English as a subject. But here again, there was a great deal of variation in the credibility of English instruction. In any case, parents had little clue about the quality of instruction offered.

(iii) Pre-primary Section

Many of the private schools surveyed had a pre-primary section and in almost all them the minimum age of admission was three or four years. This was one of the reasons behind the better academic performance of children in private schools. The extra time at school and longer teaching time per student has increased their learning preparedness.

(iv) Parental Support

Parents, on the whole, were as heavily supportive of private schools as they were dismissive of government schools and helpless and angry about the state of these schools. When they did admit their children in these private schools, they usually took care to see that children were regular and that they did their homework according to the private school teachers. PROBE survey data corroborates this. Eighty-four per cent of the children enrolled were found at school and in some schools all the children enrolled were present. One-third of the private schools said parents had made a contribution to the needs of the school in terms of labour, classroom furniture, etc. In Bhakhunkhola (Almora), the private school reported that it would never be able to run in such a poor village without the co-operation of parents. Only about four private schools had major complaints, mainly about parental indifference and delays in the payment of fees.

6. SCHOOLING DECISIONS AND PRIVATE SCHOOLS

6.1. In Search of Satisfaction

Schooling decisions are largely influenced both by the cost factor and by the quality factor. If the family was very poor and could not afford even the cost of government schooling the children may never be enrolled at all. On the other hand, the parents may decide to opt out of the schooling system because the quality does not justify the expenditure. Still, other parents in their search for a decent education incur the cost of transport and send their children to a village where the government school is functioning better. Generally, only privileged parents can take advantage of the private schools which have sprung up because of the combination of high motivation and the malfunctioning government school system.

6.2. Clientele of Private Schools

No fewer than 18 per cent of school-going children interviewed during the household survey, went to private schools. The proportion was as high as 36 per cent in Uttar Pradesh, but much lower in other states (Bihar: 7 per cent, Rajasthan: 11 per cent, and Madhya Pradesh: 5 per cent). Since private schools are fee charging, one could expect these private school students to come from prosperous families. The household survey results indicated that this was only partly true. Though the majority of children in private schools were from prosperous families, there were a few from disadvantaged families too In such cases, one child was usually sent to a private school whereas other children were sent, if at all, to a government school. The survey indicated that the parents of no less than 15 per cent of children enrolled in private schools were casual labourers. Parents with *kacchi naukree* or temporary employment (8 per cent) and the self-employed (24 per cent) perhaps also concealed some of the very poor within their numbers. About 14 per cent of the parents belonged to the SC/ST category (see Table 8).

The fact that the majority of private school students came from relatively prosperous or educated families gave the students of these schools a learning advantage, even if the schools were of an indifferent quality. Only five children in our sample of private school children (2.5 per cent) came from illiterate families. So for most families with children going to private schools, not only is motivation for education high but there was the added advantage of a supportive home environment. The whole burden of teaching was not on the school, unlike that experienced by government school teachers who struggled with large numbers of first generation learners.

7. CONCLUSION

Few issues that were raised by the schooling scenario include a poor quality government schooling system and the mushrooming of private schools of heterogeneous quality, often marginally better than the existing government schools. The emergence of these private schools is in itself yet another confirmation of high parental demand for education. But the fact that the private schools arise chiefly because of the collapse of the government schooling system is a different matter.

For one thing there is the question of access. Parents who cannot even afford the cost of government schooling are in any case out of the picture. But even for families with more resources, the financial burden of private schooling is considerably higher than that of government schooling. It is interesting that costs were very high even in the two aided schools surveyed, and there were no schools which offered to exempt students from all expenses if they were poor. When disadvantaged parents did use the private school option, differentiated demand came into play and they sent the child, usually a boy, whose education was deemed of highest priority (It is not clear from a one-point survey how far these disadvantaged families can sustain even this effort). Thus a considerable number of children are kept out of the benefits of education because of class or gender, or the cost or poor quality of government schooling. This is in spite of the emergence of private schools.

The question of quality is also important. Government schools apparently serve as a benchmark for private schools. The quality of private schools is better than that of government schools but that is not a very demanding task. It is so easy that 'quack' private schools in the PROBE states can come up and survive. A look at the Himachal Pradesh private schools tells us that these private schools are far better than those found in the PROBE villages. Since the basis for comparison in Himachal Pradesh is a government schooling system which is functioning fairly well, private schools are forced to supply even better quality if they want to survive.

Third, there is the question of equity. By allowing the government schooling system to collapse and taking refuge in the emergence of private schools, the government is continuing the process of allowing a dual schooling system to emerge—a different one for the rich, who can use the private option, and for the poor, who have to use the government schools. Therefore, there is a strong probability that this dual track will further impoverish the government schooling system by removing from it those parents with power and resources.

In allowing this situation to continue the state is also abdicating its responsibility towards a helpless and vulnerable section of parents—those who have no idea of what to expect from good schools. This is one of the reasons why private schools of good quality are so rare. The parents are satisfied with frills, which seem to indicate that the school is of good quality. Parents are impressed by the serious teaching activity but they have little understanding of teacher training, competence, and the need for other curricular activities. Even an inept teacher can maintain the appearances of good teaching without imparting much education to the children. Benches and desks, ties and uniforms and an English education all add to the confusion. So what these children receive is cram school education, of slightly better quality than that of existing government schools, which can by no means be defined as 'good education'.

Finally, with regard to the goal of UEE, high parental motivation presents immense scope for achieving this goal. However, if nothing is done to halt the decay of government schools, instead of universal elementary education we may achieve universal enrolment. The motivation could in fact become so high that all parents may send their children to some school whether it is a fruitful exercise or not. Given the condition of the schooling system, even universal literacy will be impossible.

ENDNOTES

1. The survey was the preliminary work for the Public Report on Basic Education in India (1999).
2. The NCAER's sampling procedure are described in National Council of Applied Economic Research (1996), chapters 1 and 2.
3. Access to school in terms of physical distance was not found to be a major problem in PROBE villages for two reasons: first, expansion of the government school system in recent years and second, the size of the PROBE villages (population: 300–3,000). The PROBE survey found that 6 per cent of the villages did not have a government primary school. But the problem is still very important for upper primary education (72 per cent of the PROBE villages were without upper primary schools). This acts as a great deterrent for upper primary education for disadvantaged families and for all girls.
4. This was particularly so for girls going to school: *Garibi bahut hai, kahan se padhaenge?* (How are we to educate our children amidst poverty)?

REFERENCES

Banerji, Rukmini, 1997. 'Why Don't Children Complete Primary School: A Case Study of a Low-income Neighbourhood in Delhi', *Economic and Political Weekly*, 9 August.

Kingdon, Geeta G., 1996. 'Private Schooling in India: Size, Nature and Equity-effects', *The Development Economics Research Programme*, STICERD, LSE, May 1996, mimeo.

National Council of Allied Economic Research (NCAER), 1996. *Human*

Development Profile of India: Inter-state and Inter-group Differentials, Volume 1, Main Report, New Delhi.

National Sample Survey Organization (NSSO), 1993. *Sarvekshana: Results on Participation in Education, NSS 42nd Round* (July 1986–June 87) 56th Issue, Vol. XVII, No. 1, July-September, Department of Statistics, Ministry of Planning, Government of India, New Delhi.

The PROBE Team, 1999. *Public Report on Basic Education in India*, New Delhi, Oxford University Press.

Vaidyanathan, A. 1998, 'The Rural Scene', *Seminar*, 464, April 1998.

chapter 13

Should Higher Education in India be Self-financing?

• *V.N. Kothari*

1. INTRODUCTION

The problem of financing of higher education in India can be approached from two different points of view. One view is to treat higher education as investment in human capital from a purely individualistic point of view. The other approach is to view it from a political economy perspective.

Looking at higher education from a purely individualistic point of view, one could ask 'what would happen if higher education were made self-financing?' By self-financing we would mean covering recurring as well as capital costs through fees and other private sources. At present, fees paid by the students constitute hardly 10 per cent of the recurring expenditure of colleges and universities. In government aided technical, engineering and medical colleges, fees would constitute an even smaller fraction of recurring costs. If the implicit capital costs by way of depreciation and interest on capital invested in buildings and equipment in government aided institutions of higher education are taken into account, the contribution of fees to total institutional costs would be negligible. Self-financing would in all probability imply a fee structure ranging from Rs 10,000 per year for undergraduate courses in Arts and Commerce to about Rs 50,000 per year for undergraduate courses in Medicine. Fees for other courses would range in between.

The following section outlines the practical consequences of introducing self-financing. Section 3 discusses the issue of public expenditure incurred on higher education across various departments in India. Section 4 sets out the rationale for providing government support for maintaining the quality of human capital in the economy. The last section presents the conclusions emerging from the discussion.

2. CONSEQUENCES OF SELF-FINANCING

The practical consequences of a fee structure aimed at making higher education self-financing could be the following:

(i) There will be a drastic reduction in the size of the higher education sector.

(ii) Enrolment of girls in higher education would decrease even more sharply. Parents who have to choose between education of their sons or daughters, would probably decide in favour of the son.

(iii) Reduction in enrolment of students from rural areas, from the traditionally disadvantaged classes of population and from the families of first generation learners would be proportionately greater. This is on account of their economic viability as well as expectations of benefits from education being lower as also due to their weaker labour market connections.

(iv) Enrolment in subjects with limited, meagre or uncertain market opportunities would suffer greater reduction.

(v) The 'social demand' for education, that is the demand for degrees for social status, security purposes or for cultural accomplishment would practically disappear.

(vi) The phenomenon of educational inflation, that is continuous upgradation of educational qualifications required for jobs, would be reduced due to lower rates of enrolment and consequently reduced output of graduates.

(viii) In engineering, technology and medicine courses, reduction in total enrolment may be much smaller but the composition of student population will change drastically. A large number of students of merit who cannot afford higher fees implied by self-financing will opt out of these courses and their place will be taken by less meritorious students who may be able to afford high fees. Merit ordered enrolment would be replaced to a significant extent by a system that is ordered on the basis of being able to afford enrolment in these subjects. At present there exist both government aided and unaided colleges that offer engineering and medical courses. In unaided colleges, 50 per cent seats are 'payment' seats and 50 per cent seats are the so-called 'free' seats, which charge lower fees as compared to fees charged by government aided colleges. Thus, in unaided colleges, a student on a payment seat pays for his full cost as well as for the uncovered part of the cost of one fellow student on the 'free' seat. Under the self-financing arrangement of higher education, there will be no distinction between 'payment' seats and 'free' seats. For those students who are enrolled at present, fees would decline on 'payment seats' while it would sharply rise for students on the 'free' seats. Since many students are on 'free' seats, the more meritorious students would not be able to pay the increased fees. Such seats would be filled by less meritorious students who may be able to pay the reduced level of fees for the 'payment' seats.

(viii) It is difficult to see how the policy of reservations will be implemented under the arrangement of self-financing.

(ix) The quality of education in arts, commerce and science courses is likely to improve due to reduced pressure of numbers. Presently, undergraduate courses in arts, commerce and science have an open door policy while there is a highly selective admissions policy for professional courses particularly engineering, technology and medicine. Under the self-financing fee regime, this dichotomy would end.

(x) On the whole, one would expect that the humanpower needs of the economy might not be adequately met. Shortages of educated humanpower especially for middle and high schools and middle level administrative posts might hinder economic development. Jobs and occupations requiring higher education might become more expensive and might command higher earnings. Further, the structure of relative earnings may also change and lead to widening of earning disparities. Economic and social stratification may be expected to worsen.

In the event of higher education being made self-financing, it would not then lay claims on the resources of the state. School education, particularly elementary education, would have more resources available to ensure universal enrolment of children in the age group 6 to 14. How large would these resources be?

3. PUBLIC EXPENDITURE ON HIGHER EDUCATION

As evident from Table 1, the total budgeted revenue expenditure on higher education by the education departments of the central and the state governments in 1995-6 was Rs 303.5 billion, of which over 47 per cent was spent on elementary education while over 16 per cent

TABLE 1. BUDGETARY EXPENDITURE ON EDUCATION ON REVENUE ACCOUNT FOR 1995-96 BY THE EDUCATION AND OTHER DEPARTMENTS OF THE CENTRE AND STATES

(Rs million)

Sector	*Budgeted Expenditure on Education of the Education Department*	*Budgetary Expenditure on Education of the Departments other than Education*
1	*2*	*3*
1. Elementary Education	14,296 (47.26)	—
2. Secondary Education	9,591 (31.71)	—
3. University and Other Higher Education including Technical Education	4,954 (16.38)	—
4. Adult Education, Language Development, General Education and Physical Education	1,410 (4.66)	—
Total	30,250	5,925

Note: Figures in parentheses are percentages to total expenditure.
Source: GOI (1997).

was spent on university and other higher education including technical education. Besides these amounts, departments other than education have also spent on education and training (other than training for their own personnel).[2]

Expenditure on education by other departments in 1995-6 was Rs 59.25 billion (budget estimates) on revenue account. How much of this was earmarked for higher education is not known. The other departments include agriculture, labour, home affairs, atomic energy, environment and forestry, urban development, health and family welfare, social welfare, railways, youth affairs and sports, arts and culture, and women and child welfare. Agriculture and health departments support agricultural universities and medical colleges. If it is assumed that about 50 per cent of Rs 59.25 billion (say, Rs 30 billion) were spent on higher education, the aggregate expenditure by the government on higher education would be about Rs 79.54 billion, out of a total expenditure of Rs 361.76 billion on revenue account on all stage of education and training by all the government departments.[3] This accounts for 22 per cent of total expenditure on education by all the departments of the centre and the state governments.

The observation often made that too much is being spent on higher education is not borne out by these figures. It is worth nothing that budgetary support to higher education would come to 0.8 per cent of GDP at factor cost. Total budgetary support to all levels of education and training was 3.7 per cent of GDP at factor cost, in 1995-6. Capital expenditure by education departments outside revenue account was Rs 2.230 million on higher education.

4. RATIONALE FOR PUBLIC EXPENDITURE

Within the individualistic viewpoint of higher education as investment in human capital, is it possible to make a case for government budgetary support? Is it possible to plead for public financial support on the grounds that higher education is a merit good? Since the benefits of higher education, (which is generally more specific and specialised) are captured by the individual concerned and the externalities are relatively small except at the research level, higher education cannot be considered a merit good. Public financial support for higher education through the merit good route seems difficult. However, there are other grounds for public support of higher education.

From a political economy perspective, public support makes good sense. According to the political economy perspective, higher education is a sub-system in the totality of economy, polity and society. Five objectives of the higher education system can be stated around which there is likely to be widespread agreement in our country:

(i) The higher education system should supply in adequate measure educated humanpower capable of performing varied technical and professional tasks so that economic development is not held up because of shortage of adequately trained humanpower.

(ii) The processes of higher education should prevent social stratification and promote social integration in terms of participation in higher education by women, people from rural areas, educationally backward classes that hitherto did not have access to education, etc. This would be important because higher positions in administration, professions, business and industry are likely to be filled by well-educated persons. In a democratic country, administrative personnel should be drawn from a wide spectrum of society.

(iii) The government and public sector are the major employees of educated persons. If higher education is self-financed, higher remuneration may have to be paid to qualified personnel. This may more that offset the savings on grants to higher education.

(iv) The education system should foster creative individuals capable of making a contribution to knowledge.

(v) The higher education system is needed for the cultivation of a scientific and rational attitude and acts as a repository of the growing body of knowledge.

Stated in this manner, self-financing institutions or courses are not ruled out but they will have only a minor scope. The mainstream higher education institutions should continue to be supported by the government. However, much that is in the present set up by way of what one might call a 'waiting room' role of higher education institutions, has to be ruled out. For this purpose (i) entry requirements, (ii) attendance and performance compliance, and (iii) affordable payment of fees would be required.

What do we mean by affordable payment of fees? Around 1950-1, the average fees paid per student year was Rs 156 (Table 2). In that year the per capita NNP at factor cost at current prices was Rs 239. That is to say, fees were nearly two-thirds of the average per capita income and contributed about 35 per cent to recurring higher education institutional expenditure. At that time, only about 0.7 per cent of the relevant age group was enrolled in higher education. Since 1950-1, price levels, as reflected in the implicit GDP price deflator, increased seventeen times. Can we assume that fees would have to be increased to Rs 2,600?

This is not to suggest a definite figure but to point to the potential

TABLE 2: NUMBER OF STUDENTS IN UNIVERSITIES AND COLLEGES IN INDIA IN 1950–51 AND DIRECT EXPENDITURE AND FEES PAID BY THE PUBLIC

Item	*(Rs)*
1	2
1. Number of students in Universities and Colleges (*New*)	4,03,519
2. Total Direct Expenditure on Universities and Colleges (*Rs 000's*)	1,76,778
3. Amount collected through fees (*Rs 000's*)	63,053
4. Direct expenditure per pupil	438
5. Annual fees per pupil	156

Source: GOI, 1997, Tables IV, IX, LVI, pp. 10-11, 19 and 133.

of resource mobilisation through fees for a sector that is at present facing a severe resource crunch.

Let us take into account five important respects in which the situation has changed. First, over the past forty-five years, the per capita real income has doubled. Second, families have become smaller due to declining birth rates. Third, educational institutions have spread far and wide so that the real cost of access to higher education has decreased. This is because the necessity of having to bear the expenses of stay in hostels or boarding and long distance travel for students from mofussil places has been reduced. Fourth, the marriagable age for girls has been rising; concurrently unwillingness of parents to educate their daughters is declining though gender differences in access to education still persist. Finally, longevity has increased, thereby improving the willingness to invest in human capital.

Presently, government aided institutions charge nominal fees and a self-financing sector with obligation for 'free' seats also exists. While there is scope for such self-financing institutions, it is difficult to visualise this sector meeting the manpower needs of a growing economy like ours. Increased stratification of society would be a further argument against self-financing pattern of expansion of higher education. Public sector financing, along with enhanced fees, seems to be the most desirable way out of the present impasse. With about 6 million students enrolled in higher education institutions, even a Rs 1,000 increase in fees per annum would bring in Rs 6,000 million. Let us also note that some states have made education completely free for girl students irrespective of their economic background. Unless we tackle the problem in a targeted manner, the resource crunch in higher education will persist.

Per capita income at current prices for the year 1995-6 was Rs 9,321. As noted earlier, fees at two-third of the per capita income in 1950-1 had confined higher education to only 0.7 per cent of the relevant age group. Due to five important respects in which the situation has changed during the subsequent 45 years as noted earlier, even fees at two-third of the present per capita income that is about Rs 6,000 per year, would ensure an enrolment exceeding 0.7 per cent of the relevant age group. However, enrolment of a higher fraction of the relevant age group would be desirable both for meeting the growing human power needs as well as for wider dissemination of higher education among hitherto deprived classes of population. To ensure this, it may be necessary to bring down the level of fees to one-fourth or even one-fifth of the current per capita income i.e Rs 2,300 or Rs 1,800 per year, but there is no need to make fees an insignificant item as a source of finance.

5. CONCLUSION

Theoretically, it is possible to argue that fees could be kept high enough to cover the full costs of education by making arrangements for adequate loans for those who cannot afford to pay such fees. However, loan recoveries are bound to present an intractable problem. Also, we should take into account the middle class reluctance to incur debts. A feasible fee structure should be such that the majority of aspirants for higher education (say 80 per cent) should be able to pay fees. For the remaining, there should be mechanisms and arrangements for part or full fee waivers and even a measure of financial aid towards other expenses for education.

What sections of the population at present avail higher education can be empirically ascertained through a survey. It would then be possible to arrive at a figure of affordable fees for the majority (say 80 per cent) and work out an arrangement for financial assistance for the rest. To overcome the inhibiting effect of fees for the working class and middle level agriculturists, who have started making an entry into institutions of higher education, it should be possible to invite applications during the twelfth year of school for fee waivers or relief and their claims for a three or four year waiver can be examined by school or local educational authorities. Applications of students who have attended fee charging primary schools as also those whose parents are income tax payers or those who have a registered vehicle can be rejected. Presently, higher education is confined to only about 7 per cent of the relevant age group, who might be belonging to the upper 30 per cent of the economically well-off population. If that is so, there is scope for charging higher fees.

ENDNOTES

1. I am grateful to Shri Kolhatkar for his comments.
2. The preceding figures do not include the expenditure incurred by the departments on the training of their own staff members.
3. These figures should be used cautiously. There is some double counting as what is given by the central government to the states may also be included in the expenditure by the states.

REFERENCES

Government of India (GOI), 1997. *Analysis of Budgeted Expenditure on Education 1993-4 to 1995-6*, Ministry of Human Resource Development, Department of Education, Planning and Monitoring Unit, New Delhi.

———, *Education in India 1950-5'*, Vol.1 Ministry of Education, Government of India, New Delhi.

chapter 14

Human Capital, Performance and Earnings: A Firm Level Study

• *Ramesh Datta*

1. INTRODUCTION

Renewed interest by researchers and policy planners in the field of the 'Quality of the Human Factor', or investment in social sectors in general in the 1990s, might be attributed to the following:

(i) The recent work on the endogenous growth theory which predicts that a larger stock of human capital facilitates technological progress or, for a country that is not on the technological frontier, relatively rapid acquisition of technological capability.

(ii) Globalisation and the dynamic competition that it has created based on new technologies, requiring a multi-skilled functionally flexible labour force; and

(iii) Structural adjustment programmes, and the growing recognition of development of a 'social time bomb' reflected in lack of remunerative employment opportunities, declining quality of existing employment opportunities etc., which have to be dealt with through social sector reforms.

As a result of this, there has been growing pressure on the state to not only increase allocation of resources for the hitherto neglected social sector but also to treat this social spending as an investment—one that provides economic justification for this allocation or reallocation. The fundamental theoretical concept behind this discussion

I am grateful to Dr Manohar Rao for his comments on my paper.

is that of human capital, according to which education augments cognitive and other skills, which in turn increase the productivity of labour.

Interest in this idea of human capital grew in the mid-1950s, out of the failure of traditional growth theories that could not explain more than about one-half of the total increase in economic output during a given period. Later on, T.W. Schultz ascribed Robert Solow's 'residual' of unexplained growth significantly to the improved quality of labour through investment in education. In the Presidential address to the American Economic Association in 1960, Schultz ushered in what his colleague Mary Jean Bowman subsequently termed, the 'Human Capital Revolution in Economic Thought' (Bowman, 1964).

Since then most research studies on the role played by human capital investment, particularly formal education, in explaining the level and variation in earnings in developed and developing countries, have invariably found a statistically significant positive correlation between the levels of education and earnings. These relationships are well demonstrated the world over (Psacharopoulos, 1993) by economists of education who have intensively researched on 'rates of return to education' from the individual and social points of view. These rates have been calculated on the basis of earnings differences that are presumed to reflect productivity differences due to additional educational qualifications. Although profitability estimates of investment in this new form of capital may have become an important part in research scholars' discussions and debates, most developing countries in their educational policy continue to be guided mainly by the 'social demand for education' approach.

In fact, since its inception in the 1960s, the conceptual basis of the 'rates of return' approach to investment in education has remained controversial (Merret, 1966), and further lost its effect with the emergence of the 'screening theory'. In recent years, the Indian government has been proposing an increased allocation of resources for the education sector, but has also proposed to de-link formal educational degrees from jobs in its education policy, probably acknowledging the devaluation of education.

Research conducted on economics of education and labour economics in more recent years, especially since the late 1970s (Thurow 1975; Blaug, 1976, 1985; Cain, 1976; Bowles and Gintis, 1976; Carnoy, 1978; Medoff and Abraham, 1980, 1981) has brought the 'Human Capital' theory, which forms the foundation of 'economics of education', under severe attack. It has also provided scope for new theories and alternative explanations for the existence and persistence of a number of empirical anomalies viz., educated unemployment, educational inflation, inequality in income distribution, labour-market segmentation, credentialism, and non-competing groups. The point to be noted in these alternative theories, though not necessarily mutually exclusive, is that almost none of them questions or refutes the positive association between education and income. The main area of disagreement is about the causes of this observed relationship. Attempts to answer the vexing question, 'What does education do to an individual?' has given rise to the theory of screening or signalling (Arrow, 1973; Albrecht, 1981), Marxian approach to the relationship between education and class structure (Bowles, 1972 and 1975; Bowles and Gintis, 1976), job competition or labour queue theory (Thurow, 1975), job ladder model (Bhagwati and Srinivasan, 1977), and dual or labour market segmentation theory (Doeringer and Piore, 1971).

The Human Capital theory contends that the individual's earnings in the labour market is a function of his or her personal decisions and choices regarding investment in education. In other words, skills acquired in school are directly related to the characteristics that labour needs, and thus results in improved economic performance. Therefore, performance or productivity is the intervening variable in the connection between education and earnings. This implies that efficiency and equity and therefore social welfare in society would improve if resources are allocated, within the education sector and between sectors, by taking into account the 'rates of return' to investment in education. Appropriate 'doses' of human capital, through educational opportunities and subsidised education for certain disadvantaged groups, would correct the prevailing low productivity and thus low earnings of individuals. The human capital theory thus attributes causality to the positive association between 'education and earnings'.

According to the 'screening' theorists, who disagree with this approach, education acts merely as an instrument through which the effects of some other variables, which are inherent and non-cognitive in nature, are transmitted. Under conditions of uncertainty and imperfect information, employers treat formal educational qualifications as a predictive surrogate for the employees' potential productivity. Educational achievements indicate to the employers the presence of certain personality traits viz., ability, motivation, reliability and willingness to learn, which are linked by them to an individual's potential trainability and adaptability. In the extreme case of screening theory, education conveys some information about innate pre-existing abilities and has no productivity enhancing effect. The radicals attribute this widely observed association between education and earnings to non-cognitive personality traits developed in schools rather than to cognitive skills acquired in schools, which are rarely used by employees. According to them, on the job performance is determined by behavioural traits such as punctuality, docility, compliance and ability to work in a group. Inculcation of definite values and attitudes, and the development of these traits, are among some of the principal functions of the educational system in order to preserve the capitalist order of the economic system. Some economists (see Filer, 1981) have tried include some of these personality traits like human relations skills in effective human capital.

According to the job queuing model, productivity and thus earnings of an individual in the labour market is an attribute of the job rather than that of personal characteristics acquired in schools. Prospective employers select employees from a queue formed by individuals based on their trainability with least cost trainable heading the queue. Once a worker is hired, the cognitive skills necessary to raise the worker's productivity to the requirements of the job are learned, through formal and informal training programmes. Several studies in the fields of institutional and organisational behaviour (Rosenbaum, 1981; Cascio and Ramos, 1986) have supported the queue theory. Job analysis, specifications, evaluation, performance appraisals, etc. are very important elements in fixing wages, evaluating performance on the job, giving wage increments, promotions, and hierarchical movement in the firm. The arguments put forth by the proponents of internal labour markets do not differ much from this view. The internal labour market is ultimately 'an administrative unit, such as a manufacturing plant, within which the pricing and allocation of labour is governed by a set of administrative rules and procedures' (Doeringer and Piore, 1971).

Where does all this leave us? Do earnings reflect productivity? Are the more educated more productive? Does schooling contribute to increased output or does it allocate individuals to jobs with higher training, productivity and earning possibilities? If investment in social sectors, particularly in education, is to be seen as a policy variable, and a potent weapon in the effort to improve incomes at the bottom of the scale, it is essential to validate the education-productivity link.

There have been few studies that have empirically examined the relationship between investment in education and direct measures of workers' productivity. A research study by Fuller (1972) on two electrical machinery plants in Bangalore, compared efficiency ratings and educational levels for workers. While in one plant there was no relationship between the number of years spent in formal education and efficiency ratings, there was a small positive relationship in the other. Godfrey (1977) examined the relationship between formal educational qualifications and the performance of candidates on trade tests and found a 'small significance of schooling in explaining test performance'. Medoff and Abraham (1980, 1981) found a positive relationship between experience, another important source of human capital, and earnings, but a very low association between experience and productivity as measured by supervisor's performance ratings.

With respect to the agricultural sector, in the Less Developed Countries (LDCs), where the positive linkage between education and productivity has been supported empirically, researchers have emphasised the provision of complementary factors to ensure a dynamic relationship between education in general or schooling in particular and productivity levels. In fact, Leonar (1976) emphasised that effectiveness of education in increasing production depends on what goes along with it and by itself, it is likely to be of little help. Berry (1980) suggests that there is little conclusive evidence that education has a positive effect on productivity in urban jobs and, therefore, that the relationship between education and earnings is less straightforward than what the human capital theory has posited.

Objectives

It is in this context that the present study aims to analyse the education-productivity-earnings connection at the level of the firm. Individual workers' performance ratings, which involve job analysis, evaluation and description, and performance appraisal by superiors shall be utilised as a direct measure of productivity for this purpose. The model postulates that education, work experience and formal training determine workers' productivity at the workplace. In addition, Mincerian earnings function is also tested with and without performance ratings as an intervening variable. The sequence of causation may be depicted as:

(Investment in Human Capital) $\rightarrow$ (Job Performance) $\rightarrow$ (Earnings)

The present study departs from the basic perspective of the human capital theory by including performance rating as an intervening variable. Though it attempted to incorporate the effects of other factors like motivation, human relations, skills, regularity, ability to do multi-machine operations, which are considered by the employer while promoting or giving increments to employees, employers use this method to link pay with performance. The next section presents results and analyses of the study with typical earnings and performance functions. The last section provides the conclusions of the study.

2. METHODOLOGY

A recursive model was employed for empirical analysis. The following set of equations are implied by it:

$$P = a_o + a_1 Ed + a_2 EX + A_3\ FT + U_1 \qquad (1)$$
$$Y = b_o + b_1 Ed + b_2 EX + U_2 \qquad (2)$$
$$Y = c_o + C_1 Ed + C_2 EX + C_3 P \quad + U_3 \qquad (3)$$

where P = Performance Rating
Ed = Formal education in years
Ex = Work experience (Age-Ed-6)
FT = Formal vocational training at the Training Centre. Used as Dummy
Variable FT= 1 and NOFT = 0
Y = Gross earning per annum
U_1, U_2 and U_3 are the residuals in the respective equations

The postulated relationships are assumed to be linear and may be correctly estimated by utilising ordinary least square regression technique to each of the equations. The model, however, will be expanded to allow for diminishing marginal effects of some variables.

All data are taken from the personal files of the employees of a single firm. The empirical results are based exclusively on a population of 1,802 male full-time workers working in one of the large multinational engineering firms in the Indian private sector.

3. RESULTS AND ANALYSES

The mean and standard deviation of the all-major variables appearing in the sample are presented in Table 1. The correlation matrix for all the variables, which have entered the earnings and performance functions given by the recursive model is presented in Table 2. Ex^2 term has been introduced to account for the observed Mincerian parabolic experience-earnings profiles.

TABLE 1. MEANS AND STANDARD DEVIATIONS IN THE SAMPLE

Variable	*Mean*	*S.D.*
Ed	8.520	2.593
Y	55376.407	15877.769
P	15.76	2.96
EX	17.343	6.289
EX^2	340.323	239.378
FT	.094	.293

TABLE 2. CORRELATION MATRIX

	Ed	*P*	*FT*	*EX*	*EX^2*	*LogY*
Ed	1.000	.119	.184	–.203	–.231	-.016
P		1.000	.168	.149	.140	.356
FT			1.000	–.243	–.236	0.58
EX				1.000	.972	.668
EX^2					1.000	.631
LogY						1.000

3.1 Typical Earnings Function

The typical earnings function is presented in Table 3. It indicates that formal schooling and experience explained about 46 per cent of the dispersion of earnings. Regression coefficients of both schooling and experience were statistically significant.

TABLE 3. MINCERIAN EARNINGS FUNCTIONS

Log Y = f(Ed, Ex, Ex^2)	
Variable	Coefficient
Ed	.008 (7.287)
Ex	.026 (14.489)
Ex^2	-.001 (-4.001)
Constant	10.489
R^2	.464
F-Value	658.99

Note: 't' statistics in parentheses.

Every additional year of formal education added 8 per cent into the annual earnings of a worker. Every year of on-the-job experience yielded an increase of 2.6 per cent of a worker's annual earnings. A significantly negative coefficient of Ex^2 exhibited a clearly defined parabola.

3.2 *Performance Function*

As mentioned earlier, the on-the-job performance of workers in this firm was rated every year by the management. The factors which were considered while rating on a scale of 1 to 40 were output, quality of work (rejection, etc.), ability to do a variety of jobs, orderliness and cleanliness, punctuality of work, care of tools and machinery and attendance record. On the basis of these ratings, future training needs of workers were identified.

The ratings of workers were regressed on typical human capital variables such as schooling and experience (Table 4). Although both the human capital variables were significant, the model explained only 3.5 per cent of the variation in job performances of workers.

TABLE 4. PERFORMANCE FUNCTION I

$P = f(Ed, Ex)$	
Variable	Coefficient
Ed	.175
	(5.76)
Ex	.071
	(6.07)
Constant	13.147
R^2	.035
F-value	28.9

Note: 't' statistics in parenthesis.

However, on the inclusion of in-firm training as an additional variable in the 'performance function', the explanatory power of the model changed (Table 5). While addressing the performance of an individual worker, formal education lost its significance in the presence of in-firm vocational training. On-the-job experience was significant and a year of such experience added 0.04 units to the worker's performance rating. Formal Training (FT) was also significant in determining on-the-job performance. Those with FT gained almost a unit increase in their performance rating.

TABLE 5. PERFORMANCE FUNCTION II

P= f (Ed, Ex, FT)	
Variable	Coefficient
Ed	.017
	(.842)
Ex	.048
	(5.692)
FT	.968
	(5.281)
Constant	6.033
R^2	.474
F-Value	323.7

Note: 't' statistics in parentheses.

The explanatory power of the model rose to 47 per cent, which is a little more significant than the explanatory power of typical human capital variables in the earnings function in Table 3.

The next equation includes in-firm training as a variable in Mincerian earnings function (Table 6). These results show that all the variables were statistically significant and the model explained 49 per cent of variation in earnings. Those with in-firm training increased their annual earnings by almost 10 per cent as compared to a 2.8 per cent and 0.5 per cent contribution of an additional year of on-the-

TABLE 6. EXPANDED EARNINGS FUNCTIONS

Log Y= f(Ed, FT, Ex, Ex²)	
Variable	Coefficient
ED	0.005
	(4.951)
FT	0.098
	(10.457)
Ex	0.028
	(15.968)
Ex^2	–0.002
	(–4.83)
Constant	568.54
R^2	0.493
F-value	443.22

Note: 't' statistics in parentheses.

job experience and an additional year of formal education, respectively.

It should be mentioned that Nelson and Phelps (1966), in their study, observed that more educated workers were able to adjust to disequilibria. This view has been further developed by Welch (1970) and in its most general form by Schultz (1975). In-firm training of workers seems to enable them to adapt faster to the dynamic environment. Off-the-job conceptual training on statistical process control, numerically controlled machines, techniques of total quality management and ISO 9000 are a few examples of such continuous in-firm training applied to upgrade the quality of human capital and deal with technological change.

In the next equation, an additional variable of performance-rating (P) was in the earnings function (Table 7). Inclusion of 'P' in the model increased its explanatory power to 57 per cent, viz. an increase of more than 10 percentage points.

TABLE 7. A VARIANT OF EARNINGS FUNCTION

Log Y= f(Ed, Ex, Ex², P)

Variable	Coefficient
Ed	.004
	(3.68)
Ex	.027
	(15.284)
Ex^2	.002
	(–4.982)
P	.014
	(15.228)
Constant	10.302
R^2	.573
F-value	575.8

Note: 't' statistics in parentheses.

Thus, the analysis indicates that the positive correlation observed between investment in human capital, performance on-the-job and earnings is no doubt a causal one as postulated within the theoretical framework provided by the human capital theory. However, post-schooling investment in the form of off-the-job and in-firm training played a more significant role than mere formal schooling. Thus, the correlation is turned into a causation model.

$$Y \longleftarrow f(HC) \text{ via } (P)$$

Is it worthwhile experimenting with a reversal of this paradigm? 'Earnings aimed at' represents the independent variable, suggesting that an 'anticipated increase in earnings' would elicit a better performance rating from an individual in the future (Table 8). Thus, the model fitted was as follows:

$$P \longleftarrow f(y)$$

The model explained 12 per cent of the performance variation. It also shows that every point per cent increase in earnings led to a 6-point increase in performance rating of an individual worker. Thus, 'earnings aimed at' push 'efforts' of workers upwards, by acting as wage incentives.

TABLE 8. REVERSING THE PARADIGM

Log P = f(Y)	
Variable	Coefficient
Y	6.207
	(15.78)
Constant	- 52.309
R^2	0.126
F-value	249.060

Note: 't' statistics in parentheses.

4. CONCLUSION

The results of this case study, while supporting the human capital approach to earnings determination, also show that traditional simple human capital variables viz., years of formal education and experience on-the-job, do not necessarily determine performance variation among workers. In the present era of competition, where the gap between skills required to work with new production process technologies and existing skills is constantly emerging and changing, new human capital in the form of continuous in-firm and off-the-job training to upgrade workers' skills has become imperative. This is depicted in a stylised form in the diagram in Figure 1.

Although in reality it would be observed that annual increments of workers are 'institutionalised', it seems that the employer keeps upgrading the performance of 'core' group of employees through in-firm training to pay workers such increments.

FIGURE 1. WAGES/PERFORMANCE AND SKILLS UNDER NEW COMPETITION

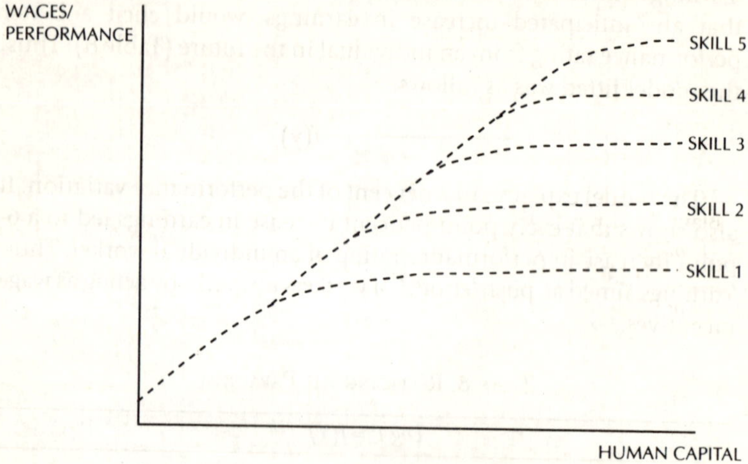

SKILL 1= WAGES–PERFORMANCE
SKILL 2 [Acquire more skills to be flexible functionally] = WAGES–PERFORMANCE
SKILL 3 [Perform multiple roles, develop broad understanding of work processes] = WAGES–PERFORMANCE
SKILL 4 [Member of self directed work team] = WAGES-PERFORMANCE
SKILL 5 [Adaptability to technological change] = WAGES–PERFORMANCE

The World Employment Report (1998–9) of the International Labour Organisation pointed to the growing evidence that upskilling and reskilling of workers is a significant determinant of economic success and failure of firms in the global world markets. Simultaneously, it also pointed out that most companies do not invest in upgrading the skills of workers. The report thus advocates investment in upgrading the vocational skills of workers at the firm level. One of the major reasons for the failure of the Government of India in giving a 'human face' to structural reforms since the early 1990s may be traced to its inability to identify the type of skills required in the market. An additional factor is the difficulty in training workers in whom the firms had never invested and who have been losing jobs due to the restructuring exercise. There is thus a need to develop close links between training institutions and firms in order to bridge the 'skill gaps' of workers.

REFERENCES

Albrecht, J.W., 1981. 'A Procedure for Testing the Signalling Hypothesis', *Journal of Public Economics*, 15: 123–32.

Arrow, K., 1973. 'Higher Education as a Filter', *Journal of Public Economics*, 2: 193–216.

Berry, A., 1980. 'Education, Income, Productivity, and Urban Poverty', in *Education and Income*, World Bank Staff Working Paper No. 402: 153–230, July.

Blaug, M., 1976. 'Human Capital Theory: A Slightly Jaundiced Survey', *Journal of Economic Literature* (Sept): 827–55.

______, 1985. 'Where Are We Now in the Economics of Education?' *Economics of Education Review*, 4(1): 17–28.

Bhagwati, J.N. and T.N. Srinivasan, 1977. 'Education in a "Job ladder" Model and the Fairness-In-Hiring Rule', *Journal of Public Economics*, 7: 1–22, February.

Bowles, S., 1972. 'Schooling and Inequality from Generation to Generation', *Journal of Political Economy*, 80(3): S219–51, May–June, Part II.

______, 1975. 'Unequal Education and the Reproduction of the Social Division of Labour', in M. Carnoy (ed.), *Schooling in a Corporate Society*, Second Edition, David McKay, New York.

______, and H. Gintis, 1976. *Schooling in Capitalist America*, Basic Books, New York.

Cain, G.C., 1976. 'The Challenge of Segmented Labour Market Theories of Orthodox Theory: A Survey', 14: 1215–57, December.

Carnoy, M., 1978. 'Can Educational Policy Equalise Income Distribution?' *Prospects*, VIII (1): 3–18.

Cascio, W.F. and R.A. Ramos, 1986. 'Development and Application of a New Method for Job Assessing Performance in Behavioural/Economic Terms', *Journal of Applied Psychology*, 71(1): 20–8.

Doeringer, P. and M. Piore, 1971. *Internal Labour Markets and Manpower Analysis*, Lexington, Mass.: D.C. Heath Lexington Books, 1971.

Filer, R.K., 1981. 'The Influence of Affective Human Capital on the Wage Equation', *Research in Labour Economics*, Vol. 4: 367–416, Jai Press, Inc.

Fuller, W.P., 1972. 'Evaluating Alternative Combinations of Education and Training for Job Preparation: An Example from Indian Industry', *Manpower Journal*, 8(1): 7–38.

Godfrey, M., 1977. 'Education, Training, Productivity and Income: A Kenyan Case Study', *Comparative Education Review*, 21(1): 29–35.

Leonor, M.D., 1976. 'Education and Productivity: Some Evidence and Implications', WEP Research Working Papers, WEP 2-18/WP 18, ILO, Geneva.

Mincer, J., 1974. 'Schooling, Experience and Earnings', NBER, New York.

Medoff, J.L. and K.G. Abraham, 1980. 'Experience Performance and Earnings', *Quarterly Journal of Economics*, 95(4): 703–36.

______, 1981. 'Are Those Paid More Really More Productive? The Case of Experience', *Journal of Human Resources*, 16(2): 186–217.

Merret, S., 1966. 'The Rate of Return to Education: A Critique', *Oxford Economic Papers*, 18(3): 289–303, November.

Nelson, R. and P. Phelps, 1966. 'Investment in Humans, Technological Diffusion and Economic Growth', *American Economic Review*, LVI: 69–76, May.

Psacharopolous, G., 1993. Bowman, ILO, 1999 'World Employment Report 1998–9'.

Rosenbaum, J.E., 1981. 'Organisational Career Tracking and Individual's Careers: The Internal Stratification of a Corporation', Academic Press, New York.

Schultz, T., 1975. 'The Value of the Ability to Deal with Disequilibria', *Journal of Economic Literature*, 13(3): 827–46, September.

Thurow, L.C., 1975. 'Generating Inequality', Basic Books, New York.

Welch, F., 1970. 'Education in Production', *Journal of Political Economy*, 78: 35–59, January/February.

ADDITIONAL REFERENCES

Datta, R.C., 1985. 'Education and the Distribution of Earnings', in *Artha Vijana*, 27(1): 1–20, March.

Deshpande, L.K., 1985. 'Segmentation of Labour Market: A Case Study of Bombay', Gokhale Institute of Politics and Economics, Pune.

Gintis, H., 1971. 'Education, Technology and Worker Productivity', *American Economic Review*, 61(2): 266–79.

Psacharopoulos, G., 1985. 'Returns to Education: A Further International Update and Implications', *Journal of Human Resources*, 20(4): 583–604.

Rao, M.J.M. and R.C. Datta, 1985. 'Human Capital and Hierarchy', in *Economics of Education Review*, 4(1): 67–76.

______, 1989. 'Rate of Return in the Indian Private Sector', in *Economics Letters*, 30(3): 373–8.

______, 1989. 'The Screening Hypothesis and the Marginal Productivity Theory', in *Economics Letters*, 30: 379–84.

Rosenbaum, J.E., 1984. 'Career Mobility in Corporate Hierarchy', Academic Press, New York.